STRUCTURE AND VARIATION
IN INFLUENZA VIRUS

DEVELOPMENTS IN CELL BIOLOGY

Volume 1—Development and Differentiation in the Cellular Slime
        Moulds, edited by P. Capuccinelli and J.M. Ashworth, 1977

Volume 2—Biomathematics and Cell Kinetics, edited by A.J. Valleron and
        P.D.M. Macdonald, 1978

Volume 3—Developmental Biology of Acetabularia, edited by S. Bonotto,
        V. Kefeli and S. Puiseux-Dao, 1979

Volume 4—Physical and Chemical Aspects of Cell Surface Events in
        Cellular Regulation, edited by Charles DeLisi and Robert
        Blumenthal, 1979

Volume 5—Structure and Variation in Influenza Virus, edited by Graeme
        Laver and Gillian Air, 1980

STRUCTURE AND VARIATION
IN INFLUENZA VIRUS

Proceedings of the International Workshop on Structure and Variation in
Influenza Virus, Thredbo, Australia, December 10-12, 1979

Editors:

GRAEME LAVER and GILLIAN AIR
*Department of Microbiology, John Curtain School of Medical Research,
Australian National University, Canberra City, A.C.T., Australia*

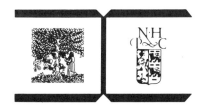

ELSEVIER/NORTH-HOLLAND
NEW YORK • AMSTERDAM • OXFORD

Published by:

Elsevier North Holland, Inc.
52 Vanderbilt Avenue, New York, New York, 10017

Sole distributors outside of the United States and Canada:

Elsevier/North-Hoiland Biomedical Press
335 Jan van Gaienstraat, P.O. Box 211
Amsterdam, The Netherlands

Library of Congress Cataloging in Publication Data

International Workshop on Structure and Variation in Influenza Virus, Thredbo
    Village, Australia, 1979.
    Structure and variation in influenza virus.
    (Developments in cell biology; v. 5)

    Includes bibliographies and index.
    1. Influenza viruses—Congresses. 2. Hemagglutinin—Analysis—
    Congresses. I. Laver, William Graeme, 1929- II. Air, Gillian. III. Title.
    IV. Series. [DNLM: 1. Orthomyxoviruses—Ultrastructure—Congresses.
    2. Orthomyxoviruses—Genetics—Congresses. 3. Variation (Genetics)—
    Congresses. W1 DE997VN v. 5 / QW168.5.07 I61s 1979]
QR201.I6157   1979   616.2'030194   80-11835
ISBN 0-444-00400-9
      0-444-41607-2 (Series)

Manufactured in the United States of America

Contents

PREFACE   xi

ACKNOWLEDGMENTS   xiii

CLONING AND DNA SEQUENCE OF DOUBLE STRANDED COPIES OF

HAEMAGGLUTININ GENES FROM H2 AND H3 STRAINS OF INFLUENZA VIRUS

     MARY-JANE GETHING, JACKIE BYE, JOHN SKEHEL AND   1

     MICHAEL WATERFIELD

THE CARBOHYDRATE SIDE CHAINS AND DISULPHIDE BONDS OF THE

HAEMAGGLUTININ OF THE INFLUENZA VIRUS A/JAPAN 305/57 (H_2N_1)

     M.D. WATERFIELD, M.J. GETHING, G. SCRACE   11

     AND J.J. SKEHEL

STRUCTURAL STUDIES ON A HONG KONG INFLUENZA HEMAGGLUTININ.

THE STRUCTURE OF THE LIGHT CHAIN AND THE ARRANGEMENT OF

THE DISULPHIDE BONDS.

     THEO A. DOPHEIDE AND COLIN W. WARD   21

THE HONG KONG (H3) HEMAGGLUTININ. COMPLETE AMINO ACID SEQUENCE

AND OLIGOSACCHARIDE DISTRIBUTION FOR THE HEAVY CHAIN OF

A/MEMPHIS/102/72

     COLIN W. WARD AND THEO A. DOPHEIDE   27

COMPLETE NUCLEOTIDE SEQUENCE OF THE FOWL PLAGUE VIRUS

HAEMAGGLUTININ GENE FROM CLONED DNA

     ALAN G. PORTER, CHRISTINE BARBER, NORMAN H. CAREY,   39

     ROBERT A. HALLEWELL, GEOFFREY THRELFALL AND

     SPENCER EMTAGE

NUCLEOTIDE SEQUENCE OF THE HA_2 REGION OF THE A/VICTORIA/3/75

HAEMAGGLUTININ GENE DETERMINED FROM A CLONED DNA TRANSCRIPT

     GEOFFREY THRELFALL, CHRISTINE BARBER, NORMAN CAREY   51

     AND SPENCER EMTAGE

CLONING AND DNA NUCLEOTIDE SEQUENCE ANALYSIS OF THE

HEMAGGLUTININ AND NEURAMINIDASE GENES OF INFLUENZA A STRAINS

      WILLY MIN JOU, MARTINE VERHOEYEN, RENE DEVOS,   63

      ERIC SAMAN, DANNY HUYLEBROECK, LUDO VAN ROMPUY,

      RONG XIANG FANG AND WALTER FIERS

THE HAEMAGGLUTININ GENE OF INFLUENZA A VIRUS: NUCLEOTIDE

SEQUENCE ANALYSIS OF CLONED DNA COPIES

      M.J. SLEIGH, G.W. BOTH, G.G. BROWNLEE, V.J. BENDER   69

      AND B.A. MOSS

A COMPARISON OF ANTIGENIC VARIATION IN HONG KONG INFLUENZA

VIRUS HAEMAGGLUTININS AT THE NUCLEIC ACID LEVEL

      G.W. BOTH, M.J. SLEIGH, V.J. BENDER AND B.A. MOSS   81

RNA SEGMENT 8 OF THE INFLUENZA VIRUS GENOME CONTAINS TWO

OVERLAPPING GENES: MAPPING THE GENES FOR POLYPEPTIDES

NS_1 AND NS_2

      ROBERT A. LAMB, PURNELL W. CHOPPIN, ROBERT M. CHANOCK   91

      AND CHING-JUH LAI

HAEMAGGLUTININ BIOSYNTHESIS

      J. MCCAULEY, J. SKEHEL, K. ELDER, M.-J. GETHING, A. SMITH   97

      AND M. WATERFIELD

NATURALLY OCCURRING RECOMBINANTS OF HUMAN INFLUENZA A VIRUSES

      WILLIAM J. BEAN, JR., NANCY J. COX AND ALAN P. KENDAL   105

DNA SEQUENCES DERIVED FROM GENOMIC AND mRNA SPECIES THAT CODE

FOR THE HEMAGGLUTININ AND THE NEURAMINIDASE OF INFLUENZA A

VIRUS

      CHING-JUH LAI, LEWIS J. MARKOFF, MICHAEL SVEDA,   115

      RAVI DHAR AND ROBERT M. CHANOCK

SEQUENCE VARIATIONS OBSERVED IN THE NEURAMINIDASES OF SEVERAL

STRAINS OF INFLUENZA VIRUS

        J. BLOK AND G.M. AIR   125

SEQUENCES FROM THE 3' ENDS OF INFLUENZA VIRUS RNA SEGMENTS

        G.M. AIR   135

THE SYNTHESIS AND CLONING OF LARGE INFLUENZA A cDNAS

USING SYNTHETIC DNA PRIMERS

        IAN CUMMINGS AND WINSTON SALSER   147

THE CLONING AND EXPRESSION IN ESCHERICHIA COLI OF AN INFLUENZA

HAEMAGGLUTININ GENE

        SPENCER EMTAGE, WILLIAM TACON AND NORMAN CAREY   157

3' -TERMINAL SEQUENCES OF HEMAGGLUTININ AND NEURAMINIDASE GENES

OF DIFFERENT INFLUENZA A VIRUSES

        ULRICH DESSELBERGER, PAUL ZAMECNIK AND PETER PALESE   169

THE 5' ENDS OF INFLUENZA VIRAL MESSENGER RNAs ARE DONATED

BY CAPPED CELLULAR MESSENGER RNAs

        ROBERT M. KRUG, MICHELE BOULOY AND STEPHEN J. PLOTCH   181

THE STRUCTURE OF THE HEMAGGLUTININ AND NEURAMINIDASE GENES

AS REVEALED BY MOLECULAR HYBRIDIZATION

        CHRISTOPH SCHOLTISSEK   191

STUDIES ON STRUCTURE - FUNCTION RELATIONSHIPS OF INFLUENZA

VIRUS GLYCOPROTEINS

        RUDOLF ROTT   201

PROCESSING OF THE HEMAGGLUTININ: GLYCOSYLATION AND PROTEOLYTIC

CLEAVAGE

        HANS-DIETER KLENK   213

STUDIES ON THE STRUCTURE AND FUNCTION OF THE OLIGOSACCHARIDES

OF THE INFLUENZA A HEMAGGLUTININ

      RICHARD W. COMPANS, KIYOTO NAKAMURA, MICHAEL G. ROTH   223

      WILLIAM L. HOLLOWAY AND MAURICE C. KEMP

IDENTIFICATION OF THE SULPHATED OLIGOSACCHARIDE OF

A/MEMPHIS/102/72 INFLUENZA VIRUS HEMAGGLUTININ

      COLIN W. WARD, JEAN C. DOWNIE, LORENA E. BROWN   233

      AND DAVID C. JACKSON

MOLECULAR IMMUNE RECOGNITION OF PROTEINS: THE PRECISE

DETERMINATION OF PROTEIN ANTIGENIC SITES HAS LED TO SYNTHESIS

OF ANTIBODY COMBINING SITES AND OTHER TYPES OF PROTEIN

BINDING SITES

      M. ZOUHAIR ATASSI   241

AN EXPERIMENTAL APPROACH TO DEFINE THE ANTIGENIC STRUCTURES

OF THE HEMAGGLUTININ MOLECULE OF A/PR/8/34

      WALTER GERHARD, JONATHAN YEWDELL AND MARK FRANKEL   273

ANTIGENIC DRIFT IN HONG KONG (H3N2) INFLUENZA VIRUSES:

SELECTION OF VARIANTS WITH POTENTIAL EPIDEMIOLOGICAL

SIGNIFICANCE USING MONOCLONAL ANTIBODIES

      ROBERT G. WEBSTER AND WILLIAM G. LAVER   283

THE ANTIGENIC SITES ON INFLUENZA VIRUS HEMAGGLUTININ.

STUDIES ON THEIR STRUCTURE AND VARIATION

      W.G. LAVER, G.M. AIR, R.G. WEBSTER, W. GERHARD,   295

      C.W. WARD AND T.A. DOPHEIDE

ANTIGENIC AND IMMUNOGENIC PROPERTIES OF INFLUENZA VIRUS

HEMAGGLUTININ FRAGMENTS

      D.C. JACKSON, L.E. BROWN, R.J. RUSSELL, D.O. WHITE,   309

      T.A. DOPHEIDE AND C.W. WARD

IN VITRO STUDIES ON THE SPECIFICITY OF HELPER T CELLS
FOR INFLUENZA VIRUS HEMAGGLUTININ

      E. MARGOT ANDERS, JACQUELINE M. KATZ, LORENA E. BROWN,   321

      DAVID C. JACKSON AND DAVID O. WHITE

ANTIGENIC DRIFT IN THE HAEMAGGLUTININ FROM VARIOUS STRAINS OF
INFLUENZA VIRUS A/HONG KONG/68 (H3N2)

      B.A. MOSS, P.A. UNDERWOOD, V.J. BENDER   329

      AND R.G. WHITTAKER

STRUCTURAL STUDIES ON THE HAEMAGGLUTININ GLYCOPROTEIN
OF INFLUENZA VIRUS

      IAN A. WILSON, JOHN J. SKEHEL AND DON C. WILEY   339

PRELIMINARY STRUCTURAL STUDIES ON TWO INFLUENZA VIRUS
NEURAMINIDASES

      P.M. COLMAN, P.A. TULLOCH AND W.G. LAVER   351

GLYCOPROTEINS OF INFLUENZA C VIRUS

      HERBERT MEIER-EWERT, GEORG HERRLER, ARNO NAGELE   357

      AND RICHARD W. COMPANS

SOMATIC CELL HYBRIDS SECRETING HUMAN ANTIBODIES TO INFLUENZA
VIRUS

      ROBERT L. RAISON, KAREN Z. WALKER, ELIZABETH ADAMS   367

      AND ANTONY BASTEN

ANTIGENIC ANALYSIS OF THE HAEMAGGLUTININ, NEURAMINIDASE
AND NUCLEOPROTEIN ANTIGENS OF INFLUENZA A VIRUSES

      G.C. SCHILD, R.W. NEWMAN, R.G. WEBSTER, DIANE MAJOR   373

      AND VIRGINIA S. HINSHAW

COMPARISON OF THE HAEMAGGLUTININ GENES OF HUMAN H2 AND H3
AND AN AVIAN Hav_1 INFLUENZA A SUBTYPE

      GEORGE G. BROWNLEE   385

INDEX   391

Preface

Influenza is still a major disease of man and the virus regularly causes epidemics of varying severity which cannot be prevented by the vaccines currently available. Our inability to control influenza by vaccination is due mainly to the capacity of the two surface antigens of the virus - the hemagglutinin and the neuraminidase - to change their structure in such a way that antibody effective against a particular strain of influenza may not be able to neutralize viruses which subsequently arise.

There are two types of variation of the surface antigens of influenza virus which seem to occur by two entirely different mechanisms. In the major antigenic shifts, "new" influenza viruses suddenly appear in the human population with hemagglutinin and, sometimes, neuraminidase antigens which are quite unlike those of viruses circulating just before the new virus appeared. Whether these viruses arise by genetic reassortment between human and animal influenza virus strains, whether they are viruses from epidemics which occurred many years previously and have existed in a dormant or latent state for long periods of time, or whether they arise by some other mechanism is not known.

In the other kind of antigenic variation - antigenic drift - which occurs following the emergence of a new (or re-emergence of an old) sub-type, the hemagglutinin and neuraminidase antigens change gradually so that a series of variants is formed, each one different from its predecessor. Successive variants differ more and more from the original member of the sub-type.

To obtain information about the changes in the structure of the antigens occurring during antigenic drift, studies on the amino acid sequence of the hemagglutinin polypeptides from two influenza virus sub-types (H2 and H3) were undertaken by Mike Waterfield and his collaborators in London and by Colin Ward and Theo Dopheide in Melbourne. These determinations, using classical sequencing techniques, were time-consuming, required relatively large amounts of material, and also failed to give information about certain regions of the molecule.

The recent developments in recombinant DNA and nucleic acid sequencing technology enable whole genes to be sequenced relatively quickly, using much smaller amounts of material. Assuming that the genetic code is the same, and checking that gene splicing does not occur, complete amino acid sequences of viral-coded proteins can be obtained by this method. This has led to the rapid accumulation of sequence data on a number of different genes and proteins from different strains of influenza virus.

At the same time techniques to produce monoclonal hybridoma antibodies became available, and such antibodies made to influenza virus allow a detailed antigenic analysis of the hemagglutinin. Furthermore, monoclonal antibodies can be used to select variants showing changes in single antigenic sites and the altered antigenicity correlated with changes in amino acid sequence of the hemagglutinin polypeptides.

X-ray diffraction data being accumulated on hemagglutinin and neuraminidase crystals should enable correlation of the sequence changes with the antigenic analyses, and the meeting at Thredbo in Australia was convened to discuss the latest developments in these areas of influenza virus research.

W.G. Laver
G.M. Air

Acknowledgments

Support for the meeting was provided by:

Australian National University

Commonwealth Scientific and Industrial Research Organization

National Institute of Allergy and Infectious Diseases, U.S.A.

Center for Disease Control, Atlanta, Georgia, U.S.A.

Bureau of Biologics, FDA, U.S.A.

Fogarty International Center, NIH, U.S.A.

Commonwealth Serum Laboratories

G.D. Searle and Co. Ltd.

Australian Overseas Telecommunications Commission

Qantas Airways

STRUCTURE AND VARIATION
IN INFLUENZA VIRUS

CLONING AND DNA SEQUENCE OF DOUBLE STRANDED COPIES OF HAEMAGGLUTININ GENES FROM H2 AND H3 STRAINS OF INFLUENZA VIRUS

MARY-JANE GETHING, JACKIE BYE, JOHN SKEHEL[+] AND MICHAEL WATERFIELD
Imperial Cancer Research Fund, Lincoln's Inn Fields, London, WC2A 3PX, UK; [+]Division of Virology, National Institute for Medical Research, Mill Hill, London, NW7, UK.

INTRODUCTION

Approximately 70% of the amino acid sequence of the Haemagglutinin (HA) glycoprotein from Influenza strain A/Japan/307/57 (H2) has been determined in our laboratory using classical protein chemistry techniques[1]. However analysis of certain regions of the molecule, including the hydrophobic membrane associated peptides has proved difficult. Thus complementary cDNA copies of HA virion RNA have been cloned and sequenced in order to complete the determination of the primary structure of the molecule. The HAs chosen for analysis were from Influenza strains A/Japan and A/X-31 (H3). Sequence data for X-31 HA are now required for interpretation of X-ray crystallographic data of Wiley[2] in order to determine the 3-dimensional structure of the protein. Virion RNAs from these strains have been purified and double stranded (ds) cDNAs have been synthesized using reverse transcriptase and DNA polymerase I. The cDNAs were inserted into plasmid pAT153 or pBR322 at the Pst I restriction site and cloned and propagated in E. coli X1776. Recombinant plasmids containing HA gene sequences have been amplified, purified and analysed using restriction endonuclease digestion. One such plasmid contained an insert comprising approximately 95% of the nucleotide sequence of the Japan HA gene. A restriction fragment from the distal end of this insert has been utilized to prime synthesis of a ds cDNA copy and to clone the missing portion of the HA sequence. Another recombinant plasmid contained approximately 45% of the X-31 HA gene. DNA sequence analysis of these inserts provides the complete primary structure of the Japan HA molecule and allows comparison of the protein and nucleotide sequences of HAs from different pandemic strains of Influenza virus.

MATERIALS AND METHODS

It is not appropriate to give a detailed description of methods in this communication. General protocols have been described and referenced in the Results section. A full account of the materials and methods employed will be the subject of a future publication.

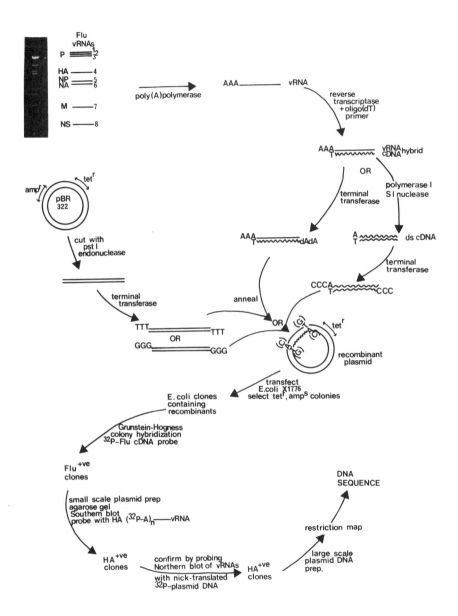

Fig. 1. Strategy for cloning Influenza nucleotide sequences.

3

RESULTS

Our strategy for cloning Influenza nucleotide sequences is illustrated in Figure 1. The individual steps in this protocol are described below.

Total virion RNAs from Influenza strains A/Japan and A/X-31 were purified and polyadenylated at their 3'-termini using poly(A)polymerase[3]. An average of approximately 50 adenylate residues were added to each molecule.

The polyadenylated vRNAs were then used as templates for reverse transcription of DNA copies using oligo(dT)$_{12-18}$ as primer[4]. When the products were separated by denaturing agarose gel electrophoresis 8 discrete bands were resolved (Figure 2) and their sizes indicated that they were essentially full length copies of the RNA genome segments.

At this point the strategies for cloning Japan and X-31 nucleic acid sequences diverged. Cloning of X-31 involved direct insertion[5] of poly(dA) tailed[6] cDNA-vRNA hybrids into the Pst I site of the plasmid vector pBR322[7], after poly(dT) tailing[6] of the linearized plasmid. However no full length cloned copies of the HA gene were obtained and this method also has the disadvantage that cloned inserts are not easily cleaved from the plasmid vector. Subsequent experiments with the Japan strain involved the production of double stranded DNA copies before insertion into the Pst I site of plasmid pAT153 (a derivative of pBR322 with a 622 base deletion (D. Sharratt, unpublished results)).

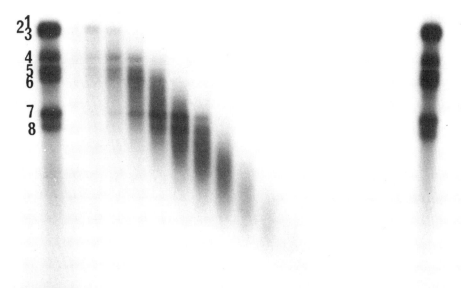

Fig. 2. Japan ds cDNAs were separated on a 10-30% sucrose gradient. Individual fractions were analysed by electrophoresis on alkaline agarose gels and autoradiographed. Side tracks are of ss cDNAs made by reverse transcription of vRNAs.

4

Single stranded DNA copies of Japan vRNAs were converted to the double stranded form utilizing the ability of the cDNA to form 3'-terminal hairpin loops[8] to prime DNA polymerase I[9]. Subsequent cleavage of the hairpin loops with S1 nuclease yielded non-covalently joined ds cDNAs. These were separated on a 10-30% sucrose gradient (Figure 2) and fractions containing full length ds cDNAs were selected. Poly(dC) tailed[6] ds cDNAs were inserted[6] into the Pst I site of pAT153 after poly(dG) tailing[6] of the linearized plasmid.

Transfection of hybrid plasmids into E. coli X1776[10] was carried out under Category III (and subsequently Category II) containment under a program of research approved by the British Genetic Manipulation Advisory Group using the procedure of Hanahan[11]. This method yields 3-5 x 10^7 transformants per μg of supercoiled plasmid DNA. The transformation efficiency obtained with tailed, annealed DNA was approximately 5 x 10^4 transformants per μg DNA. Tetracycline^R, ampicillin^S bacterial colonies containing recombinant plasmids were grown on nitrocellulose filters and screened by a modification[11] of the Grunstein - Hogness[12] in situ colony hybridization technique. The ^{32}P-labelled probe for Influenza sequences was prepared by reverse transcription of Influenza vRNAs using calf thymus oligomers as random primers[13]. In order to identify which gene segments were represented in the cloned recombinant plasmids, Japan and X-31 vRNAs were separated on agarose gels, transferred to and immobilized on diazotized paper[14] and probed by hybridization with ^{32}P-labelled recombinant plasmid DNA prepared by nick translation[15] (Figure 3).

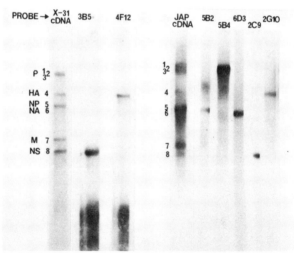

Fig. 3. ^{32}P-labelled recombinant DNA preparations from the numbered clones were hybridized to fractionated vRNAs immobilized on diazotized paper[14]. A, X-31 vRNA B, Japan vRNA. The positions of the 8 vRNA genes were identified by hybridization with the appropriate total ^{32}P cDNA.

Restriction endonuclease mapping of plasmids which had been identified as containing HA sequences indicated that clone 2G10 had an insert corresponding to approximately 95% of the HA gene from the Japan strain and clone 4F12 contained approximately 45% of the X-31 HA gene. This insert corresponds to the NH_2-terminal portion of the coding sequence.

In order to determine the sequence of the missing portion of the Japan HA gene a restriction fragment from the distal end of the 2G10 clone was used to prime synthesis of a cDNA copy from Japan vRNA template. The ss cDNA was poly(dA) tailed and oligo(dT) primer was utilized to prime second strand synthesis by DNA polymerase I to circumvent the loss of terminal sequences resulting from hairpin priming [16]. Using the methods described above a clone containing the missing Japan sequences was identified and mapped by restriction endonuclease digestion.

Determination of the DNA sequence of the cloned inserts was carried out using the procedures of Maxam and Gilbert[17]. Figure 4 shows restriction enzyme maps of the inserts and indicates the distances sequenced on various fragments. Figure 5 provides the completed nucleotide sequences of the complementary RNA strands corresponding to the message coding sequences and shows for comparison the Fowl Plague (FP) virus sequence determined by Porter et al.[16]. Finally Figure 6 lists the amino acid sequences derived for Japan, X-31, A/Memphis/102/72 (H3) (from the protein sequence analysis of Ward and Dopheide[18]) and Fowl Plague[16] viruses.

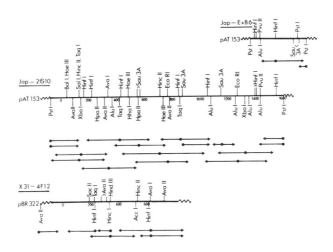

Fig. 4. Restriction enzyme maps of 2G10, ExB6 and 4F12 HA gene inserts. The distances and direction sequenced are shown by arrows.

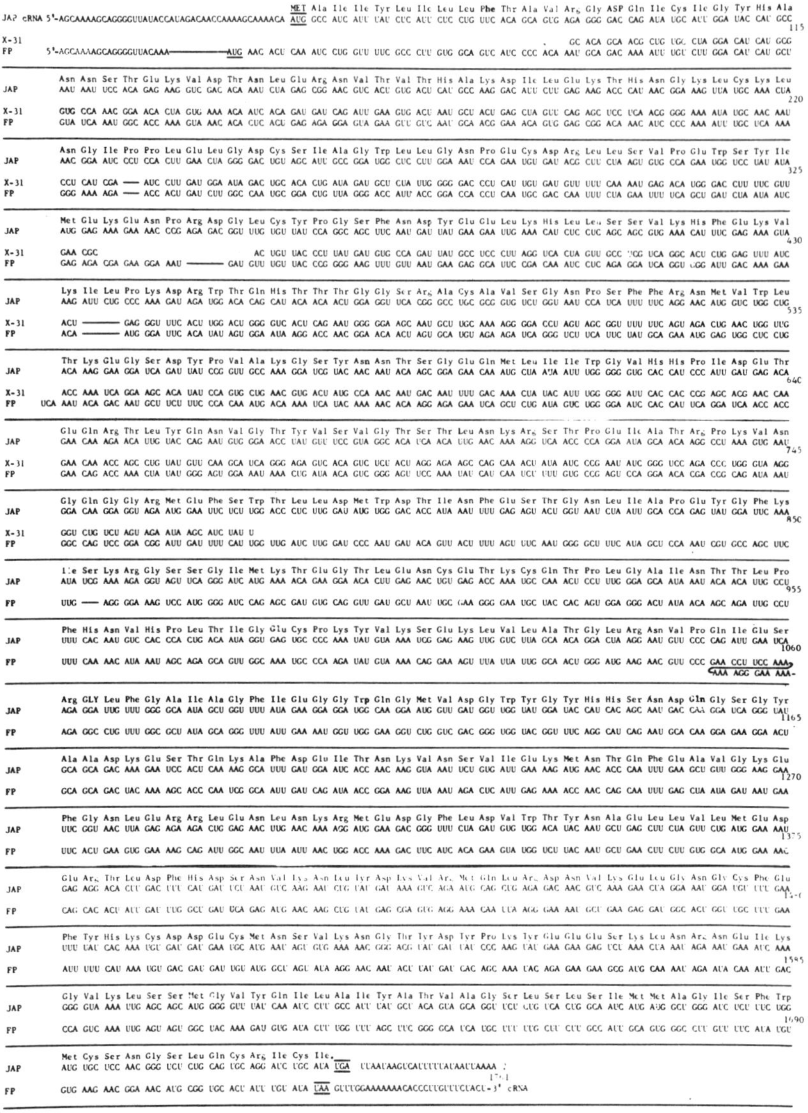

Fig. 5. Complementary RNA sequences of Japan, X-31 and FP[16] HA genes. The predicted amino acid sequence for Japan HA is shown above the RNA sequence. The sequences have been aligned according to the positions of the cysteines.

7

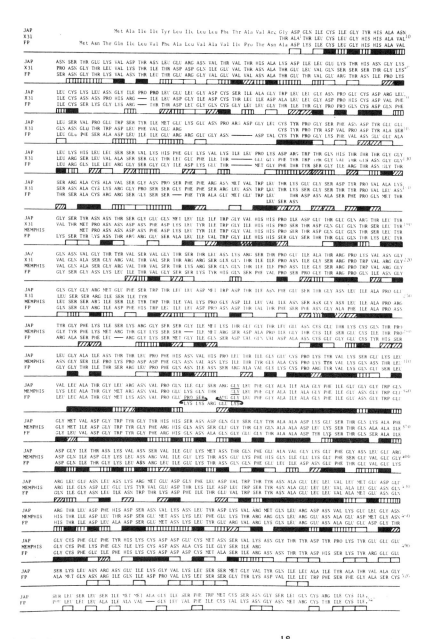

Fig. 6. Amino acid sequences of Japan, X-31, Memphis[18] and FP HAs. The sequences have been aligned according to the positions of cysteines. Homology is shown between: ▬▬ , Japan, X-31/Memphis and FP; ▭ , Japan and FP; ▨ Japan and X-31/Memphis; ▥ , FP and X-31/Memphis.

DISCUSSION

Double stranded copies of the RNA gene coding for HA from Influenza strains A/Japan/307/57 (H2) and A/X-31 (H3) have been inserted in recombinant plasmids and cloned in bacteria. One plasmid contained 95% of the nucleotide sequence of Japan HA, and the missing sequence is contained in another plasmid. DNA sequence analysis of these cloned inserts provides the complete coding sequence of the Japan HA gene, which is the first reported for the HA of an H2 pandemic strain of Influenza virus. Using these two clones it will now be possible to construct a recombinant plasmid containing the entire HA gene. We have also cloned 45% of the HA gene from strain A/X-31 (H3) corresponding to the NH_2-terminal amino acid sequence of the protein. This sequence overlaps by 66 amino acids with the published amino acid sequence of the HA from A/Memphis/102/72 (H3) and together the data provide 88% of the sequence of H3 HA. Only 2 amino acid differences which could be due to single base changes have been noted in the overlapping region.

When the amino acid sequences of the HAs from Japan, X-31, Memphis and Fowl Plague virus are compared (Figure 6) considerable sequence homology between all 3 HA types (30%) is shown. There is a greater degree of conservation in HA2 (47%) than in HA1 (21%). The similarity is even more marked between Japan and FP (43%), Japan and X-31/Memphis (41%) and FP and X-31/Memphis (47%). The amino acid sequences have been aligned to place cysteine residues in corresponding positions. The sequence homologies have been calculated for this alignment and thus are maximum estimates for HA_1. Even without this artificial alignment the positions of cysteine residues are closely conserved, probably because of constraints on the folding of the molecule and the formation of disulphide bridges. The conservation of glycosylation sites has been discussed by Waterfield et al., (this volume). As noted previously by Porter et al., the overlapping nature of homologies between the three HAs implies that the corresponding HA genes have evolved from one and not from two or more distinct ancestors.

HA glycoprotein is synthesized in infected cells as a single polypeptide precursor which is proteolytically cleaved into 2 disulphide bonded subunits HA_1 and HA_2[19,20]. This cleavage is required for the formation of infectious virus. The data reported here shows that the mature Japan HA consists of 547 amino acids and that a single Arg residue is removed during formation of HA_1 (324 amino acids) and HA_2 (222 amino acids). In this respect Japan HA differs markedly from FP HA where activation cleavage removes a sequence of 6 charged amino acids of which 5 are sensitive to cleavage by trypsin. This difference may explain why FP virus is more susceptible to cleavage activation[21].

The HA molecules contain 3 hydrophobic regions which are conserved in all the virus strains. These are the prepeptide or signal sequence, the NH_2-terminus of HA_2 and the membrane insertion sequence at the COOH-terminus of HA_2.

We have previously shown that the nascent Japan HA polypeptide chain contains a hydrophobic prepeptide [1,22,23] which is probably responsible for transport of the polypeptide through the membrane of the endoplasmic reticulum. This polypeptide is cleaved off when the process of membrane insertion is complete. The DNA sequence reported here defines a 15 amino acid prepeptide containing 14 uninterrupted non-polar amino acids before the known NH_2-terminus of mature HA_1[1]. The sequence agrees with the data of Air[24], with our previous data from direct RNA sequencing[23] and with the partial amino acid sequence obtained by radiochemical micro-sequence analysis[23]. FP HA also has an 18 amino acid prepeptide containing a core of 11 hydrophobic amino acids[16]. However this sequence shows no homology with the Jap prepeptide indicating that it is the hydrophobicity and not specific sequence that is important for membrane transport. The size and non-polar character of these prepeptides is similar in other secreted proteins[25].

The second hydrophobic sequence at the NH_2-terminus of HA_2 is highly conserved in Influenza HAs. We have previously suggested that this sequence may have a functional role in interaction with and penetration of the cell membrane during infection[1] and have also noted a high degree of homology with the NH_2-terminus of the F_1 subunit of Sendai virus[26] which is exposed after cleavage activation of infectivity and fusion activity.

The third hydrophobic sequence at the COOH terminus of HA_2 is probably involved in anchoring the HA in the lipid envelope. Japan HA has a stretch of 41 non-polar amino acids and FP HA[16] has 27 non-polar amino acids preceding charged amino acids near the COOH terminus. There is some homology within these sequences but it is not greater than the degree of similarity exhibited elsewhere in HA_2. It may be that as in the case of the prepeptide, it is hydrophobicity and not specific sequence that defines the interaction with the membrane.

The 5'-non coding regions of Japan (43 nucleotides) and FP (21 nucleotides)[16] are identical for the first 17 positions. The prokaryotic-like binding site noted by Porter et al.,[16] is retained in the Japan sequence.

REFERENCES

1.	Waterfield, M.D., Espelie, K., Elder, K. and Skehel, J.J. (1979) British Medical Bulletin, 35, 57-64.
2.	Wiley, D. This volume.
3.	Sippel, A.E. (1973) Eur. J. Biochem. 37, 31-40.
4.	Buell, G.N., Wickens, M.P., Payvar, F. and Shimke, R.T. (1978) J. Biol. Chem. 253, 2471-2482.
5.	Wood, K.O. and Lee, J.C. (1976) Nucl. Acid Res. 3, 1961-1971.
6.	Roychoudhury, R., Jay, E. and Wu, R. (1976) Nucleic Acids Res. 3, 863-877.
7.	Bolivar, F., Rodriguez, R. L., Green, P.J., Betlach, M.L., Heyneker, H.L. and Boyer, H.W. (1977) Gene 2, 95-113.
8.	Seeburg, P.H., Shine, J., Martial, J.A., Baxter, J.D. and Goodman, H.M. (1977) Nature 270, 486-494.
9.	Wickens, M.P., Buell, G.N. and Shimke, R.T. (1978) J. Biol. Chem. 253, 2483-2495.
10.	Curtiss, R., III, Innoue, M., Pereira, D., Hsu, J., Alexander, L. and Rock, L. (1977) In Molecular Cloning of Recombinant DNA, Proceedings of the Miami Winter Symposium, Scott, W.A. and Werner, R. ed., New York; Academic Press pp. 99-111.
11.	Hanahan, D. (1979) Nucleic Acids Res. In press.
12.	Grunstein, M. and Hogness, D.S. (1975) Proc. Nat. Acad. Sci. USA, 72, 3961-3965.
13.	Taylor, J.M., Illmensee, R. and Summers, J. (1976) Biochim. Biophys. Acta, 442, 324-330.
14.	Alwine, J.C., Kemp, D.J. and Stark, G.R. (1977) Proc. Nat. Acad. Sci. USA, 74, 5350-5354.
15.	Rigby, P.W.J., Dieckmann, M., Rhodes, C. and Berg, P. (1977) J. Mol. Biol. 113, 237-251.
16.	Porter, A.G., Barber, A., Carey, N.H., Hallewell, R.A., Threlfall, G. and Emtage, J.S. (1979) Nature, 282, 471-477.
17.	Maxam, A. and Gilbert, W. (1977) Proc. Nat. Acad. Sci. USA, 74, 560-564.
18.	Ward, C.W. and Dopheide, T.A.A. (1979) British Medical Bulletin, 35, 51-56.
19.	Klenk, H-D., Rott, R., Orlich, M., and Blodorn, J. (1975) Virology 68, 426-439.
20.	Lazarowitz, S.G., and Choppin, P.W. (1975) Virology 68, 440-454.
21.	Rott, R., Klenk, H-D., and Scholtissek, C. (1978) In The Influenza Virus Haemagglutinin (eds. Laver, W.G., Bachmayer, H. and Weil, R.) pp. 69-81 (Springer, New York).
22.	Elder, K.T., Bye, J.M., Skehel, J.J., Waterfield, M.D. and Smith, A.E. (1979) Virology 95, 343-350.
23.	McCauley, J., Bye, J., Elder, K., Gething, M-J., Skehel, J.J., Smith, A.E. and Waterfield, M.D. (1979) Febs Letters. In Press.
24.	Air, G. (1979) Virology 97, 468-472.
25.	Strauss, A.W., Bennett, C.D., Donohue, A.M., Rodkey, J.A. and Alberts, A.W. (1977) J. Biol. Chem. 252, 6846-6855.
26.	Gething, M.J., White, J.M. and Waterfield, M.D. (1978) Proc. Nat. Acad. Sci. USA, 75, 2732-2740.

THE CARBOHYDRATE SIDE CHAINS AND DISULPHIDE BONDS OF THE HAEMAGGLUTININ OF THE INFLUENZA VIRUS A/JAPAN 305/57 (H$_2$ N$_1$)

M.D. WATERFIELD, M.J. GETHING, G. SCRACE AND J.J. SKEHEL[+]

Protein Chemistry Laboratory, Imperial Cancer Research Fund Laboratories, Lincoln's Inn Fields, London; and [+]Virology Division, National Institute of Medical Research, London.

INTRODUCTION

The Haemagglutinin (H) is initially synthesised as a single polypeptide of about 580 amino acids with an apparent molecular weight of 65000 on SDS polyacrylamide gels [1,2,3,4]. Subsequently the polypeptide is glycosylated and the apparent molecular weight increases to 75000 [5,6]. At some stage during biosynthesis disulphide bonds are formed, and three identical H molecules through non-covalent interactions form a trimer of apparent molecular weight 210,000[7]. On virus particles each H monomer is found to be cleaved to form two disulphide bonded polypeptides HA$_1$ and HA$_2$[8], and this cleavage has been shown to be essential for the virus to become infectious [9,10]. For A-type viruses both HA$_1$ and HA$_2$ polypeptides are glycosylated, the amount of carbohydrate varying from 16-25% on HA$_1$ and 4.7 - 12.5% on HA$_2$[11,6]. These authors also show that the side chains are linked by N-glycosidic bonds to asparagine residues and that the relative proportions of the constituent sugars can vary from strain to strain.

In this paper we present data which shows the location and composition of the carbohydrate side chains on the H molecule of an Asian strain of virus and we make a comparison between this data and that obtained for the Hs of other strains [11,12].

The location of the disulphide bonds and any free sulphydryl groups in the H molecule is also under investigation in our laboratory and here we report the initial stages of these studies.

MATERIALS AND METHODS

Viruses were grown in the allantoic cavity of embryonated fowl eggs, harvested and purified as previously described[13]. The Bromelain released fragment (BH) was purified on sucrose gradients [14], and the detergent released H by cellogel electrophoresis[8]. The separation of component polypeptide chains and of cyanogan bromide fragments of these chains was as described in [13] or [6]. High pressure liquid chromatography (HPLC) was carried out using 2 Waters M6000 A pumps, a model 660 solvent programmer, a U6K injector and 2 LKB Uvicord S monitors with HPLC flow cells. Size separations were made using 2 Waters I-125 columns mounted in series, in solutions of 6M urea (deionized) containing 0.2 M formic acid at 0.5ml/min, and reverse phase separations on a Waters C$_{18}$ column using ammonium acetate (10mM pH 6.5) buffers and gradients of acetonitrile at

1.5ml/min, 5-30%. Amino acid analysis were performed by the method of Smyth et al [15] using a D500 amino acid analyser and carbohydrate analyses by the method of Clamp and Johnson [16].

RESULTS

Carbohydrate attachment sites. The primary amino acid sequence of the H of the Asian strain A/Japan/305/57 (H_2N_1) has been partially determined by structural studies of the protein [6], and completed by DNA sequence of cloned DNA copies of the RNA segment which codes for the H (Gething et al. this volume). This sequence predicts possible carbohydrate attachment sites at residues 10,11,23,139,164,165,185 and 479. The amino acid sequence at these sites and the location of these sites within the cyanogen bromide fragments and enzymatic fragments of BHA_1 and BHA_2 are shown in Fig. 1.

Amino acid sequence	Chain & CNBr Peptide	Glycopeptides isolated	Method of isolation
10 11 NH$_2$- Asn Asn Ser Thr	1-C$_2$	DQICIGYHANNSTE	V8/C$_2$ HPLC(4)
23 NH$_2$- Asn Val Thr	1-C$_2$	RMVTVTHAKDILE	V8/C$_2$ HPLC(7)
139 NH$_2$- Asn Pro Ser	1-C$_4$	AVSGNPSFFR (not glycosylated)	V8, Tryptic/C4 HPLC (63)
164 165 NH$_2$- Asn Asn Thr Ser	1-C$_6$	GSYNNTSGEQM	BHA$_1$-Tryptic Cation 5- Anion F
185 NH$_2$- Asn Thr Thr	1-C$_3$	CQTPLGAINTTLPFH- NVHPLTGE	V8/C$_3$ HPLC (F)
479 NH$_2$- Asn Gly Thr	2-C$_3$	C$_3$ only	

Fig. 1. The amino acid sequence of the glycopeptides used to establish the carbohydrate side chains of BH.

The assignment of the carbohydrate at residues 10 or 11 was made by analysis of the whole BHA$_1$ chain in the Edman sequencer. It was found that asparagine was recovered at step 10 while no residue was recovered at step 11. This result is to be expected if glycosylation is confined to the asparagine residue at 11 because the PTH derivative of asparagine linked to a carbohydrate side chain is not recovered from the sequencer. The assignment of the carbohydrate side chain at position 164 or 165 has not yet been resolved. The putative site on C$_4$ is not glycosylated.

The disulphide bonds of H. Amino acid analysis of the component polypeptides of H and BH which have been reduced with DTT and alkylated with Iodoacetamide indicated that HA_1 contained 9.6 cysteines and HA_2, 5 cysteines[6]. Sequence analysis (Gething et.al. this volume) suggests that HA_1 contains 9, BHA_2 contains 3 and HA_2 contains 6 cysteines. Recalculation of the data from Waterfield et al. (1979) using 323 residues instead of 339 for BHA_1, reduces the cysteine content to 9.1 residues and similar recalculation of the BHA_2 composition using 170 residues instead of 158 gives a value of 2.9 cysteines. These values are thus similar to the predicted results for these 2 chains obtained from sequence analysis. The analysis of HA_2 suggests that 2-3 additional cysteines are located in the hydrophobic tail. The precise nature of the -SH or S-S groups in this region has not yet been deduced.

Cyanogen bromide cleavage of H. To determine the intra and interchain disulphide bonds of the H, the polypeptide was digested with cyanogen bromide in 70% formic acid for 24 hours and the digest was lyopholised. The digest was redissolved in dilute formic acid and insoluble material in the H digest which was not present in the BH digest was removed by centrifugation. Both digests were fractionated by HPLC using 2 I-125 columns (Waters) in series equilibrated in 6 M urea containing 0.2 M formic acid. These columns separate polypeptides by size[17] and the elution profile of the BH digest is shown in Fig. 2a. The profile for the H digest was identical.

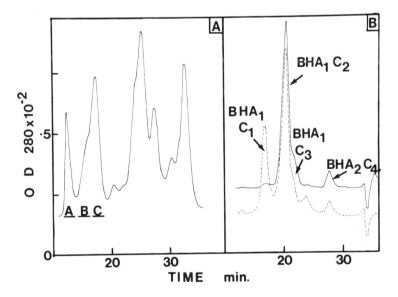

Fig. 2. Separation of CNBr fragments of CB before (A) and after (B) full reduction

Eluates were pooled on the basis of optical density, dialyzed to remove urea or desalted on Sep-Pak cartridges[17], and aliquots were oxidised with performic acid and subjected to amino acid analysis. Pools A, B and C contained cysteic acid. Peak A could not be redissolved after desalting and lypholisation, and analysis on SDS polyacrylamide gels containing urea showed that this peak contained a heterogeneous mixture which could be partial cleavage products. Aliquots of peaks B and C were fully reduced and alkylated (FRA) and rerun on the gel exclusion columns. The elution profiles are shown in Fig. 2b. After reduction of disulphide bonds and alkylation peak B was resolved into 3 distinct components which were identified by their elution positions relative to the known elution positions of the cyanogen bromide fragments of BHA_1 and BHA_2. Thus peak B contains C_1, C_2 and C_3 from BHA_1 and C_4 of BHA_2 while peak C contains C_2 and C_3 from BHA_1 and C_4 of BHA_2. It is known from previous studies that cyanogen bromide peptide C_1 of BHA_1 is a partial cleavage product made up of C_2 and C_4 which results from incomplete cleavage of a methionine - glutamic acid bond [6]. It should be noted that Peak B also contains a small amount of a peptide which elutes in a position similar to that of C_5 of BHA_1 - we have not yet identified this fragment. This result suggests that C_2 and C_3 of BHA_1 are disulphide bonded to C_4 of BHA_2 while C_4 of BHA_1 which has been shown to contain 2 cysteine residues by amino acid analysis is not linked to any other cyanogen bromide fragments.

Protease cleavage of cyanogen bromide fragment C of BH. In order to determine the precise location of the disulphide bonds in peak C the fragment was digested first with Staphlococcus aureus V8 enzyme in ammonium bicarbonate, under which conditions the enzyme cleaves at the carboxy-terminus of glutamic acid residues. Peptides obtained after eighteen hour digestion were fractionated by HPLC under reverse phase conditions and eluted peaks identified by amino acid analysis of performic acid oxydised aliquots. The elution profile is shown in fig. 3(a). Two V8 peptides which eluted late from the column were clearly identified by compositional analysis. The first was the peptide:

(A)   LGDCSIAGWLLGNPECDRLLSVPE

and the second peptide:

(B)   CPKYVKSE
         TKCQTPLGAINTTLPFHNVHPLTIGE

It was also possible to tentatively identify a third peptide which was not pure:

(C)   DQICIGYHANNSTE
         LGNGCFEFYHKCDDECM

This V8 digest was then further digested with trypsin for 2 hours to obtain cleavage of lysine and arginine residues in addition to the previous cleavages at glutamic acid residues. This digest was fractionated by HPLC under identical conditions to the previous one and the elution profile is shown in Fig. 3(b).

A comparison of the 2 profiles (Fig. 3a and b) reveals several peaks which migrate in identical positions. These peaks are given by V8 peptides which lack basic residues and are uncleaved by trypsin. The peptide WSYIHsn(E) which elutes late from the column as 2 peaks in both chromatograms is an example of such a peptide. In this case the 2 forms are probably due to one peptide with C-terminal homoserine and one with C-terminal homoserine lactone. Amino acid analysis of performic acid oxidized aliquots of the eluted peaks was used to identify peptides. The last 2 peaks eluted were found to be tryptic peptides derived from the V8 peptides identified in the V8 digest.

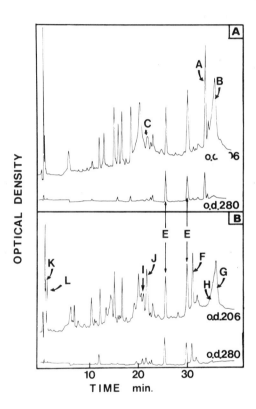

Fig. 3. Fractionation of V8 (A), and V8 plus trypsin (B) digests of peak C from CNBr BH on reverse phase columns.

The peptide:

(A)   LGDCSIAGWLLGNPECDRLLSVPE

was found as the tryptic cleavage product

(F)   LGDCSIAGWLLGNPECDR

and the peptide:

(B)   CPKYVKSE
            |
        TKCQTPLGAINTTLPFHNVHPLTIGE

was recovered in 2 forms:

(G)   CPK
            |
        TKCQTPLGAINTTLPFHNVHPLTIGE

and:

(H)   CPK
        |
        CQTPLGAINTTLPFHNVHPLTIGE

It was also possible to identify the following peptides as partially pure products:

(I)   DQICIGYHANNSTE   and   (J)   DQICIGYHANNSTE
        | |
        LGNGCFE   LGNGCFEYHK

Two other peptides which were eluted at the beginning at the column which were impure were also tentatively identified as:

(K)   CDDE   and   (L)   LCK
        | |
        CM   GTLENCE

However peptide (K) requires further analysis before this composition can be confirmed.

Protease cleavage of cyanogen bromide fragment B of BH. Fragment B contains at least 3 peptides which are disulphide bonded together - these include the partial cleavage product C_2 and C_4 of BHA_1, C_3 of BHA_1 and C_4 of BHA_2. Protease cleavage with V8 and with trypsin was carried out as described for fragment C of BH and the mixture of peptides again fractionated by HPLC using reverse phase conditions.   An additional cysteine containing peptide which is believed to be derived from C_4 of BHA_1 was isolated in an impure form which appears to be:

                DGLCK
                |
        HTTTGGSRACAVSGNPSFFR

However this assignment awaits further purification before the disulphide bond can be firmly established.

DISCUSSION

The amino acid sequence of H reported by Gething et al (this volume) contains 8 regions in which the recognition sequence for N-glycosidic attachment of carbohydrate side chains as predicted by Neuberger et al.[18] occurs. From isolation of six peptides using chemical cleavage and enzymatic cleavage and column chromatography we have shown that carbohydrate side chains are present on 5 distinct peptides (see Fig. 1). It is clear that the sequence -Asn Pro Ser- is not glycosylated. Three of these peptides contain unique sequences which fit the -Asn-X-Thr or Ser-rule while the other two contain sequences - Asn- -Asn- -Ser or Thr.- We have been able to show by sequence analysis in the Edman sequencer that carbohydrate is found only on residue 11 and thus the second asparagine is the one which has the carbohydrate side chain. The second place where this sequence occurs is at residue 164 and 165 but we have not yet established which asparagine carries the carbohydrate. A similar sequence has been reported in the B chain of haptoglobin[19] and it is evident that in this case the carbohydrate is also on the second asparagine residue of -Asn Asn Ser Thr.- It is interesting to note that the analogy between the sequences of these 2 proteins in this region also includes 2 other residues as shown in Fig. 4.

		Residue No. 46								
B chain of Human[19] Haptoglobin	-L	H	E	N	N*	S	T	A	K	B -
Japan 305/57 HA$_1$	-Y	H(8)	A	N	N*	S	T	E	K	V -
Fowl Plague HA$_1$[12]	-H	H(8)	A	V	S	N*	G	T	K	V -

Fig. 4. A comparison of the amino acid sequences of the B chain Haptoglobin & H.

A comparison with the Fowl plague amino acid sequence (Fig. 5) predicted by the DNA sequence of a cloned DNA copy of segment 4 of the virion RNA[12] shows that the glycosylation would occur at residue 12 rather than 11 and that the sequence similarity with Haptoglobin is confined to the His and Lys residues. A comparison of the location of the established carbohydrate attachment sites on the H$_2$ sequence of A Japan/305/57, and the predicted attachment sites on the fowl plague amino acid sequence is shown in Fig. 5.

NH$_2$ —11— 23 —————— 165— 285 ————————— 479 ———COOH
NH$_2$ —12— 28 ——————————— 231 ————— 406* 479 ———COOH

Fig. 5. Location of carbohydrate side chains found on the H of A Japan 305/57 compared with those predicted on the H of FPV virus (The FPV sequence is from Porter et al[12]).

*probably not glycosylated[20]

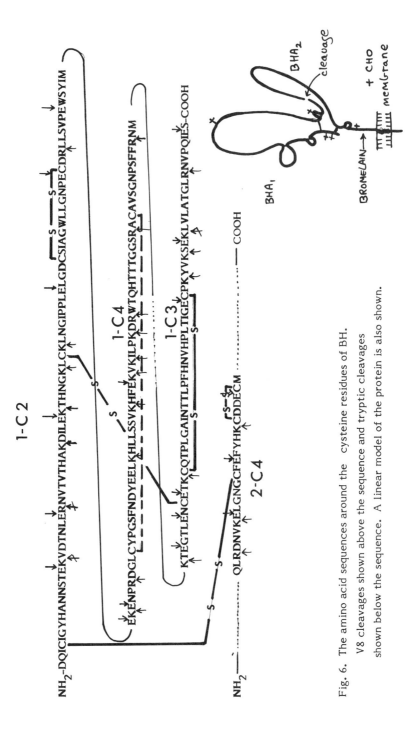

Fig. 6. The amino acid sequences around the cysteine residues of BH. V8 cleavages shown above the sequence and tryptic cleavages shown below the sequence. A linear model of the protein is also shown.

A comparison of the amino acid sequence of the BHs of FPV[12] and A Japan/305/57 (H_2 N_1) Gething et al. (this volume) with the partial sequence data available for the memphis (H_3 N_2) strain[11] shows that the cysteine residues are conserved. It remains to be seen if this conservation is found in all Hs. The additional cysteine residues at the carboxyl terminus of the H found in the H of FPV have not yet been sequenced for the H_2 strain we have studied, but since these may be under different selection pressures due to their unique position near the membrane associated region it may be expected that these could vary from strain to strain.

The study of the disulphide bonds reported here is preliminary since we have not yet purified and partially sequenced the relevant peptides. However it is clear that for the H_2 strain the interchain bonds involve the amino terminal cysteine of HA_1 at position 4 and a cysteine near the bromelain cleavage point of HA_2.

Three disulphide bonds have been found and 2 tetatively established. It is clear from our data that the molecule must fold in several loops since the amino terminus is disulphide bonded to a region near the carboxyl terminus and also to a region near the protease cleavage site which forms HA_1 and HA_2 during maturation of the protein.

A summary of the location of the peptides and possible arrangement of the molecule is shown in Fig. 6. This linear model implies very little about the true folding of the protein but simply serves as a working model for study.

References

1. Lazarowitz, S.G., Compans, R.W., and Choppin, P.W. (1971) Virology, 46, pp 830-843.
2. Skehel, J.J. (1972) Virology, 49 pp. 23-26.
3. Klenk, H.D., and Rott, R. (1973) J. Virol. 11 pp. 823-831.
4. Nakamura, K. and Compans, R.W. (1978) Virology, 86, pp 432-442.
5. Elder, K.T., Bye, J.M. Skehel, J.J., Waterfield, M.D. and Smith, A.E. (1979) Virology 95, pp. 343-350.
6. Waterfield, M.D., Espelie, K., Elder, K. and Skehel, J.J. (1979). British Medical Bulletin 35, pp 57-64.
7. Wiley, D.C., Skehel, J.J. and Waterfield, M.D. (1977) Virology 79 pp. 446-448.
8. Laver, W.G. (1971) Virology, 45 pp 275-288.
9. Klenk, H.D., Rott, R., Orlich, M. and Blödorn, J. (1975) Virology, 68 pp. 426-439.
10. Lazarowitz, S.G. and Choppin, P.W. (1975) Virology, 68 pp. 440-454.

20

11. Ward, C.W. and Dophiede T.A. (1979) British Medical Bulletin, 35 pp. 51-56

12. Porter, A.G., Barber, C. Carey, N.H. Hallewell, R.A., Threlfall, G. and Emtage, J.S. (1979) Nature, In press.

13. Skehel, J.J. and Waterfield, M.D. (1975) Proc. Natl. Acad. Sci. USA. 72 pp 93-97.

14. Brand, C.M. and Skehel, J.J. (1972) Nat. New Biol. 238 pp. 145-147.

15. Smyth, D.G., Stein, W.H. and Moore (1963) J. Biol. Chem. 246 pp. 227-234.

16. Clamp, J.R. and Johnson, I. (1922) In Gottschalk, A, ed. The glycoproteins: their composition, structure and function, 2nd ed., pt A, pp 612-652. Elsevier, Amsterdam.

17. Waterfield, M.D. and Scrace, G. (1980) In Hawk, G.L., ed. Biological Biomedical Applications of Liquid Chromatography, 3, In press Marcell Dekker.

18. Newberger, A. Gottschalk, A., Marshall, R.D. and Spiro, R.G. (1972). In: Gottschalk, A. ed. The glycoproteins: their composition, structure and function, 2nd ed, pt A, pp 450-490. Elsevier, Amsterdam.

19. Barker, W.C., and Dayhoff, M.O. (1976) In: Dayhoff. M.O., ed. Atlas of Protein sequence and structure, vol. 5, suppl. 2, pp. 96. National Biomedical Research Foundation, Maryland, USA.

20. Clamp, J.R. (1975) In The Plasma Proteins (Putnam, F.W., ed.) 2nd Ed., Vol II pp 163-211. Academic Press, New York.

ACKNOWLEDGEMENT

We would like to thank Miss E. Yiangou for invaluable help in typing this manuscript and Dr. R. Faulkes for carrying out carbohydrate analyses.

STRUCTURAL STUDIES ON A HONG KONG INFLUENZA HEMAGGLUTININ.

THE STRUCTURE OF THE LIGHT CHAIN AND THE ARRANGEMENT OF THE DISULPHIDE BONDS

THEO A. DOPHEIDE and COLIN W. WARD
CSIRO, Division of Protein Chemistry, 343 Royal Parade, Parkville, Vic., 3052.
Australia.

INTRODUCTION

The hemagglutinin of influenza virus occurs as trimeric spikes[1,2] projecting from the viral proteolipid envelope. It is the major antigenic protein, against which neutralising antibodies are directed[3,4] and is quantitatively the most important glycoprotein on the viral surface.[5]

It consists of two disulphide-linked peptide chains,[6] a heavier (HA1) chain, M.W.47,000[7,8] and a lighter (HA2) chain, M.W.30,000.[7,8] Both of these chains appear to have definite functions; the HA1 chain, especially the amino-terminal half, seems to be the main contributor to the antigenic properties of the native protein[9] while it also carried nearly all of the carbohydrate.[7,8] The HA2 chain is the anchor holding the hemagglutinin to the viral surface, via hydrophobic interactions involving the carboxyl-terminal part of HA2.[10]

As a contribution to an understanding of the antigenic variation, which makes influenza such an unpredictable and intractable disease, we have studied the structure of the hemagglutinin peptide chains from the Hong Kong variant A/Mem/72 (H_3N_2), and also the manner in which these chains are cross-linked by disulphide bonds.

This paper will discuss the structure of HA2 and the pattern of disulphide bonding within the hemagglutinin molecule.

1. The structure of the light chain

HA2 was obtained in an aggregated form from density-gradient separations of HA1 and HA2. It does not contain any proline, contains very little carbohydrate, four methionines and seven ½-cystines.

Cyanogen bromide cleavage gave four peptides (CN1-4), which were separated by Sephadex gel chromatography (Fig. 1). Five peptides were expected on the basis of the methionine content, but the fourth methionine has been found unmodified within the highly aggregated CN1.[11] The analyses of whole HA2 and the individual cyanogen bromide peptides is shown in Table 1.

Because of the extreme aggregation of CN1, it was very difficult to purify, and its composition reflects this difficulty. The structure of CN2, CN3 and

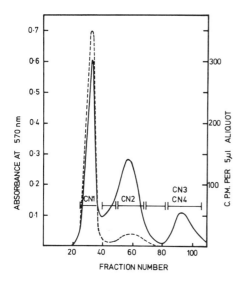

Fig. 1. The separation of cyanogen bromide peptides derived from Hong Kong HA2, on G-100 Sephadex (130 x 2.2 cm) in 50% formic acid. Peptides were quantitated with ninhydrin after alkaline hydrolysis, and radioactivity was measured by scintillation counting of 5 µl aliquots. Fraction size 5 ml.

TABLE 1

AMINO ACID COMPOSITIONS OF THE CYANOGEN BROMIDE PEPTIDES FROM A/MEM/72 HEMAGGLUTININ HA2, WHOLE HA2 AND THE RESIDUAL TRYPTIC PEPTIDE (T) REMAINING AFTER EXHAUSTIVE TRYPTIC DIGESTION OF HA2-CN1.

Amino Acid	CN1	CN2	CN3	CN4	HA2	T*
Aspartic acid	15	14	3	1	30	3
Threonine	1	6	1	–	8	–
Serine	5	5	–	–	10	3
Glutamic acid	6	19	4	2	29	2
Proline	–	–	–	–	–	–
Glycine	10	6	–	5	22	4
Alanine	4	6	1	2	13	2
Valine	3	4	–	–	8	–
Methionine	1	–	–	–	4	1
Isoleucine	12	8	–	2	20	5
Leucine	7	8	2	1	19	5
Tyrosine	4	3	–	–	7	1
Phenylalanine	5	3	1	2	11	2
Lysine	7	7	2	–	15	2
Histidine	2	3	–	–	5	–
Arginine	4	3	3	–	10	1
Homoserine	–	1	1	1	–	–
Cysteic acid	7	–	–	–	7	1*
Tryptophan	ND	2	–	1	4	ND
Glucosamine	3.3	–	–	–	4	–
Total amino acids					222	

MEM |Gly-Leu-Phe-Gly-Ala-Ile-Ala-Ala-Gly-Phe-Ile-Glu-Asn-Gly-Trp-Glu-Gly-Met-Ile-Asp-Gly-Trp-Tyr-Gly-Phe-Arg-His-**Gln**-Asn-
10   20

JAP |Gly-Leu-Phe-Gly-Ala-Ile-Ala-Gly-Phe-Ile-Glu-Glu|Gly-Trp-Glu-Gly-Met|Val|Asp-Gly-Trp-Tyr-Gly|Tyr

MEM Ser-Glu-Gly-Thr-Gly-Gln-Ala-Ala-Asp-Leu-Lys-Ser-Thr-Gln-Ala-Ala-Ile-Asp-Gln-Ile-Asp-Gly-Lys-Leu-Asn-Arg-Val-Ile-
30   40   50

MEM Glu-Lys-Thr-|Asn-Glu-Lys-|Phe-|His-Gln-Ile-Glu-|Lys-Glu-Phe-Ser-Glu-Val-Glu-Gly-Arg-Ile-Gln-Asp-Leu-Glu-Lys-Tyr-Val-
60   70   80

JAP   Met-Asn-|Thr-Gln-|Phe-Gln-Ala-Val-Gly-Lys|

MEM Glu-Asp-Thr-Lys-Ile-Asp-Leu-Trp-Ser-Tyr-Asn-Ala-Glu-Leu-Leu-Val-Ala-Leu-|Glu-Asn-Gln-|His-|Thr-Ile-|Asp-|Glu-Thr-Asp-
90   100   110

JAP   Met-|Glu-Asx-Glx-|Arg-|Thr-|Leu-Asx-|Phe-His

MEM Ser-Glu-Met-Asn-Lys-Leu-Phe-Glu-Lys-Thr-Arg-Arg-|Gln-Leu-Arg-|Glu-Asn-Ala-Glu-Asp-Met-|Gly-Asn-Gly-Cys-Phe-|Lys-|Ile-
120   130   140

JAP   Met-|Gln-Leu-Arg-|Asx-Asx-Val-Lys-Glx-|Leu-Gly-Asx-Gly-Cys-Phe-|Gln-Phe-

MEM |Tyr-His-Lys-Cys-Asp-Asn-Ala-|Cys-|Ile-|Gly-|Ser-|Ile-Arg-Asn-Gly-Thr-Tyr-Asp-His-|Asp-Val-Tyr-Arg-Asp-Glu-Ala-Leu-Asn-
150   *   160

JAP |Tyr-His-Lys-Cys-Asx-Asx-|Glx-|Cys-|Met-Asn-|Ser-|Val-Lys

MEM Asn-Arg-Phe-Gln-Ile-Lys-Gly-Val-Glu-Leu-Lys-Ser-Gly-Asp-Lys-(Ala-Ile-Ser-Cys-Phe)-indigestible residue peptides-
170   180

MEM Gly-Asn-Ile-Glu-Cys-Asn-Ile-Cys-Ile.
~222

Fig. 2. The amino acid sequence of A/Mem/72 hemagglutinin light chain. It is compared with available data relating to the A/Jap/57 light chain[13] which we arranged so as to maximise the homology. Boxes indicate identical residues. Asn* indicates the glycosylated asparagine in Mem HA2. Brackets indicate an unplaced peptide.

CN4 have been reported previously.[11,12]

Peptide CN1 is the most interesting part of HA2, since it carries the single glycosylated asparagine and all the seven ½-cystines. Its insolubility and aggregation make it a challenge for the protein chemist. It has an N-terminal glycine and a C-terminal isoleucine.[11] Digestion with trypsin, chymotrypsin or thermolysin gave a series of overlapping soluble peptides comprising the first fifty residues of CN1. In addition, two non-overlapped peptides, both containing ½-cystine, contributed another 14 residues. One of these, a tryptic peptide, represents the C-terminal sequence of HA2, while the other, a chymotryptic one, remains unplaced. All enzymic digests gave, besides these soluble peptides, very insoluble residues, which were heterogeneous by end group determination. The composition of one such insoluble mixture T, derived from a trypsin digest and given in Table 1, shows the hydrophobic nature of these aggregated residues.

In Fig. 2, the sequence of A/Mem/72 HA2 is set out, and compared with the known sequence details of A/Jap/57.[13] The only carbohydrate moiety in HA2 we have found to contain 4 glucosamines only; the sequence in which it occurs again reinforces the empirical rule requiring a 3-hydroxy amino acid one residue removed C-terminally from the asparagine for glycosylation.[14]

It is evident that shift between strains involves considerable differences in hemagglutinin structure, but it is interesting to see preservation of certain details, which must be key-features, notably the amino terminal sequence[15] and the area around the ½-cystine residues.

2. The disulphide-bond pattern of HA.

We have used the Brown and Hartley diagonal method[16] to separate thermolysin-derived disulphide peptides as their oxidised pairs. Micro sequencing[17] was used to identify most pairs, while some peptides were identified by composition alone.

In this manner, eight ½-cystines on HA1 could be divided into three intra-chain bridges and two interchain bonds with two of the three proximal HA2 ½-cystines. A third interchain bond (involving HA2 Cys 148 and HA Cys 97) was inferred, but only the HA2 partner was isolated. However, it is possible to free the hemagglutinin from the viral surface with bromelain,[10] to give a truncated HA2 lacking the C-terminal 70 or so residues;[15] this missing part includes the C-terminal four ½-cystines, which therefore cannot be linked to any ½-cystine except themselves. This virtually proves the existence of the inferred third HA1-HA2 link. We have no knowledge of the state of these terminal ½-cystines because the drastic procedures needed to investigate this

TABLE 2

CYSTEIC ACID - CONTAINING PEPTIDES, OBTAINED FROM A$_2$/MEM/72 INFLUENZA
HEMAGGLUTININ THROUGH A DIAGONAL MAPPING PROCEDURE: THEIR MOBILITIES BEFORE[1]
AND AFTER[2] PERFORMIC ACID OXIDATION, AND THEIR SEQUENCE.

Pair	Mob[1]	Mob[2]	Sequence	Source
1a	−0.35	−0.65	Leu-Cys^{14}	HA1
1b		−0.55	Leu-Arg-Glu-Asn-Ala-Glu-Asp-(Met O$_2$- Gly-Asn-Gly-Cys^{137})	HA2
2a	0.40	neutral	Ile-Cys^{52}-Asn-Asn-(Pro-His-Arg)	HA1
2b		−0.45	Ile-Gly-Thr-Cys^{277}	HA1
3a	−0.60	−0.40	Ile-Asp-Cys^{64}-Thr	HA1
3b		−0.70	Leu-Gly-Asp-Pro-His-(Cys^{76}-Asp-Gly)	HA1
4a	neutral		Ile-Ser-Glu-Cys^{281}	HA1
4b			Gly-Ala-Cys^{305}-(Pro-Lys-Thr)	HA1
5a	0.20	−0.55	(Lys-Cys^{144}-Asp)	HA2
5b		−0.05	(Ala-Cys^{139}-Lys-Arg-Gly-Pro-Asp)	HA1
6	neutral	−0.60	(Asn-Ala-Cys^{148})	HA2
			Partner not resolved.	

Mobilities are given with respect to the mobility of aspartic acid (−1.0 at
pH 6.5).
The numbers over the ½-cystine residues correspond with the numbers of the
½-cystines in the chains (Fig. 2).

area were not conducive to the survival of disulphide bonds. Figure 3 shows a
schematic arrangement of the disulphide bonds of HA. Although the basis for
sequence comparisons is small at this stage, the published details of a
hemagglutinin from A/Jap/57[13,15] show a 55% difference with the sequences of
A/Mem/72 hemagglutinin chains. On the other hand, the relative location of
those ½-cystines which we can compare, four on HA1 and three on HA2, are all
invariant.

This argues for the importance of the disulphide bonds in providing
structural integrity necessary for the functionality of the hemagglutinin.

REFERENCES

1. Laver, W.G. and Valentine, R.C. (1969) Virology, 38, 105-119.

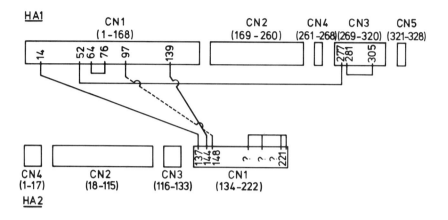

Fig. 3. Diagrammatic structure of influenza hemagglutinin. The cyanogen bromide fragments are indicated as boxes, with the numbers within the boxes giving the positions of the ½-cystine residues in the sequence. Bracketed numbers refer to the position of each cyanogen bromide fragment in the chains. The dotted bridge is assumed, and question marks indicate unplaced ½-cystine residues.

2. Griffiths, I.P. (1975) in Negative Strand Viruses, Mahy, B.H.J. and Barry, R.D. ed., Academic Press, London, pp.121-132.
3. Drzeniek, R., Seto, J.T. and Rott, R. (1966) Biochim. Biophys. Acta, 128, 547-558.
4. Laver, W.G. and Kilbourne, E.D. (1966) Virology, 30, 493-501.
5. White, D.O. (1974) Curr. Top. Microbiol. Immunol., 63, 1-48.
6. Laver, W.G. (1971) Virology, 45, 275-288.
7. Dopheide, T.A.A. and Ward, C.W. (1978) in The Influenza Virus Hemagglutinin, Laver, W.G., Bachmayer, H. and Weil, R. ed., Springer, Vienna, pp.193-201.
8. Ward, C.W. and Dopheide, T.A.A. (1976) FEBS Lett., 65, 365-368.
9. Jackson, D.C., Dopheide, T.A.A., Russell, Robyn J., White, D.O. and Ward, C.W. (1979) Virology, 93, 458-465.
10. Skehel, J.J. and Waterfield, M.D. (1975) Proc. Natl. Acad. Sci. U.S.A., 72, 93-97.
11. Dopheide, T.A.A. and Ward, C.W. (1979) Virology, 92, 230-235.
12. Ward, C.W. and Dopheide, T.A.A. (1979) Virology, 95, 107-118.
13. McCauley, J., Skehel, J.J. and Waterfield, M.D. (1978) in The Influenza Virus Hemagglutinin, Laver, W.G., Bachmayer, H. and Weil, R. ed., Springer, Vienna, pp.181-192.
14. Neuberger, A., Gottschalk, A., Marshall, R.D. and Spiro, R.G. (1972) in 'Glycoproteins', Gottschalk, A. ed., Elsevier, Amsterdam, 2nd Ed., Part A, pp.450-490.
15. Waterfield, M.D., Espelie, K., Elder, K. and Skehel, J.J. (1979) Br. Med. Bull. 35, 57-63.
16. Brown, J.R. and Hartley, B.S. (1966) Biochem. J. 101, 214-228.
17. Bruton, C.J. and Hartley, B.S. (1968) Biochem. J. 108, 281-288.

THE HONG KONG (H3) HEMAGGLUTININ.   COMPLETE AMINO ACID SEQUENCE AND
OLIGOSACCHARIDE DISTRIBUTION FOR THE HEAVY CHAIN OF A/MEMPHIS/102/72

COLIN W. WARD AND THEO A. DOPHEIDE
CSIRO, Division of Protein Chemistry, 343 Royal Parade, Parkville, 3052,
Victoria, Australia.

INTRODUCTION

Effective vaccination against influenza is still an unattained goal despite
the fact that the virus was first isolated almost fifty years ago and can be
readily cultivated in the laboratory. This is in part due to the inappropriate-
ness of current vaccination procedures,[1,2] but also to the unique ability of
influenza virus to undergo frequent and often dramatic antigenic change.
Although both viral coat proteins (hemagglutinin and neuraminidase) undergo
independent major (antigenic shift) and minor (antigenic drift) changes, the
hemagglutinin, because of its central role in the infection process, is
considered the more important antigen.[3-6] Peptide maps[7,8] have shown that
these antigenic changes in the hemagglutinin reflect alterations in its amino
acid sequence and there has been considerable speculation concerning the number
and nature of antigenic determinants on the hemagglutinin and the way these
change during antigenic shift and drift.[9-13']

In order to establish the chemical basis of this antigenic variation we
have determined the amino acid sequence of the hemagglutinin from the Hong
Kong variant A/Memphis/102/72 while Waterfield and co-workers[14,15] have
established most of the sequence of the hemagglutinin from the Asian variant
A/Jap/305/57. In this article we describe the complete amino acid sequence of
A/Mem/72 heavy chain (HA$_1$) including data on the location and composition of
its six constituent oligosaccharides. The structure is discussed in relation
to the available data on the hemagglutinins from other influenza strains and
recent developments in the analysis of antigenic shift and drift.

MATERIALS AND METHODS

Virus strain and protein preparation. The virus strain used, the procedures
employed in virus cultivation, purification, hemagglutinin isolation and
separation into HA$_1$ and HA$_2$ have been previously described.[16,17]

Peptide fragmentation. The procedures employed in reduction, carboxymethyl-
ation with 2-^{14}C-iodoacetic acid, cyanogen bromide cleavage and chromatographic
separation of the resultant peptides;[18] enzymic hydrolysis and peptide

purification by gel chromatography and high-voltage paper electrophoresis[17,19] have been fully described.

Amino acid sequence determination. Automated sequence analyses, manual dansyl-Edman degradations, amino acid analyses and C-terminal amino acid analyses were as previously described.[17,19]

RESULTS AND DISCUSSION

Molecular weight. The hemagglutinin monomer is coded for by a single segment of RNA[20] and is synthesized as a single polypeptide chain. Post-translational processing results in the proteolytic removal of an N-terminal signal sequence[21] and, depending on the virus strain, host cell type and culture conditions,[22] the proteolytic cleavage into HA_1 and HA_2.

The reported molecular weights for HA_1 polypeptides from the same, as well as from different, virus strains exhibit considerable variation (see refs. 16 and 23). Values ranged from 65,000 to 46,000 and were believed to reflect true differences in the number of amino acids present in the proteins as well as differences in the amount of carbohydrate attached to the polypeptide chains. Subsequently we were able to demonstrate that a large part of this variation was due to differences in the experimental conditions employed.[16] Most of these molecular weight estimates were based on relative mobilities in SDS gels, a technique known to result in over-estimations when applied to glycoproteins

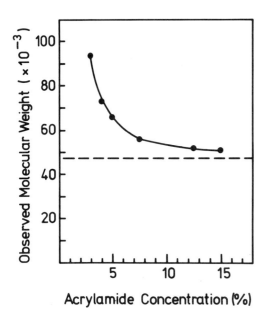

Fig. 1. Observed molecular weight of A/Mem/72 HA_1 in SDS gels of different acrylamide concentrations (based on ref. 16). The true molecular weight based on ultracentrifugal analysis is 47,000 (----)

containing more than 10% carbohydrate, and these over-estimations increase as the gel concentration used is decreased.[24] When A/Mem/72 HA_1 was examined under a variety of gel concentrations its apparent molecular weight fell from 92,000 in 3% gels to 51,000 in 15% gels as shown in Figure 1. Ultracentrifugal analysis indicated that the true molecular weight was approximately 47,000.[16]

Amino acid sequence. Carbohydrate and amino acid analyses indicated that A/Mem/72 HA_1 contained approximately 67 residues (MW 11,500) of carbohydrate and 330 amino acid residues (MW 35,500) including 4 methionines.[16] Cyanogen bromide cleavage at the 4 methionine residues yielded 5 peptides CN1 to CN5[18] and their amino acid compositions are shown in Table 1. Peptides CN1 and CN3 are glycopeptides with CN1 containing most of the carbohydrate. The two small peptides CN4 and CN5 were sequenced directly[18] while the structures of the larger peptides CN1,[17] CN2[25] and CN3,[18] were established by analysis of tryptic and chymotryptic peptides.

TABLE 1

AMINO ACID COMPOSITIONS OF A/MEM/72 HA_1 AND ITS CYANOGEN BROMIDE PEPTIDES

Residue	HA_1	CN1	CN2	CN3	CN4	CN5
CM-cysteine	9	6		3		
Aspartic acid	46	27	11	7		1
Threonine	28	15	6	5	1	1
Serine	30	15	10	3	2	
Glutamic acid	22	11	6	3		
Proline	20	8	6	5		2
Glycine	27	15	7	4	1	1
Alanine	13	8	2	3		
Valine	20	10	7	2		1
Methionine	4					
Isoleucine	23	7	10	5	1	
Leucine	22	15	5	2		
Tyrosine	11	5	4	2		
Phenylalanine	11	8	2	1		
Histidine	6	4	2			
Lysine	16	5	4	5	1	1
Arginine	14	5	6	1	1	1
Tryptophan	6	3	3			
Homoserine		1	1	1	1	
Total Amino Acid Residues	328	168	92	52	8	8
Sequence Position		1–168	169–260	269–320	261–268	321–328

Values are expressed as residues per mole and are taken from refs. 16-18,25. Peptides CN1 and CN3 carry carbohydrate.

The complete amino acid sequence of A/Mem/72 HA$_1$ is shown in Figure 2. This Hong Kong HA$_1$ was found to contain 328 amino acid residues, which is very close to the 330 residues predicted from our molecular weight and chemical composition data.[16]

CN1 contains 168 residues and accounts for the N-terminal half of this Hong Kong HA$_1$. It has a blocked N-terminus characteristic of all Hong Kong strains examined to date as well as the two putative progenitors of the human Hong Kong pandemic.[15,23,26,27] This N-terminal blocking group in Mem/72 HA$_1$ was found to be pyroglutamic acid.[17] CN1 contains five glycosylated asparagine residues at positions 8,22,38,81 and 165. CN1 also contains six half-cystine residues at positions 14,52,64,76,97 and 139.

CN2 contains 92 amino acids and extends from residue 169 to 260. It does not contain any half-cystine residues or carbohydrate.[25] Peptides CN4 (residues 261-268), CN3 (residues 269-320) and CN5 (residues 321-328) account for the C-terminal 68 amino acids in A/Mem/72 HA$_1$.[18] CN3 contains one glycosylated asparagine residue at position 285 and three half-cystines at positions 277, 281 and 305 (Figure 2). CN5 contains no methionine or homoserine and is the C-terminal peptide of HA$_1$. As discussed previously[18,23,27] the presence of Thr as the C-terminal residue rather than the expected Lys or Arg strongly suggested that the infectivity-enhancing[22,28] cleavage of HA into HA$_1$ and HA$_2$ was not a simple cleavage of a Thr-Gly bond, but more likely involved the sequential removal of a small trypsin susceptible connecting peptide. Nucleotide sequences of the hemagglutinin genes from fowl plague virus[29] and some Hong Kong strains[30-32] shows that this is so. With fowl plague the connecting peptide contains a sequence of five residues Lys-Arg-Glu-Lys-Arg while in the Hong Kong strains there is only a single arginine.

Figure 2 also includes the partial amino acid sequence of HA$_1$ from the early Hong Kong variant A/Aichi/2/68 (X-31). As found with A/Mem/72 HA$_1$, five peptides are produced on reaction with cyanogen bromide. The two small octapeptides CN4 and CN5 are identical in both strains, while CN3 (residues 269-320) shows only 1 sequence change, Asp for Gly, at position 275. The Thr/Ser substitutions at positions 270 and 279, found by Waterfield et al.[15] were not

---

Fig. 2. Amino acid sequence of HA$_1$ polypeptides of A/Mem/72 and A/Aichi/2/68 (X-31). Methionine residues occur at positions 168,260,268 and 320. Oligosaccharide units are attached in both strains at residues 8,22,38,81,165 and 285. A/Mem/72 data (upper case lettering) is from ref. 17; X-31 data is from Ward and Dopheide, unpublished.

```
Aichi/2/68 (X-31)  Glx-Tyr-Leu-Pro-Gly-Asn-Asp-Asn-Ser-Thr-Ala-Thr-Leu-Cys-Leu-
                                                 *
Mem/102/72         GLX-ASP-PHE-PRO-GLY-ASN-ASP-ASN-SER-THR-ALA-THR-LEU-CYS-LEU-
                                                 *           10

                                         *
Gly-His-His-Ala-Val-Pro-Asn-Gly-Thr-Leu-Val-Lys-Thr-Ile-Thr-Asn-Asp-Gln-Ile-Glu-
GLY-HIS-HIS-ALA-VAL-PRO-ASN-GLY-THR-LEU-VAL-LYS-THR-ILE-THR-ASN-ASP-GLN-ILE-GLU-
            20            *                      30

             *
Val-Thr-Asn-Ala-Thr-Glu-Leu-Val-Gln-Ser-Ser-Ser-Thr-Gly-Lys-Ile-Cys-Asn-Asn-Pro-
VAL-THR-ASN-ALA-THR-GLU-LEU-VAL-GLN-SER-SER-SER-THR-GLY-LYS-ILE-CYS-ASN-ASN-PRO-
        *        40                             50

His-Arg-Ile-Leu-Asp-Gly-Ile-Asp-Cys-Thr-Leu-Ile-Asp-Ala-Leu-Leu-Gly-Asp-Pro-His-
HIS-ARG-ILE-LEU-ASP-GLY-ILE-ASP-CYS-THR-LEU-ILE-ASP-ALA-LEU-LEU-GLY-ASP-PRO-HIS-
                    60                          70

                         *
Cys-Asp-Gly-Phe-Gln-Asn-Glu-Thr-Trp-Asp-Leu-Phe-Val-Glu-Arg-Ser-Lys-Ala-Phe-Ser-
CYS-ASP-GLY-PHE-GLN-ASN-GLU-THR-TRP-ASP-LEU-PHE-VAL-GLU-ARG-SER-LYS-ALA-PHE-SER-
                80   *                          90

Asn-Cys-Tyr-Pro-Tyr-Asp-Val-Pro-Asp-Tyr-Ala-Ser-Leu-Arg-Ser-Leu-Val-Ala-Ser-Ser-
ASN-CYS-TYR-PRO-TYR-ASP-VAL-PRO-ASP-TYR-ALA-SER-LEU-ARG-SER-LEU-VAL-ALA-SER-SER-
                100                             110

Gly-Thr-Leu-Glu-Phe-Ile-Thr-Glu-Gly-Phe-Thr-Trp-Thr-Gly-Val-Thr-Gln-Asn-Gly-Gly-
GLY-THR-LEU-GLU-PHE-ILE-ASN-GLU-GLY-PHE-THR-TRP-THR-GLY-VAL-THR-GLN-ASN-GLY-GLY-
                120                             130

Ser-Asn-Ala-Cys-Lys-Arg-Gly-Pro-Gly-Ser-Gly-Phe-Phe-Ser-Arg-Leu-Asn-Trp-Leu-Thr-
SER-ASP-ALA-CYS-LYS-ARG-GLY-PRO-ASP-SER-GLY-PHE-PHE-SER-ARG-LEU-ASN-TRP-LEU-TYR-
                140                             150

                                 *
Lys-Ser-Glu-Ser-Thr-Tyr-Pro-Val-Leu-Asn-Val-Thr-Met-Pro
LYS-SER-GLY-SER-THR-TYR-PRO-VAL-LEU-ASN-VAL-THR-MET-PRO-ASN-ASN-ASP-ASN-PHE-ASP-
            160              *                  170

LYS-LEU-TYR-ILE-TRP-GLY-VAL-HIS-HIS-PRO-SER-THR-ASP-GLN-GLU-GLN-THR-SER-LEU-TYR-
                180                             190

VAL-GLN-ALA-SER-GLY-ARG-VAL-THR-VAL-SER-THR-LYS-ARG-SER-GLN-GLN-THR-ILE-ILE-PRO-
                200                             210

ASN-ILE-GLY-SER-ARG-PRO-TRP-VAL-ARG-GLY-LEU-SER-SER-ARG-ILE-SER-ILE-TYR-TRP-THR-
                220                             230

ILE-VAL-LYS-PRO-GLY-ASP-ILE-LEU-VAL-ILE-ASN-SER-ASN-GLY-ASP-LEU-ILE-ALA-PRO-ARG-
                240                             250

                 Met-Arg-Thr-Gly-Lys-Ser-Ser-Ile-Met-Arg-Ser-Asp-Ala-Pro-Ile-Asp-
GLY-TYR-PHE-LYS-MET-ARG-THR-GLY-LYS-SER-SER-ILE-MET-ARG-SER-ASP-ALA-PRO-ILE-GLY-
                260                             270

Thr-Cys-Ile-Ser-Glu-Cys-Ile-Thr-Pro-Asn-Gly-Ser-Ile-Pro-Lys-Pro-Asp-Asp-Phe-Gln-
THR-CYS-ILE-SER-GLU-CYS-ILE-THR-PRO-ASN-GLY-SER-ILE-PRO-LYS-PRO-ASP-ASP-PHE-GLN-
                280          *                  290

Asn-Val-Asn-Lys-Ile-Thr-Tyr-Gly-Ala-Cys-Pro-Lys-Tyr-Val-Lys-Gln-Asn-Thr-Leu-Lys-
ASN-VAL-ASN-LYS-ILE-THR-TYR-GLY-ALA-CYS-PRO-LYS-TYR-VAL-LYS-GLN-ASN-THR-LEU-LYS-
                300                             310

Leu-Ala-Thr-Gly-Met-Arg-Asn-Val-Pro-Glu-Lys-Gln-Thr-COOH
LEU-ALA-THR-GLY-MET-ARG-ASN-VAL-PRO-GLU-LYS-GLN-THR-COOH
                320          325
```

present in our isolate of X-31. The 92 residue CN2 from X-31 has the same end group, Pro, as in A/Mem/72 but has not been studied further. The N-terminal CN1 from X-31 contains 168 residues and five oligosaccharide units attached at the same positions as in A/Mem/72, but shows several changes in amino acid sequence. These substitutions occur at positions 2,3,122,144,155 and 158 (see Fig. 2). The changes at 144 and 155 have been reported previously[36] in a study of the amino acid sequence changes occurring in the soluble peptides of nine different Hong Kong variants.

When compared with the amino acid sequence data available for other influenza strains[15,29] these Hong Kong HA_1 polypeptides contain an additional 10 residues at their N-termini. All other influenza sub-type HA_1 chains start at residue 11. This extended sequence contains few hydrophobic residues and bears no homology with the N-terminal signal sequence of the Asian variant R15-.[21] Since this extended sequence appears to be a characteristic feature of the Hong Kong hemagglutinin it will be of great interest to see if both A/duck/Ukraine/ 63 and A/equine/Miami/63 [33] contain this extended N-terminal sequence. As shown in Figure 3 the relative locations of the half-cystine residues in A/Mem/ 72, A/Jap/57 and A/FPV are invariant, while the positions of the methionine and glycosylated asparagine residues are not. A/Jap/57 contains only four

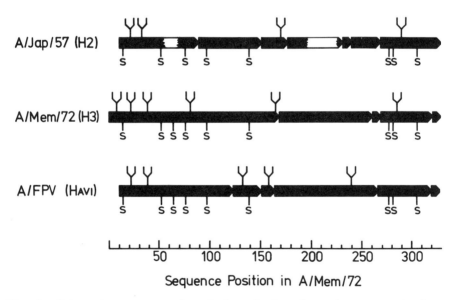

Fig. 3. Schematic representation of the relative size and arrangement of cyanogen bromide peptides of A/Jap/57, A/Mem/72 and A/FPV HA_1 polypeptides. The positions of the half-cystine residues and glycosylated asparagine residues are indicated.

oligosaccharide units attached at positions 21,33,170 and 289 (numbers refer to Hong Kong sequence) residues which are close to, but not identical with, some of the glycosylated residues in the Hong Kong strain. Furthermore, the carbo- hydrate groups in similar regions are of different types. That present on Asn_{285} in A/Mem/72 is simple[18] containing 2 N-acetylglucosamine residues and 5 mannose, while that on Asn_{289} in A/Jap/57 is complex and contains all four sugars.[15] Fowl plague virus HA_1 is predicted to contain five oligosaccharide units, two of which occur at identical positions to two in the Hong Kong strain (residues 22 and 38), a third which is near the position of another in A/Mem/72, while the remaining two occur in quite different regions. Fowl plague virus HA_1 has been reported to contain only complex oligosaccharide chains.[34,35] These comparisons illustrate that the major differences in the distribution of oligosaccharide side chains on the various hemagglutinins are primarily influenced by alterations in the amino acid sequence. Mutations which affect the occurrence of Asn-x-$\frac{Ser}{Thr}$ sequences will subsequently affect both the type and locations of attached carbohydrate.

Comparison of the amino acid sequences of A/Jap/57, A/Mem/72 and the predicted sequence of A/FPV reveals over 55% differences between them. This is in marked contrast to the small number (approximately 7%) of changes that accumulated in the Hong Kong strains isolated between 1968 and 1977.[36] Such large differences between sub-types in conjunction with the low base sequence homologies observed for the corresponding HA-coding RNA segments[37] indicate that antigenic drift does not involve the mutation of pre-existing variants via so-called bridging strains.[9]

Location and composition of oligosaccharides. Since the carbohydrate on the influenza hemagglutinin is attached by host cell transferases these oligo- saccharides would be expected to resemble normal host glycoproteins in their mechanism of synthesis and general structures. Like glycoproteins from other sources[38] the influenza hemagglutinin is glycosylated by the transfer of glucosamine-mannose cores from glycolipid intermediates[39] followed by the attachment of peripheral galactose and fucose units. As shown for vesicular stomatitis virus glycoprotein, glycosylation commences while the polypeptide is still being synthesized, continues in several discrete steps and is completed at approximately the same time as the polypeptide backbone.[40]

Numerous qualitative studies using radiolabelled sugars have been carried out to assess the number and type of oligosaccharide units attached to HA_1 and HA_2[34,35,41,42] but few quantitative studies.[15,16,43] All these studies show that both chains are glycosylated with most carbohydrate being on HA_1. The

34

TABLE 2

CARBOHYDRATE COMPOSITIONS OF DIFFERENT INFLUENZA A VIRUS HA$_1$ POLYPEPTIDES

Residue	Bel/42 (HO)	Weiss/43 (HO)	FMI/47 (H1)	Jap/57 (H2)	Aichi/68 (H3)	Mem/72 (H3)	Port Ch/73 (H3)
N-Acetyl-glucosamine	28	20	12	29	22	19	15
Mannose	∿8	19	12	16	24	33	24
Galactose	∿6	22	13	17	12	10	12
Fucose	∿5	6	4	5	5	5	3
Total	∿47	67	41	67	67	67	54

Data for Bel/42 is from ref. 43; for Weiss/43, FMI/47, Jap/57, Aichi/68 and Port Chalmers/73 from ref. 15 and for Mem/72 from ref. 16.

sugar compositions for several HA$_1$ polypeptides are shown in Table 2. Four strains, Weiss/43, Jap/57, X-31 and Mem/72 contain approximately the same amount of total carbohydrate, although the molar ratios of the individual sugars differ. The other strains examined have considerably less carbohydrate on HA$_1$. All strains contain the same four sugars N-acetylglucosamine, mannose, galactose and fucose, known since 1956 to be present on whole virions[44] and as pointed out previously[16] should thus contain only oligosaccharide chains attached in N-glycosidic linkage to asparagine residues. In a recent paper Keil et al.[35] reached the same conclusion. As shown in Figure 2 all six oligosaccharide chains on Mem/72 HA$_1$ are attached to asparagine residues (positions 8,22,38,81, 165 and 285) as is the single oligosaccharide unit in A/Mem/72 HA$_2$.[45] As

TABLE 3

TRIPEPTIDE SEQUENCE AND CARBOHYDRATE COMPOSITION OF THE SIX GLYCOSYLATED REGIONS OF A/MEM/72 HA$_1$

Asn Position	Sequence	GlcNAc	Man.	Gal.	Fuc.	Carbohydrate Type
8	Asn Ser Thr	4	4	5	2	Complex
22	Asn Gly Thr	4	2	2	1	Complex
38	Asn Ala Thr	4	6	3	1	Complex
81	Asn Glu Thr	3	3	2	1	Complex
165	Asn Val Thr	2	6			
285	Asn Gly Ser	2	5			Simple

Data from Ward, Gleeson and Dopheide unpublished.

expected, no carbohydrate was found attached in O-glycosidic linkage to serine or threonine. Examination of the structure in Figure 2 shows that all potential glycosylation sites (Asn-X-$^{Ser}_{Thr}$ sequences) do have carbohydrate attached.

The compositions of each of these oligosaccharide units on A/Mem/72 are shown in Table 3. Those on residues 8,22,38 and 81 are complex containing all four sugars, while those on residues 165 and 285 are of the simple type containing just 2 residues of N-acetylglucosamine and 5 or 6 residues of mannose. The carbohydrate moiety on Asn_8 is the only one that is sulphated[46] and is presumably the host antigen.[47]

Structural implications of the primary sequence

The sequence data for A/Mem/72 has recently been used to characterise the changes occurring during antigenic drift in the Hong Kong sub-type. Chemical and antigenic analysis of 10 variants selected with monoclonal hybridoma antibodies indicated that there were at least four distinct non-overlapping regions on the Hong Kong HA_1.[48] When extended to an analysis of nine Hong Kong field strains[36] isolated between 1968 and 1977 the same tryptic peptides that showed substitutions in the monoclonal variants also changed in the field strains but in each case the substitutions found were different. These and similar studies on the HO variant A/PR/8/34[49] have led to the conclusion that the widespread survival of new strains which arise by antigenic drift would require changes in every antigenic region.

To fully characterize the number and nature of antigenic regions on the influenza hemagglutinin comparative amino acid sequences and three-dimensional crystal structures are going to be required. Using the algorithm and parameters of Chou and Fasman[50,51] some tentative predictions of local secondary structure can be made and these are summarized in Table 4. As has been found for other proteins[52] the glycosylated asparagine residues on HA_2 and four of those on HA_1 (residues 8,22,81 and 285) occur at β-bends. Antigenic regions would also be expected to involve residues at or near β-bends. As shown in Table 4 the residues found to change during antigenic drift[36] in the Hong Kong sub-type (residues 53,54,122,133,143-146,155,158,207,208,217-224,225-229) do occur at or near predicted β-bends. The most striking feature in Table 4 is the contrast between the predicted structures for HA_1 and HA_2. HA_1 is very rich in potential β-structure. It contains 19 β-strands several of which are found in sheets of 3 or more anti-parallel strands connected by hairpin β-bends (residues 10-38,108-133,174-214 and 222-246). In contrast the light chain is

TABLE 4

PREDICTED SECONDARY STRUCTURE FOR A/MEM/72 HA_1 AND HA_2

| | HA_1 | | | HA_2 | |
α-helix	β-sheet	β-turn	α-helix	β-sheet	β-turn
	10-16	3-6, 6-9	2-11		10-14
	24-30	20-23, 30-33			18-22
39-45	33-38	46-50, 52-55			26-29
65-71		61-64, 73-76			28-31
	83-88	76-79, 81-84	34-40		31-34
89-94		94-97, 98-101	41-48		48-51
	108-113	102-105,114-117	57-74	52-56	
	117-122	122-125	77-92		93-96
	125-133	133-136,135-138	96-103	104-111	
		139-142,142-145	112-123		
	150-155	144-147,155-158	125-133		133-137
	163-168	158-162,168-171		137-144	144-147
	175-184	171-174,184-187			148-151
	191-198	198-201			152-156
	201-207	206-209			157-160
	209-214	214-217,216-219			162-165
	222-226	219-222,227-230		170-173	168-171
	230-238	238-241	174-180		179-182
	242-246	246-249,253-257			182-185
		260-263,263-266		185-211	210-213
	273-279	268-272,278-281		214-221	
		283-286,288-291			
	294-298	291-294,296-300			
	300-305	305-308			
313-318	308-312	323-326			

Data from Ward and Dopheide, unpublished.

predicted to be highly helical particularly in the region between residues 35
and 133. Here 77 of the 99 residues occur in seven sections of α-helix. Even
more striking is the observation that the heptad distribution of polar and non-
polar residues in this helical region is very similar to that found in some
fibrous proteins[53-55] and raises the possibility that the filamentous appearance of the influenza hemagglutinin may be due in part to the presence of a
coiled-coil.

REFERENCES

1. Mims, C.A. (1976) in Influenza, Virus, Vaccines, Strategy. Selby, P. ed.,
   Academic Press, London, pp.95-105.
2. Tyrrell, D.A.J. (1979) Br. Med. Bull. 35, 77-85.
3. Drzeniek, R., Seto, J.T. and Rott, R. (1966) Biochim. Biophys. Acta, 128,
   547-558.

4. Laver, W.G. and Kilbourne, E.D. (1966) Virology, 30, 493-501.
5. Klenk, H-D., Rott, R., Orlich, M. and Blödorn, J. (1975) Virology, 68, 426-439.
6. Lazarowitz, S.G. and Choppin, P.W. (1975) Virology, 68, 440-454.
7. Laver, W.G. and Webster, R.G. (1968) Virology, 34, 193-202.
8. Laver, W.G. and Webster, R.G. (1972) Virology, 48, 445-455.
9. Fazekas de St. Groth, S. (1978) in The Influenza Virus Hemagglutinin, Laver, W.G., Bachmayer, H. and Weil, R. ed., Springer-Verlag, Vienna, pp.15-24.
10.Virelezier, J.L., Postlethwaite, R., Schild, G.C. and Allison, A.C. (1974) J. Expl. Med. 140, 1559-1570.
11.Gerhard, W. (1978) in The Influenza Virus Hemagglutinin, Laver, W.G., Bachmayer, H. and Weil, R. ed., Springer-Verlag, Vienna, pp.15-24.
12.Webster, R.G. and Laver, W.G. (1975) in The Influenza Viruses and Influenza, Kilbourne, E.D. ed., Academic Press, New York, pp.209-314.
13.Russell, R.J., Burns, W.H., White, D.O., Anders, E.M., Ward, C.W. and Jackson, D.C. (1979) J. Immunol. 123, 825-831.
14.Waterfield, M.D., Skehel, J.J., Nakashima, Y., Gurnett, A. and Bilham, T. (1978) in The Influenza Virus Hemagglutinin, Laver, W.G., Bachmayer, H. and Weil, R., ed., Springer-Verlag, Vienna, pp.181-192.
15.Waterfield, M.D., Espelie, K., Elder, K. and Skehel, J.J. (1979) Br. Med. Bull. 35, 57-63.
16.Ward, C.W. and Dopheide, T.A. FEBS. Lett. 65, 365-368.
17.Ward, C.W. and Dopheide, T.A. (1980) Virology, In press.
18.Dopheide, T.A. and Ward, C.W. (1978) Eur. J. Biochem. 85, 393-398.
19.Ward, C.W. and Dopheide, T.A. (1979) Virology, 95, 107-118.
20.Scholtissek, C. (1978) in Current Topics Microbiol. Immunol. 80, 139-169.
21.Air, G.M. (1979) Virology 97, 468-472.
22.Choppin, P.W., Lazarowitz, S.G. and Goldberg, A.R. (1975) in Negative Strand Viruses, Academic Press, London, Vol. 1, pp.105-119.
23.Dopheide, T.A. and Ward, C.W. (1978) in The Influenza Virus Hemagglutinin, Laver, W.G., Bachmayer, H. and Weil, R. ed., Springer-Verlag, Vienna, pp.193-201.
24.Segrest, J.P. and Jackson, R.L. (1972) Methods Enzymol. 28, 54-63.
25.Ward, C.W., Dopheide, T.A., and Inglis, A.S. (1980) Aust. J. Biol. Sci. In press.
26.Laver, W.G. and Webster, R.G. (1977) Virology 81, 482-485.
27.Ward, C.W. and Dopheide, T.A. (1979) Br. Med. Bull. 35, 51-56.
28.Klenk, H-D., Rott, R., and Orlich, M. (1977) J. Gen. Virol. 36, 151-161.
29.Porter, A.G., Threlfall, G., Carey, N.H., Smith, J.C. and Emtage, J.S. (1980). This volume.
30.Sleigh, M.J., Both, G.W., Brownlee, G.G., Bender, V.J. and Moss, B.A. (1980). This volume.
31.Threlfall, G. (1980). This volume.
32.Min-Jou, W. (1980). This volume.
33.Laver, W.G. and Webster, R.G. (1973) Virology 51, 383-391.
34.Schwarz, R.T., Schmidt, F.G., Anwer, V. and Klenk, H-D. (1977) J. Virol. 23, 217-226.
35.Keil, W., Klenk, H.-D., and Schwarz, R.T. (1979) J. Virol. 31, 253-256.
36.Laver, W.G., Air, G.M., Dopheide, T.A. and Ward, C.W. (1980) Nature. In press.
37.Scholtissek, C., Rohde, W., Harms, E. and Rott, R. (1977) Virology, 79, 330-336.
38.Waechter, C.J. and Lennarz, W.J. (1976) Ann. Rev. Biochem. 45, 95-112.
39.Klenk, H.-D., Schwarz, R.T., Schmidt, M.F. and Wollert, W. (1978) in The Influenza Virus Hemagglutinin, Laver, W.G., Bachmayer, H. and Weil, R. ed., Springer-Verlag, Vienna, pp.83-99.

40. Elder, K.T., Bye, J.M., Skehel, J.J., Waterfield, M.D. and Smith, A.E. (1979) Virology, 95, 343-350.
41. Nakamura, K. and Compans, R.W. (1978) Virology, 86, 432-442.
42. Nakamura, K. and Compans, R.W. (1979) Virology, 95, 8-23.
43. Laver, W.G. (1971) Virology, 45, 275-288.
44. Ada, G.L. and Gottschalk, A. (1956) Biochem. J. 62, 686-689.
45. Dopheide, T.A. and Ward, C.W. (1980). This volume.
46. Ward, C.W., Downie, J.C., Brown, L. and Jackson, D.C. (1980). This volume.
47. Downie, J.C. (1978) J. Gen. Virol. 41, 283-293.
48. Laver, W.G., Air, G.M., Webster, R.G., Gerhard, W., Ward, C.W. and Dopheide, T.A. (1979) Virology, 98, 226-237.
49. Yewdell, J.W., Webster, R.G. and Gerhard, W.V. (1979) Nature (London) 279, 246-248.
50. Chou, P.Y. and Fasman, G.D. (1977) J. Mol. Biol. 115, 135-175.
51. Chou, P.Y. and Fasman, G.D. (1978) Ann. Rev. Biochem. 42, 251-276.
52. Aubert, J-P. and Loucheux-Lefebvre, M.H. (1976) Arch. Biochem. Biochem. Biophys. 175, 400-409.
53. McLachlan, A.D. and Stewart, M. (1975) J. Mol. Biol. 98, 293-304.
54. Parry, D.A.D., Crewther, W.G., Fraser, R.D.B. and MacRae, T.P. (1977) J. Mol. Biol. 113, 449-454.
55. Doolittle, R.F., Goldbaum, D.M. and Doolittle, L.R. (1978) J. Mol. Biol. 120, 311-325.

COMPLETE NUCLEOTIDE SEQUENCE OF THE FOWL PLAGUE VIRUS HAEMAGGLUTININ GENE FROM
CLONED DNA

ALAN G. PORTER, CHRISTINE BARBER, NORMAN H. CAREY, ROBERT A. HALLEWELL,
GEOFFREY THRELFALL AND SPENCER EMTAGE
Searle Research & Development, Division of G. D. Searle & Co. Ltd.,
P. O. Box 53, Lane End Road, High Wycombe, Bucks, HP12 4HL, England.

INTRODUCTION

Fowl plague virus (FPV) like other influenza viruses is a negative strand
virus with a genome of eight separate and unique RNA segments[1], two of which
code for the surface antigens, haemagglutinin (gene 4)[2,3] and neuraminidase.
The haemagglutinin (HA) is responsible for attaching the virus to cell
receptors[4] and for initiating infection[5,6]. It is firmly established that host
antibodies are directed against the haemagglutinin[7,8], and that the virus can
escape neutralisation by spontaneous mutation, resulting in amino acid changes
in the haemagglutinin. These changes may be major and cause pandemics
(antigenic shift) or relatively minor and cause epidemics (antigenic drift)[9].
The minor antigenic changes occur more frequently, but their precise nature and
location remain unknown.

Due to the difficulty of RNA sequencing with a molecule the size of the HA
gene, peptide sequencing was, until recently, the best method of studying
antigenic variation of influenza viruses. Ward and Dopheide[10] and Waterfield
and Skehel[11] have determined most of the peptide sequence of the mature HA of a
Hong Kong strain (H3N2) and an Asian strain (H2N2) respectively. With the
introduction of gene cloning and rapid DNA sequencing greater speed is obtained,
and certain problems such as the difficulty of sequencing hydrophobic peptides
are overcome. In addition, the gene sequence not only predicts the complete
amino acid sequence of the mature protein, but will also indicate the sequence
of any peptides that are discarded during its maturation and perhaps also if
untranslated sequences (introns) interrupt the coding region of the gene.

Gene sequences can also provide information about the structure of genes not
evident from the protein sequence, and a means of comparing different virus
strains in even greater detail than techniques such as hybridisation[12], gel
electrophoretic mobility[13] and oligonucleotide mapping[14].

In this chapter we describe the determination of the complete nucleotide
sequence of the FPV haemagglutinin gene using recombinant DNA techniques. The
predicted sequence of the HA allows us to correlate some of the known functions

with specific structures in the molecule and to compare the amino acid sequence with partial sequences of human influenza haemagglutinins[10,11].

MATERIALS AND METHODS

A full description of all methods is presented in reference 15, on which this chapter is based.

RESULTS

Gene 4 sequences in plasmid pBR322-FPV$_{4-10}$

We chose to polyadenylate the eight virion RNA segments of unfractionated FPV RNA, and reverse transcribe the mixture with an oligo(dT) primer, since the resultant transcripts included substantial numbers of full length or almost full length copies of all eight genes[16].

To clone individual genes, the S$_1$-nuclease-treated double-stranded FPV cDNA was ligated to Hind III cut plasmid pBR322 DNA using the Hind III linker method. The mixture was then used to transform Escherichia coli K12 HB101. Thirteen tetracycline-sensitive colonies were obtained most of which contained plasmids with small gene inserts as judged by agarose gel electrophoresis. One plasmid, named pBR322-FPV$_{4-10}$, contained a large insert of about 1,700 nucleotides and the plasmid DNA specifically hybridised to a ^{32}P-labelled gene 4 probe. 59.7% of gene 4 probe was hybridised compared with not more than 3.1% for probes derived from genes 1-3 and 5-8, demonstrating the presence of gene 4 sequences in pBR322-FPV$_{4-10}$. This plasmid was chosen for sequence analysis as the insert was calculated[16] to be an almost full length copy of gene 4.

Restriction enzyme mapping and sequence determination

As a first step to sequence analysis of pBR322-FPV$_{4-10}$ the cleavage sites for a number of restriction enzymes were mapped. Remarkably, all the six base-pair enzymes tested (except SacI, Hind III and Hpa I) were found to cut the gene 4 insert at least once (Fig. 1). Some of these enzymes were used in the DNA sequence analysis. The lettered arrows in Fig. 1 refer to the distances sequenced and this procedure was usually done twice[18].

The first sequences to be established for the gene 4 insert were at the extremities (Fig. 2). The left end of the insert (adjacent to the Eco RI site of pBR322 DNA) has the sequence corresponding exactly to the 3'-end of the virion RNA (5'-end of cRNA), while the right end overlaps the published sequence at the 5'-end of the vRNA at nucleotide 47 (ref. 20). There are five base differences between the RNA sequence and the sequence near the right hand of the insert determined on both cloned DNA strands[15]. These differences are not due to

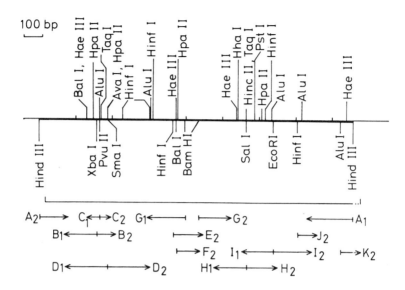

Fig. 1 Restriction enzyme map of the FPV gene 4 insert in pBR322.   The insert is the thicker line, beneath which are shown the restriction sites labelled in the sequence analysis.   The cloned gene 4 is 46 nucleotides shorter than full length gene 4 at the right hand end which corresponds to the 5'-terminal region of the virion RNA.   The distances sequenced are shown by arrows; those pointing to the left denote sequences derived from the virion RNA strand, and those pointing to the right from the cRNA strand.   The vertical line interrupting each arrow indicates the restriction site used for labelling. The dotted line in distance K_2 refers to the 5'-terminal 46 nucleotides of gene 4 missing from the plasmid.   The line above the arrows indicates the position of full length gene 4 relative to the insert.

sequencing errors or mistakes by the reverse transcriptase[15,20].   A compelling model to account for the base changes has been proposed[15].

The nucleotide sequence of FPV gene 4

The FPV gene 4 is 1,742 nucleotides long (Fig. 2).   This is about 300 nucleotides shorter than a previous estimate[16] of 2,060 nucleotides based on migration rate of RNA in formamide-polyacrylamide gels.   The coding region begins with an AUG and is terminated by a single nonsense codon (UAA).   Around nucleotides 1,030-1,050 there is an unusual sequence in the mRNA- an uninterrupted stretch of purines most of which code for the peptide connecting the two HA subunits, HA_1 and HA_2 (ref 10).

```
vRNA   3'-UCGUUUUCGUCCCCAAUGUUU UAC UUG UGA GUU UAG GAC CAA AAG CGG GAA CAC CGU CAG UAG GGG UGU UUA CGU CUG UUU
                                                                    50
cRNA   5'-AGCAAAAGCAGGGGUUACAAA AUG AAC ACU CAA AUC CUG GUU UUC GCC CUU GUG GCA GUC AUC CCC ACA AAU GCA GAC AAA
          A/FPV                 Met-Asn-Thr-Gln-Ile-Leu-Val-Phe-Ala-Leu-Val-Ala-Val-Ile-Pro-Thr-Asn-Ala-Asp-Lys-(20)
                               └─────────────────────── Precursor peptide ────────────────────────────┘
       A/Japan                                                                                          -Asp-Gln-
```

```
UAA ACA GAA CCU GUA GUA CGA CAU AGU UUA CCG UGG UUU CAU UGU GAG UGA CUC UCU CCU CAU CUU CAA CAG UUA CGU UGC
                        100                                          150
AUU UGU CUU GGA CAU CAU GCU GUA UCA AAU GGC ACC AAA GUA AAC ACA CUC ACU GAG AGA GGA GUA GAA GUU GUC AAU GCA ACG
Ile-Cys-Leu-Gly-His-His-Ala-Val-Ser-Asn-Gly-Thr-Lys-Val-Asn-Thr-Leu-Thr-Glu-Arg-Gly-Val-Glu-Val-Val-Asn-Ala-Thr-(48)
          ···········
Ile-Cys-Ile-Gly-Tyr-His-Ala-Asx-Asn-
```

```
CUU UGU CAC CUC GCC UGU UUG UAG GGG UUU UAA ACG AGU UUU CCC UUU UCU UGG UGA CUA GAA CCG GUU ACG CCU GAC AAU CCC
                        200                                          BalI, HaeIII         250
GAA ACA GUG GAG CGG ACA AAC AUC CCC AAA AUU UGC UCA AAA GGG AAA AGA ACC ACU GAU CUU GGC CAA UGC GGA CUG UUA GGG
Glu-Thr-Val-Glu-Arg-Thr-Asn-Ile-Pro-Lys-Ile-Cys-Ser-Lys-Gly-Lys-Arg-Thr-Thr-Asp-Leu-Gly-Gln-Cys-Gly-Leu-Leu-Gly-(76)
```

```
UGG UAA UGG CCU GGU GGA GUU ACG CUG GUU AAA GAU CUU AAA AGU CGA CUA GAU UAU UAG CUC UCU GCU CUU CCU UUA CUA CAA
    HpaII                          XbaI          PvuII 300              TaqI
ACC AUU ACC GGA CCA CCU CAA UGC GAC CAA UUU CUA GAA UUU UCA GCU GAU CUA AUA AUC GAG AGA CGA GAA GGA AAU GAU GUU
Thr-Ile-Thr-Gly-Pro-Pro-Gln-Cys-Asp-Gln-Phe-Leu-Glu-Phe-Ser-Ala-Asp-Leu-Ile-Ile-Glu-Arg-Arg-Glu-Gly-Asn-Asp-Val-(104)
```

```
ACA AUG GGC CCC UUC AAA CAA UUA CUU CUC CGU AAC GCU GUU GAG UCU CCU AGU CCA CCC UAA CUG UUU CUU UGU UAC CCU
    AvaI, SmaI    350                                          400                              HinfI
UGU UAC CCG GGG AAG UUU GUU AAU GAA GAG GCA UUG CGA CAA CUC AGA GGA UCA GGU GGG AUU GAC AAA GAA ACA AUG GGA
Cys-Tyr-Pro-Gly-Lys-Phe-Val-Asn-Glu-Glu-Ala-Leu-Arg-Gln-Ile-Leu-Arg-Gly-Ser-Gly-Gly-Ile-Asp-Lys-Glu-Thr-Met-Gly-(132)
```

```
AAG UGU AUA UCA CCU UAU UCC UGG UUG CCU UGU UGA UCA ACA UCU UCU AGU CCC AGA AGU AAG AUA CGU CUU UAC CUC ACC
                        450                                          500
UUC ACA UAU AGU GGA AUA AGG ACC AAC GGA AGA GCA UGU AGU AGA UCA GGG UCU UCA UUC UAU UAU GCA GAA AUG GAG UGG
Phe-Thr-Tyr-Ser-Gly-Ile-Arg-Thr-Asn-Gly-Thr-Thr-Ser-Ala-Cys-Arg-Arg-Ser-Gly-Ser-Ser-Phe-Tyr-Ala-Glu-Met-Glu-Trp-(160)
                        ···········
                                                                     -Asx-Met-Val-Trp-
```

```
GAG GAC AGU UUA UGU CUG UUA CGA AGA AAG GGU GUU UAC UGU UUU AGU AUG UUU UUG UGU UCC UCU CUU AGU CGA GAC UAU CAG
                        550                                          HinfI, AluI
CUC CUG UCA AAU ACA GAC AAU GCU UCU UUC CCA CAA AUG ACA AAA UCA UAC AAA AAC ACA AGG AGA GAA UCA GCU CUG AUA GUC
Leu-Leu-Ser-Asn-Thr-Asp-Asn-Ala-Ser-Phe-Pro-Gln-Met-Thr-Lys-Ser-Tyr-Lys-Asn-Thr-Arg-Arg-Glu-Ser-Ala-Leu-Ile-Val-(188)
                                          ···········
Leu ───── Thr-Lys-                                          -Gly-Ser-Tyr-Thr-Asn(Asn,Ser,Gly,Glx)Met ─── Leu-Ile-Ile-
       A/Memphis                          -Met-Pro-Asn-Asn-Asp-Asn-Phe-Asp-Lys-Leu-Tyr-Ile-
```

```
ACC CCU UAG GUG GUA AGU CCU AGU UGG UGG ── CUU GUC UGG UUU GAU AUA CCC UCA CCU UUA UUU GAC UAU UGU CAG CCC UCA
    HinfI      600                                          650
UGG GGA AUC CAC CAU UCA GGA UCA ACC ACC ── GAA CAG ACC AAA CUA UAU GGG AGU GGA AAU AAA CUG AUA ACA GUC GGG AGU
Trp-Gly-Ile-His-His-Ser-Gly-Ser-Thr-Thr ── Glu-Gln-Thr-Lys-Leu-Tyr-Gly-Ser-Gly-Asn-Lys-Leu-Ile-Thr-Val-Gly-Ser-(215)
Trp-Gly-Val-His-His-Pro-Ile-Asp-Glu-Thr ── Glu-Gln-Arg-
Trp-Gly-Val-His-His-Pro ── Ser-Thr-Asp-Gln-Glu-Gln-Thr-Ser-Leu-Tyr-Val-Gln-Ala-Ser-Gly-Arg-Val-Thr-Val-Ser-Thr-
```

```
AGG UUU AUA GUA GUU AGA AAA CAC GGC UCA GGU CCU UGU GCU GGC GUC UAU UUA CCG GUC AGG CCU GCC UAA CUA AAA GUA ACC
                                          HinfI 700              BalI, HaeIII HpaII         750
UCC AAA UAU CAU CAA UCU UUU GUG CCU AGU CCA GGA ACA CGA CCG CAG ACA CGG CCA CAG UCC GGA CGG AUU GAU UUU CAU UGG
Ser-Lys-Tyr-His-Gln-Ser-Phe-Val-Pro-Ser-Pro-Gly-Thr-Arg-Pro-Gln-Ile-Asn-Gly-Gln-Ser-Gly-Arg-Ile-Asp-Phe-His-Trp-(243)
                                                                     Met-Gln-Phe-Ser-Trp-
Lys-Arg-Ser-Gln-Gln-Thr-Ile-Ile-Pro-Asn-Ile-Gly-Ser-Arg-Pro-Trp-Val-Arg-Gly-Leu-Ser-Ser-Arg-Ile-Ser-Ile-Tyr-Trp-
```

```
AAC UAG AAC CUA GGG UUA CUA UGU CAA UGA AAA UCA AAG UUA CCC CGA AAG UAU CGA GGU UUA GCA CGG UCG AAG AAC ───────
    BamHI                                          800
UUG AUC UUG GAU CCC AAU GAU ACA GUU ACU UUU AGU UUC AAU GGG GCU UUC AUA GCU CCA AAU CGU GCC AGC UUC UUG ───────
Leu-Ile-Leu-Asp-Pro-Asn-Asp-Thr-Val-Thr-Phe-Ser-Phe-Asn-Gly-Ala-Phe-Ile-Ala-Pro-Asn-Arg-Ala-Ser-Phe-Leu ─── (269)
Thr-Leu-Leu-Asp-Met-Trp-Asp-Thr-Ile-Asn-Phe-Glu-Ser-Thr-Gly-Asn-Leu-Ile-Ala-Pro-Glu ── Tyr-Phe-Lys-Ile-Ser-Lys-
Thr-Ile-Val-Lys-Pro-Gly-Asp-Ile-Leu-Val-Ile-Asn-Ser-Asx-Gly-Asx-Leu-Ile-Ala-Pro-Arg-Gly-Tyr-Phe-Lys-Met-
```

```
UCC ─── CCU UUC AGG UAC CCC UAG GUC ─── UCG CUA CAC GUC CAA CUA CGA UUA ACG CUU CCC CUU ACG AUG GUG UCA CCU CCC
        BamHI 850                                                              900
AGG ─── GGA AAG UCC AUG GGG AUC CAG ─── AGC GAU GUG CAG GUU GAU GCU AAU GCA UGU GGG GAA UGC UAC CAC AGU GGA GGG
Arg ─── Gly-Lys-Ser-Met-Gly-Ile-Gln ─── Ser-Asp-Val-Gln-Val-Asp-Ala-Asn-Cys-Glu-Gly-Glu-Cys-Tyr-His-Ser-Gly-Gly-(295)
Arg ─── Gly ── Ser-Ser-Gly-Ile-Met-Lys ── Thr-Glu-Gly-Thr-Leu-Glu-Asn-Cys-Glu-Thr-Lys-Cys-Glu-Thr-Pro-Leu-Gly-
Arg-Thr-Gly-Lys-Ser-Ser ── Ile-Met-Arg-Ser-Asp-Ala ── Pro-Ile-Gly-Thr-Cys-Ile-Ser-Glu-Cys-Ile-Thr-Pro-Asn-Gly-
```

```
UGA UAU UGU UCG UCU AAC GGA AAA GUU UUG UAU UUA UCG UCU CGU CAA CCG UUU ACG GGU UCU AUA CAU UUU GUC CUU UCA AUU
                                          950
ACU AUA ACA AGC AGA UUG CCU UUU CAA AAC AUA AAU AGC AGA GCA GUU GGC AAA UCC CCA AGA UAU GUA AAA CAG GAA AGU UUA
Thr-Ile-Thr-Ser-Arg-Leu-Pro-Phe-Gln-Asn-Ile-Asn-Ser-Arg-Ala-Val-Gly-Lys-Cys-Pro-Arg-Tyr-Val-Lys-Gln-Glu-Ser-Leu-(323)
Ala-Ile-Asn-Thr-Thr-Leu-Pro-Phe-His-Asx-Val-His-Pro-Leu-Thr-Ile-Gly-Glx-Cys-Pro-Lys-Tyr-Ser ── Glu-Lys ── Leu-
Ser-Ile-Pro-Lys-Pro-Asp-Asp-Phe-Gln-Asn-Val-Asn-Lys-Ile-Thr-Tyr-Gly-Ala-Cys-Pro-Lys-Tyr-Val-Lys-Gln-Asn-Thr-Leu-
```

```
AAU AAC CGU UGA CCC UAC UUC UUG CAA GGG CUU GGA AGG UUU UUU UCC CUU UUU UCU CCG GAC AAA CCG CGA UAU CGU CCC AAA
      1000                                                        HaeIII 1,050        HhaI
UUA UUG GCA ACU GGG AUG AAG AAC GUU CCC GAA CCU UCC AAA AAA AGG GAA AAA AGA GGC CUG UUU GGC GCU AUA GCA GGG UUU
Leu-Leu-Ala-Thr-Gly-Met-Lys-Asn-Val-Pro-Glu-Pro-Ser-Lys-Lys-Arg-Glu-Lys-Arg-Gly-Leu-Phe-Gly-Ala-Ile-Ala-Gly-Phe-(351)
Val-Leu-Ala-Thr-Gly-Leu-Arg-Asx-Val-Pro-Glx-Ser-Glx-Ile-Connecting peptide.-Gly-Leu-Phe-Gly-Ala-Ile-Ala-Gly-Phe-
Lys-Leu-Ala-Thr-Gly-Met-Arg-Asn-Val-Pro-Glu-Lys-Gln-Thr-                  -Gly-Leu-Phe-Gly-Ala-Ile-Ala-Gly-Phe-
```

```
UAA CUU UUA CCA ACC CUU CCA GAC CAG CUG CCC ACC AUG CCA AAG UCC GUA GUC UUA CGU GUU CCU CUU CCU UGA CGU CGU CUG
                                          1,100 SalI, HincII                                          1,150 PstI
AUU GAA AAU GGU UGG GAA GGU CUG GAC GGG UGG UAC GGU UUC AGG CAU CAG AAU GCA CAA GGA GAA GGA ACU GCA GCA GAC
Ile-Glu-Asn-Gly-Trp-Glu-Gly-Leu-Val-Asp-Gly-Trp-Tyr-Gly-Phe-Arg-His-Gln-Asn-Ala-Gln-Gly-Glu-Gly-Thr-Ala-Ala-Asp-(379)
Ile-Glu-Gly-Gly-Trp-Glu-Gly-Met-Val-Asp-Gly-Trp-Tyr-Gly-Tyr-
Ile-Glu-Asn-Gly-Trp-Glu-Gly-Met-Ile-Asp-Gly-Trp-Tyr-Gly-Phe-Arg-His-Gln-Asn-Ser-Glu-Gly-Thr-Gly-Gln-Ala-Ala-Asp-
```

```
AUG UUU UCG UGG GUU AGC CGU UAA CUA GUC UAU UGG CCU UUC AAU UUA UCU GAG UAA CUC UUU UGG UUG GUC GUU AAA CUC GAU
                     HpaII 1,200          HinfI                                                        AluI
UAC AAA AGC ACC CAA UCG GCA AUU GAU CAG AUA ACC GGA AAG UUA AAU AGA CUC AUU GAG AAA ACC AAC CAG CAA UUU GAG CUA
Tyr-Lys-Ser-Thr-Gln-Ser-Ala-Ile-Asp-Gln-Ile-Thr-Gly-Lys-Leu-Asn-Arg-Leu-Ile-Glu-Lys-Thr-Asn-Gln-Gln-Phe-Glu-Leu-(407)
Leu-Lys-Ser-Thr-Gln-Ala-Ala-Ile-Asp-Gln-Ile-Asp-Gly-Lys-Leu-Asn-Arg-Val-Ile-Glu-Lys-Thr-Asn-Glu-Lys-Phe-His-Gln-
```

```
UAU CUA UUA CUU AAG UGA CUU CAC CUU UUC GUC UAA CCG UUA AAU UAA UUG ACC UGG UUU CUG AAG UAG UGU CUU CAU ACC AGA
     1,250  EcoRI                                                    1,300
AUA GAU AAU GAA UUC ACU GAA GUG GAA AAG CAG AUU GGC AAU UUA AUU AAC UGG ACC AAA GAC UUC AUC ACA GAA GUA UGG UCU
Ile-Asp-Asn-Glu-Phe-Thr-Glu-Val-Glu-Lys-Gln-Ile-Gly-Asn-Leu-Ile-Asn-Trp-Thr-Lys-Asp-Phe-Ile-Thr-Glu-Val-Trp-Ser-(435)
                                  -Met-Glu-Asx-Glx-Arg-Thr-Leu-Asx-Phe-His-
Ile-Glu-Lys-Glu-Phe-Ser-Glu-Val-Glu-Gly-Arg-Ile-Gln-Asp-Leu-Glu-Lys-Tyr-Val-Glu-Asp-Thr-Lys-Ile-Asp-Leu-Trp-Ser-
```

```
AUG UUA CGA CUU GAA GAA CAC CGU UAC CUU UUG GUC GUG UGA UAA CUA AAC CGA CUA AGU CUC UAC UUG UUC GAC AUA CUC GCU
                     1,350                              HinfI          AluI 1,400
UAC AAU GCU GAA CUU CUU GUG GCA AUG GAA AAC CAG CAC ACU AUU GAU UUG GCU GAU UCA GAG AUG AAC AAG CUG UAU GAG CGA
Tyr-Asn-Ala-Glu-Leu-Leu-Val-Ala-Met-Glu-Asn-Gln-His-Thr-Ile-Asp-Leu-Ala-Asp-Ser-Glu-Met-Asn-Lys-Leu-Tyr-Glu-Arg-(463)
               -Glx-Met-Asn-Thr-Gln-Phe-Gln-Ala-Val-Gly-Lys-
Tyr-Asn-Ala-Glu-Leu-Leu-Val-Ala-Leu-Glu-Asn-Gln-His-Thr-Ile-Asp-Leu-Thr-Asp-Ser-Glu-Met-Asn-Lys-Leu-Phe-Glu-Lys-
```

```
CAC UCC UUU ——— GUU AAU UCC CUU UUA CGA CUU CUC CUA CCG UGA CCA ACG AAA CUU UAA AAA GUA UUU ACA CUG CUA CUA ACA
                                                        1,450
GUG AGG AAA ——— CAA UUA AGG GAA AAU GCU GAA GAG GAU GGC ACU GGU UGC UUU GAA AUU UUU CAU AAA UGU GAC GAU GAU UGU
Val-Arg-Lys ——— Gln-Leu-Arg-Glu-Asn-Ala-Glu-Glu-Asp-Gly-Thr-Gly-Cys-Phe-Glu-Ile-Phe-His-Lys-Cys-Asp-Asp-Asp-Cys-(490)
         -Met-Gln-Leu-Arg-Asx-Asx-Val-Lys-Glx-Leu-Gly-Asx-Gly-Cys-Phe-Gln-Phe-Tyr-His-Lys-Cys-Asx-Asx-Glx-Cys-
Thr-Arg-Arg ——— Gln-Leu-Arg-Glu-Asn-Ala-Glu-Asp-Met-Gly-Asn-Gly-Cys-Phe-Lys-Phe-Gln-Ile-Lys-Cys-Asp-Asn-Ala-Cys-
```

```
UAC CGA UCA UAU UCC UUG UUA UGA AUA CUA GUG UCG UUU AUG UCU CUU CUU CGC UAC GUU UUA UCU UAU GUU UAA CUG GGU CAG
     1,500                                              1,550
AUG GCU AGU AUA AGG AAC AAU ACU UAU GAU CAC AGC AAA UAC AGA GAA GAA GCG AUG CAA AAU AGA AUA CAA AUU GAC CCA GUC
Met-Ala-Ser-Ile-Arg-Asn-Asn-Thr-Tyr-Asp-His-Ser-Lys-Tyr-Arg-Glu-Glu-Ala-Met-Gln-Asn-Arg-Ile-Gln-Ile-Asp-Pro-Val-(518)
Met-Asn-Ser-Val-Lys-
Ile-Gly-Ser-Ile-Arg-
```

```
UUU AAC UCA UCA CCG AUG UUU CUA CAC UAU GAA ACC AAA UCG AAG CCC CGU AGU ACG AAA AAC GAA GAA CGG UAA CGU CAC CCG
               1,600                        AluI                                   1,650        HaeIII
AAA UUG AGU AGU GGC UAC AAA GAU GUG AUA CUU UGG UUU AGC UUC GGG GCA UCA UGC UUU UUG CUU CUU GCC AUU GCA GUG GGC
Lys-Leu-Ser-Ser-Gly-Tyr-Lys-Asp-Val-Ile-Leu-Trp-Phe-Ser-Phe-Gly-Ala-Ser-Cys-Phe-Leu-Leu-Leu-Ala-Ile-Ala-Val-Gly-(546)
                                                                 —————— Hydrophobic tail ——————
```

```
GAA CAA AAG UAU ACA CAC UUC UUG CCU UUG UAC GCC ACG UGA UAA ACA UAU AUU CAAACCUUUUUUUGUGGGAACAAAGAUGA-5'  vRNA
                                                  |  1,700
CUU GUU UUC AUA UGU GUG AAG AAC GGA AAC AUG CGG UGC ACU AUU UGU AUA UAA GUUUGGAAAAAACACCCUUGUUUCUACU-3'  cRNA
Leu-Val-Phe-Ile-Cys-Val-Lys-Asn-Gly-Asn-Met-Arg-Cys-Thr-Ile-Cys-Ile.(563)
  Hydrophobic tail                       C-terminus HA₂
```

(See caption on following page)

Fig. 2. Nucleotide sequence of the FPV HA gene and comparison of the predicted amino acid sequence of the HA with human HA sequences. The virus RNA (with the 3'-end to the left) is shown above the complementary RNA. Boxes show the initiation codon (AUG) and termination codon (UAA). The positions of the restriction enzyme sites (Fig. 1.) found in the corresponding plasmid DNA are indicated by a bar above the cRNA. The heavy underlining near the initiation codon shows two areas of homology with prokaryotic ribosome binding sites. The underlined purine-rich sequence in the cRNA (nucleotides 1,029-1,049) spans the region coding for the peptide connecting HA_1 to HA_2. The vertical line to the left of the termination codon shows the position corresponding to the attachment of the Hind III linker to the incomplete DNA copy of gene 4. To the left of this line is shown the actual sequence of the RNA gene. The predicted amino acid sequence of the immature FPV HA is immediately below the cRNA. The A/Japan/305/57 (H2N2) partial sequence is shown below the complete FPV sequence, and the third line has the A/Memphis/102/72 (H3N2) partial sequence. In maximising homology (underlining) the sequences of these HAs have been aligned according to the positions of the cysteines. Dotted lines below the FPV HA sequence indicate asparagines which may be glycosylated in the mature HA.

During in vivo transcription of viral RNA, host mRNAs prime the synthesis of influenza mRNAs adding an extra 10-15 nucleotides to each 5'-end[21] (not shown). At the other end, transcription terminates prematurely, probably at the U_7 sequence 17-23 nucleotides from the 5'-end of the virion RNA template. Thus the 5'- and 3'-non-coding regions (including the UAA) are 31-36 and approximately 9 nucleotides long, respectively. The length of the 3' region is therefore short compared with the corresponding region of other mRNAs found in eukaryotic cells[23,24]. A putative signal sequence of 5'AAUAAA3' has been found in the 3'-non-coding region of many different types of eukaryotic mRNA[23,24]. It is absent from FPV gene 4 (Fig. 2) and this resembles the situation in some picornaviruses[25] and one of the mRNAs of vesicular stomatitis virus[26].

The 3'-ends of the cRNA and virion RNA of gene 4 can be aligned so that 12 out of 15 nucleotides are the same. This is significant as a possible signal for the initiation of replication on both these RNAs as has already been noted [19,22]. Homology between 3'-ends also means that the 5'- and 3'- ends of either virion RNA or cRNA are complementary[19], but there is no known function for such an interaction.

A striking feature of the 5'-non-coding region near the AUG (underlined in Fig. 2) is the homology with some prokaryotic ribosome binding sites. These include the R17 replicase[27], T7 early mRNA[28] and E. coli Trp E sites[29]. In FPV gene 4, there is a characteristic purine-rich sequence, AGGGG, which interacts with the 3'-end of 16S rRNA in prokaryotes[30], followed immediately by UUACA. The latter sequence is present in the prokaryotic sites as UUAC and U ACA. There is even greater homology between the gene 4 site and a spurious ribosome binding site in Qβ RNA which lacks an AUG[31]. Here at least 12 out of 16 nucleotides are the same. Support for the idea that the gene 4 site is prokaryotic in character comes from experiments on the expression of FPV gene 4 in E. coli[32].

Codon usage

The choice between degenerate codons in many mRNAs is frequently non-random, with markedly different preferences in different mRNAs[23,24]. In some mRNAs, the most frequently used codons correlate with the abundant species of isoaccepting tRNA[33], while in others the usage reflects the base composition[34]. FPV gene 4 is U-rich (34.3%) and has a low G content (18.5%). Reflecting this, there is a significant bias for codons with A in the third position (notably GAA, AGA and AAA), and against codons with third position C (Table 1).

Gene 4 has an overall deficiency of CG relative to the other 15 dinucleotides. This is not due only to the low G content, since GG sequences are almost twice as abundant. Again reflecting the base composition of the virion RNA, codons with CG in first and second or second and third position rarely occur (Table 1). There is also a deficiency of CG in the eukaryotic genome[35]. In this case it has been suggested that the frequency of CG has been kept to a minimum since cytosine in CG is a major site of DNA methylation, and methylated nucleotides are 'hot spots' for mutation[24]. But this cannot be true for influenza, an RNA virus with no known DNA intermediate in its replication.

TABLE 1

USE OF CODONS IN FPV GENE 4

Phe UUU 13	Ser UCU 4	Tyr UAU 7	Cys UGU 7
UUC 13	UCC 4	UAC 8	UGC 9
Leu UUA 6	UCA 13	Ochre UAA 1	Opal UGA 0
UUG 9	UCG 1	Amber UAG 0	Trp UGG 8
Leu CUU 9	Pro CCU 3	His CAU 7	Arg CGU 1
CUC 4	CCC 1	CAC 4	CGC 0
CUA 4	CCA 8	Gln CAA 14	CGA 4
CUG 8	CCG 4	CAG 11	CGG 3
Ile AUU 17	Thr ACU 13	Asn AAU 23	Ser AGU 11
AUC 8	ACC 12	AAC 14	AGC 8
AUA 15	ACA 15	Lys AAA 22	Arg AGA 14
Met AUG 11	ACG 1	AAG 7	AGG 8
Val GUU 9	Ala GCU 12	Asp GAU 17	Gly GGU 5
GUC 6	GCC 3	GAC 9	GGC 10
GUA 5	GCA 17	Glu GAA 28	GGA 20
GUG 10	GCG 1	GAG 10	GGG 15

Note: Codons with CG are underlined. 20.0% of codons used end in C, 32.9% end in A, 19.0% end in G and 28.1% end in U.

Amino acid sequence organisation of the FPV haemagglutinin

The immature FPV HA consists of 563 amino acids, of which 18 form the N-terminal 'pre-peptide', 319 are in HA_1, 5 are in a connecting peptide and 221 are in HA_2 (Fig. 2). The amino acid composition shows similarities to human haemagglutinins; for example in the high proline content of HA_1 compared to HA_2, and in the number and distribution of cysteine residues[10,11]. The positions of the cysteines have been highly conserved, perhaps to help give each molecule a basically similar overall shape by disulphide bridging.

Existing evidence suggests that immature HA has a short N-terminal leader sequence which is cleaved off when the process of membrane insertion is complete[11]. The DNA sequence predicts that the FPV leader consists of 18 amino acids, none of which is polar (Fig. 2). From the fifth residue, there is a core of 11 consecutive hydrophobic amino acids. The leader sequence of another influenza A haemagglutinin (Rl/5‾/57) is 15 residues in length and shows almost no sequence homology with the FPV leader, but like FPV has an uninterrupted sequence of hydrophobic amino acids[36]. The size and non-polar character of these N-terminal peptides is very similar in other secreted proteins[37], which lends strong support to the signal peptide hypothesis[38]. This states that the process of membrane transport is initiated by insertion of a hydrophobic pre-peptide, which is subsequently cleaved off.

Cleavage of HA into HA_1 and HA_2 usually takes place either on smooth internal membranes or at the plasma membrane[39]. This step is essential for infectivity[6] and apparently also for pathogenicity[40]. It is carried out by an unknown host protease with a similar specificity to trypsin[39]. In FPV, the sequence around the cleavage site is Lys-Lys-Arg-Glu-Lys-Arg-Gly (Fig. 2), where the first residue becomes the C-terminus of HA_1 and the last residue the N-terminus of HA_2. The basic nature of these residues accounts for the in vitro trypsin cleavage of HA into HA_1 and HA_2, but it is not known whether only some or all the basic residues are cut either in vitro or in vivo. In contrast to FPV, the C-terminal amino acid of HA_1 of A/Japan/305/57 is isoleucine[11] and A/Memphis/102/72 has C-terminal threonine[10]. These differences could explain why the susceptibility of HA to cleavage depends on the virus strain[39] as well as on the cell type[40].

In human influenza A strains, the C-terminal part of HA_2 has not yet been sequenced owing to the insolubility of the peptides derived from it, indicating the presence of an extensive hydrophobic region[10,11]. In FPV this begins at residue 527 and extends for 26 amino acids to residue 552 (Fig. 2). Of these, 20 residues are hydrophobic, and are probably involved in anchoring the HA to the viral lipoprotein envelope[11].

There are five potential sites for carbohydrate attachment in HA_1 and two in HA_2 (Fig. 2). This conclusion is based on the presence of the sequences Asn-X-Ser and Asn-X-Thr, which are known to occur in other glycoproteins (including haemagglutinins[10,11]) at sites of N-glycosidic linkage of asparagine to oligosaccharides[11]. Previous studies on the HA from FPV (Dutch) have indicated that there are five or six separate oligosaccharide units, but their exact location was not determined[41]. In A/Japan/305/57, the approximate location of carbohydrate side chains is known to be residues 11, 23, 192 and 303 in mature HA_1 and very near the bromelain cleavage site in HA_2 (ref. 11). In FPV, the sites at residues 30 and 46 in HA_1, and residue 496 in HA_2 seem to correspond to the known A/Japan sites at 11 and 23 in mature HA_1 and the single site in HA_2, respectively.

In Fig. 2, the FPV HA sequence is compared with published partial HA sequences for an H2N2 strain (A/Japan/305/57) and an H3N2 strain[10,11] (A/Memphis/102/72). There is considerable sequence homology (38%) between all strains. This occurs to an even greater extent between FPV and Japan (48%). Conservation of sequence appears to be greater in HA_2 than HA_1, which is not surprising as only HA_1 is thought to undergo antigenic variation.

As pointed out previously, the N-terminal 24 residues of several HA_2 molecules are highly conserved[11], and this now extends to FPV. The cleavage into HA_1 and HA_2 may expose the hydrophobic sequence at the N-terminus of HA_2, which then enables the HA to penetrate the cell membrane[11]. In at least 63% of positions where there is an amino acid difference between any two HAs (Fig. 2), the change can be accounted for by a single nucleotide substitution. This is significantly higher than the value of 38% for all possible pairs of amino acids. This consideration, together with the overlapping nature of the homologies between the three HAs (Fig. 2) implies that the corresponding HA genes have evolved from one and not from two or more distinct ancestors.

CONCLUDING REMARKS

Gene 4 of FPV is the first influenza virus gene to be completely sequenced and it predicts for the first time the complete amino acid sequence of a viral HA. The gene has some interesting features. The most notable of these are seen in the mRNA – a short 3' non-coding region, a prokaryotic-like ribosome binding site and an apparent lack of introns.

The HA of influenza viruses is a remarkable multifunctional protein. Our results and those of others have built up a picture of several functionally

48

important domains in the molecule. These are the three hydrophobic regions
with distinct functions, the connecting peptide and the carbohydrate
attachment sites.

The region of HA that interacts with cell receptors at an early stage in
infection remains to be determined, as do the antigenic sites, now known to be
in the N-terminal half of HA_1 in a Hong Kong strain[42]. The FPV sequence does,
however, provide a framework for determining these sites in combination with
other approaches. For example, it will now be possible to determine the
primary structure of HA genes from influenza strains that differ only in their
reactivity towards monoclonal antibodies[43]. A single nucleotide change
would show which amino acid had changed and pinpoint the antigenic site.
Ultimately, these methods may enable us to predict which amino acid changes will
produce influenza viruses capable of causing epidemics.

We thank Mr. G. Catlin and Mr. B. Jenkins for technical help, Dr. M.
Waterfield for useful discussions, Drs. G. Air and J. Robertson for FPV RNA and
Dr. A. J. Hale for providing research facilities. The material in this
chapter is reproduced with the permission of Nature, as it is based on
reference 15. All cloning experiments were done in a Category III
laboratory inspected and approved by GMAG.

REFERENCES

1. McGeoch, D. et al. (1976) Proc. natn. Acad. Sci. U.S.A. 73, 3045-3049.
2. Scholtissek, C. et al. (1976) Virology, 74, 332-344.
3. Almond, J.W. and Barry, R.D. (1979) Virology 92, 407-415.
4. Hirst, G.K. (1942) J. exp. Med. 75, 49-64.
5. Klenk, H.D. et al. (1975) Virology 68, 426-439.
6. Lazarowitz, S.G. and Choppin, P.W. (1975) Virology 68, 440-454.
7. Drzeniek, R. et al. (1966) Biochim, biophys. Acta 128, 547-558.
8. Laver, W.G. and Kilbourne, E.D. (1966) Virology 30, 493-501.
9. Laver, W.G. and Webster, R.G. (1979) Br. med. Bull. 35, 29-33.
10.Ward, C.W. and Dopheide, T.A. (1979) Br. med. Bull. 35, 51-56.
11.Waterfield, M.D. et al. (1979) Br.med.Bull. 35, 57-63.
12.Scholtissek, C. et al. (1978) Virology 87, 13-20.
13.Palese, P. and Schulman, J.L. (1976) J. Virol. 17, 876-884.
14.Nakajima, K. et al. (1978) Nature 274, 334-339.
15.Porter, A.G. et al. (1979) Nature 282, 471-477.
16.Emtage, J.S. et al. (1979) Nucleic Acids Res. 6, 1221-1240.
17.Scheller, R.H. et al. (1977) Science 196, 177-180.
18.Maxam, A. and Gilbert, W. (1977) Proc. natn. Acad. Sci. U.S.A. 74, 560-564.
19.Skehel, J.J. and Hay, A.J. (1978) Nucleic Acids Res. 5, 1207-1219.
20.Robertson,J.S. (1979) Nucleic Acids Res. 6, 3745-3757.
21.Plotch, S.J. et al. (1979) Proc. natn. Acad. Sci. U.S.A. 76, 1618-1622.
22.Skehel, J.J. and Hay,A.J. (1978) J. gen. Virol, 39, 1-8.
23.Seeburg, P.H. et al. (1977) Nature 270, 486-494.
24.Heindell, H.C. et al. (1978) Cell 15, 43-54.
25.Porter, A.G. et al. (1978) Nature 276,298-301.

26. McGeoch, D.J. and Turnbull, N.T. (1978) Nucleic Acids Res. 5, 4007-4024.
27. Steitz, J.A. (1969) Nature 224, 957-964.
28. Arrand, J.R. and Hindley, J. (1973) Nature new Biol. 244, 10-13.
29. Squires, C. et al. (1976) J. molec. Biol. 103, 351-381.
30. Shine, J. and Dalgarno, L. (1975) Nature, 254, 34-38.
31. Steitz, J.A. (1973) J. molec. Biol. 73, 1-16.
32. Emtage, J.S. et al. Nature (in press)
33. Post, L.E. et al. (1979) Proc. natn. Acad. Sci. U.S.A. 76, 1697-1701.
34. Nakanishi, S. et al. (1979) Nature, 278, 423-427.
35. Subak-Sharpe, J.H. (1967) Br. med. Bull. 23, 161-168.
36. Air, G. (1979) Virology 97, 468-472.
37. Strauss, A.W. et al. (1977) J. biol. Chem. 252, 6846-6855.
38. Blobel, G. and Dobberstein, B. (1975) J. cell. Biol. 67, 835-851.
39. Rott, R. et al. (1978) in The Influenza Virus Hemagglutinin, Laver, W.G.
    Bachmayer, H. and Weil, R. Eds., Springer, New York, pp 69-81.
40. Bosch, F.X. et al. (1979) Virology 95, 197-207.
41. Klenk, H.D. et al. (1978) in The Influenza Virus Hemagglutinin, Laver, W.G.
    Bachmayer, H. and Weil, R. Eds., Springer, New York, pp 83-99.
42. Jackson, D.C. et al. (1979) Virology 93, 458-465.
43. Gerhard, W. (1978) in The Influenza Virus Hemagglutinin, Laver, W.G.
    Bachmayer, H. and Weil, R. Eds. Springer, New York, pp 15-24.

DISCUSSION

Sleigh: Regarding the cloning artifacts generated near the 5' end of the second
strand in Gene 4, do you think that the mismatched nucleotides on the 'loop'
structure you drew would be recognised and cut by S1 nuclease under the
conditions you used?

Porter: We have to assume that on some molecules they weren't cut.

NUCLEOTIDE SEQUENCE OF THE HA$_2$ REGION OF THE A/VICTORIA/3/75 HAEMAGGLUTININ GENE DETERMINED FROM A CLONED DNA TRANSCRIPT

GEOFFREY THRELFALL, CHRISTINE BARBER, NORMAN CAREY AND SPENCER EMTAGE
Searle Research and Development, Division of G.D. Searle & Co. Ltd.,
P.O. Box 53, Lane End Road, High Wycombe, Bucks HP12 4HL, England.

INTRODUCTION

The continual variation in the structure of the two surface antigens of influenza virus, haemagglutinin (HA) and neuraminidase, enables the virus to evade the immune response of the host and to cause chronic or repeated infections. Haemagglutinin is involved in the initiation of infection[1,2], and is the antigen against which neutralising antibodies from the host cell are directed[3,4]. One form of antigenic variation is known as "drift" and is presumed due to accumulation of point mutations arising in the viral genome during transmission of the virus; peptide maps show only small differences in primary structure of the haemagglutinins of related strains[5,6].

A knowledge of the complete amino acid sequence of haemagglutinins from the various strains of influenza virus within a sub-type, e.g. A/Hong Kong/68 (H3N2), should allow a better understanding of the changes occurring during antigenic drift. This information can now be gained using techniques available for the synthesis of double-stranded DNA copies of RNA molecules and the cloning and amplification of these synthetic genes in suitable host-vector systems to provide adequate quantities of purified DNA for analysis by rapid DNA sequencing methods. The nucleotide sequence allows accurate prediction of the amino acid sequence and also provides information on the mechanism by which the immature protein is processed to its HA$_1$ and HA$_2$ sub-units, a necessary step for the infectious process to occur[2,7].

This paper describes the cloning of an almost full length copy of the haemagglutinin gene of A/Victoria/3/75 (H3N2) and the nucleotide sequencing of the region of the gene encoding the HA$_2$ protein, including its connection with HA$_1$ in the immature HA. Comparisons are made between the amino acid sequence predicted for the HA$_2$ of A/Victoria and the known amino acid sequence of the HA$_2$ of A/Memphis/102/72 (H3N2)[8], an earlier strain of the series derived from A/Hong Kong/68. Further comparisons are made with the HA$_2$ sequence of Fowl Plague Virus (Rostock)[9], an avian influenza virus strain (Havl Neql).

MATERIALS AND METHODS

Materials

The viral RNA used in this work was isolated from the laboratory-produced recombinant strain X-47, which contains the haemagglutinin and neuraminidase genes of A/Victoria/3/75; the remainder of the genes are from A/PR/8/34(HON1). AMV reverse transcriptase was from the National Cancer Institute, U.S.A. All restriction enzymes and T_4 polynucleotide kinase were from New England Biolabs, terminal transferase was from P-L Biochemicals and bacterial alkaline phosphatase from Worthington. S1 nuclease was purified from α-amylase[10].

Synthesis of complementary DNA (cDNA) by self-priming of the HA gene (gene 4)

[32]P-labelled cDNA was synthesised as described previously[11], with the following modifications: the RNA template (total viral RNA) was not poly-adenylated and no oligo(dT) primer was added. Under these conditions only gene 4 is efficiently copied by reverse transcriptase to give a near full-length transcript. Double-stranded DNA (dsDNA) was synthesised from this cDNA, treated with S1 nuclease, purified and characterised as described previously[11].

Tailing of dsDNA and plasmid DNA by terminal transferase[12]

Terminal addition of poly (dC) tails to the 3' ends of dsDNA and poly (dG) tails to the 3' ends of pBR322 (linearised with Hind III) was carried out in a reaction volume of 200 μl containing 20 mM Hepes buffer, pH 7.1, 1 mM $CoCl_2$, 1 mM β-mercaptoethanol, 100 μg/ml gelatin and either 0.1 mM dCTP and dsDNA (0.5 μg) or 0.1 mM dGTP and pBR322 DNA (1 μg). Incubation was at 37°C for a time which allowed the addition of 20-30 dC or dG residues to each 3' end.

The tailed dsDNA was electrophoresed on a 1.4% agarose gel, autoradiographed and the full-length band cut out, eluted from the gel slice and concentrated by ethanol precipitation.

Annealing of dsDNA with plasmid DNA

Approximately 5 ng of poly (dC)-tailed dsDNA was mixed with 50 ng of poly(dG)-tailed pBR322 DNA in 100 μl of 0.1 M NaCl, 10 mM Tris-HCl pH 8.0, 1 mM EDTA. This solution was heated at 56°C for 2', then annealed at 42°C for 2 hr.

Transformation and growth of E. coli for DNA purification

The DNA was then used to transform E. coli K12 HB101. Colonies were grown on ampicillin plates and those containing gene 4 inserts detected by colony hybridisation[13]. For DNA purification, single colonies were picked and cultures grown. Chloramphenicol was used to amplify plasmid DNA which was purified from cell lysates by centrifugation in caesium chloride-ethidium bromide gradients.

Restriction mapping and nucleotide sequencing of gene 4

Restriction mapping was carried out using 1% agarose or 5% acrylamide gels to separate restriction fragments produced by single or double restriction digests. Fragments were detected by ethidium bromide staining and their sizes calibrated by comparison with restriction fragments of known size from pBR322[14] DNA.

For nucleotide sequencing, primary restriction fragments were dephosphorylated with bacterial alkaline phosphatase and 5' end-labelled using γ^{32}P-ATP and T_4 polynucleotide kinase[15]. After cleavage with a second restriction enzyme (or in some cases, strand-separation), the required labelled fragments were separated on acrylamide or agarose gels, their positions located by autoradiography and the DNA recovered from the gel slices. The DNA was then partially degraded by chemical means[15] and the products analysed on polyacrylamide/urea gels[16].

RESULTS

Self-priming of the A/Victoria HA gene for reverse transcriptase

Initial observations indicated that after very brief polyadenylation the A/Victoria gene 4 was efficiently transcribed by reverse transcriptase, whereas the other genes were not[11]. Further experiments showed that gene 4 was a good template for reverse transcriptase in the absence of polyadenylation (and without added oligo(dT) primer).

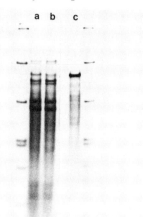

a b c

Fig. 1. cDNA was synthesised from polyadenylated and non-poly-adenylated X-47 vRNA[11]. Samples were electrophoresed on an alkaline 1.4% agarose gel. Gels were dried and autoradiographed. Lanes (a) and (b) are cDNA from vRNA polyadenylated for 4' and 2' respectively (mean rate of poly-adenylation, 15 A's per 3' end); lane (c) is cDNA from non-poly-adenylated vRNA. The two outer lanes show ^{32}P-labelled Hind III fragments of PM2 DNA, their sizes being 5400, 2350, 475, 450, 270 and 110 nucleotide pairs.

Figure 1 compares the cDNA products obtained with and without poly-adenylation after electrophoresis on a denaturing gel. In the former case (Fig. 1a and 1b), bands corresponding to all eight genes are evident and the relationship between these bands and the individual genes has already been shown[11]. When non-polyadenylated viral RNA was transcribed, the cDNA product (Fig. 1c) was seen as a major band migrating slightly faster than the transcript of polyadenylated gene 4 RNA. There is no evidence for major bands corresponding to transcripts of other viral genes.

The size of the cDNA, approximately 1700 nucleotides, suggests it is a copy of gene 4 and other results based on hybridisation support this conclusion. The 1700 nucleotide ^{32}P-cDNA was isolated from a gel and hybridised with the individual RNA genes under conditions of RNA excess. The results of this experiment (Table 1) show that the ^{32}P-cDNA was rendered resistant to Sl nuclease only by gene 4 RNA and by unfractionated viral RNA.

TABLE 1

HYBRIDISATION OF ^{32}P-cDNA TO VIRAL RNA GENES

RNA gene	^{32}P-cDNA resistance to Sl nuclease (%)	^{32}P-cDNA was synthesised and the 1700 nucleotide band isolated from an alkaline agarose gel. RNA genes 1-8 were isolated[11]. 0.5 ng of ^{32}P-cDNA was hybridised to 5 ng of each RNA gene or 20 ng unfractionated vRNA. Hybridisation was in 50% formamide, 0.3 M NaCl (pH 7), at 45°C for 16 hrs. Aliquots were removed for TCA precipitation and others for Sl nuclease treatment followed by TCA precipitation.
–	5.6	
1	4.3	
2	4.1	
3	8.6	
4	71.4	
5 & 6	12.3	
7	8.4	
8	8.0	
vRNA	99.6	

Cloning of the gene 4 transcript

dsDNA for cloning was prepared from cDNA using reverse transcriptase, for which the cDNA acted as a template without added primer[11]. After second strand synthesis, the molecular weight of the DNA product was found to have doubled to about 3400 nucleotides, as seen on a denaturing gel; after Sl nuclease treatment the strand corresponding in size to the original cDNA was detected by gel electrophoresis. These results indicate the formation of a near full-length copy of the gene into dsDNA.

Preliminary restriction mapping of the gene 4 transcript indicated the presence of cleavage sites for EcoRI, Hind III and Bam HI, which precluded the use of linker molecules for insertion into the cloning vector[9]. Instead the method of addition of homopolymeric tails to the dsDNA and to the appropriately restricted vector was used[17]. In several cases where the tailed region of cloned DNA was sequenced, the length of the poly(dG).poly(dC) double-stranded region was 30-40 base pairs, in good agreement with the estimate of 20-30 bases added per 3' end in the terminal transferase reaction.

Transformation of E. coli with 5 ng of the recombinant plasmid produced by annealing poly (dC)-tailed dsDNA with poly (dG)-tailed, Hind III-restricted pBR322 DNA produced 13 ampicillin-resistant transformant colonies. Screening by colony hybridisation with a ^{32}P-RNA probe made from fractionated viral RNA revealed 8 colonies reacting positively with the HA gene probe.

The plasmid pV-HA$_{10}$ contained the longest gene 4 insert, estimated at approximately 1800 base pairs including the homopolymer tail region, and was used for complete characterisation by nucleotide sequencing.

Restriction map of gene 4

A map of the major restriction sites of gene 4 is shown in Figure 2. The gene 4 transcript contains no cleavage sites for Hinc II, HpaI, SalI or PvuII. Interestingly, it contains two EcoRI sites extremely close together, within a sequence of 28 base pairs. These, in turn, are within a sequence of 165 nucleotides bounded by two BglII sites in the HA$_2$ region.

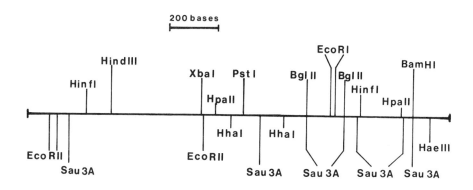

Fig. 2. Map of the major restriction sites of the A/Victoria/3/75 haemagglu-tinin gene. It was necessary to use an isoschizomer BstNI to cleave at EcoRII sites, which contain a modified cytosine.

Figure 3 shows a map of the HA$_2$ region indicating the restriction sites used for sequencing and also the sequence lengths determined from each gel. As can be seen, almost all sequences were determined at least twice, sometimes on both strands. Also, most importantly, the sequence was read through each restriction site from a different adjacent restriction site. This eliminated the

possibility of not detecting one of a pair of identical sites separated by less
than about 30 base pairs, e.g. the two EcoRI sites referred to above.

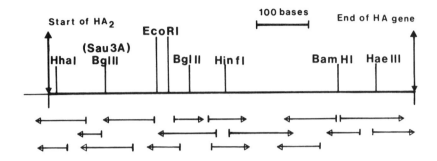

Fig. 3. Restriction map of the HA_2 region of the A/Victoria/3/75 haemagglutinin gene, indicating sites from which sequencing was begun. Horizontal
arrows indicate the length and direction of sequence data determined from each
gel.

Nucleotide sequence of the HA_2 region

Figure 4 shows the nucleotide sequence of the region coding for the HA_2
protein and also the sequence encoding the -COOH terminal 5 amino acids of HA_1
and the single arginine residue which connects HA_1 and HA_2. In addition the
sequence of 35 untranslated nucleotides corresponding to the 5' terminus of the
viral RNA is shown. This sequence was determined using the BamHI - HaeIII
restriction fragment from the gene 4 copy as a primer for elongation on the
viral RNA template by reverse transcriptase, as described previously[9]. This
sequence overlapped the end of the cloned DNA and could be read to within 2
nucleotides of the end of the gene; assuming the latter 2 nucleotides to be
the same as in FPV, the 5' terminal 21 nucleotides of the FPV and A/Victoria HA
genes are identical. This experiment also indicated that no mutations had
occurred in this region of the cloned DNA, in contrast to FPV[9].

In other experiments (not shown), the sequence at the "start" of the gene 4
DNA copy, i.e. corresponding to the 3' end of the viral RNA, was determined for
two different plasmids, pV-HA_{10} and pV-HA_2. The sequences appear to begin at
an almost identical point, within 2 nucleotides of each other, suggesting the
self-priming mechanism of A/Victoria gene 4 directs initiation of transcription
of the DNA copy from a specific point, or very short region, near the 3' end of

```
              End of HA₁          ↓Connecting Peptide↓  Start of HA₂
A/Vic    5'...CCA GAG AAA CAA ACT                AGA GGC ATA TTC GGC GCA ATA GCA GGT TTC ATA GAA AAT
                                                                                              10
A/Vic    -Pro-Glu-Lys-Gln-Thr————————————————————Arg-Gly-Ile-Phe-Gly-Ala-Ile-Ala-Gly-Phe-Ile-Glu-Asn-

A/Mem    -Pro-Glu-Lys-Gln-Thr                        Gly-Leu-Phe-Gly-Ala-Ile-Ala-Gly-Phe-Ile-Glu-Asn-

A/FPV    -Pro-Glu-Pro-Ser-Lys-Lys-Arg-Glu-Lys-Arg-Gly-Leu-Phe-Gly-Ala-Ile-Ala-Gly-Phe-Ile-Glu-Asn-


         GGT TGG GAG GGA ATG ATA GAC GGT TGG TAC GGT TTC AGG CAT CAA AAT TCC GAG GGC ACA GGA CAA GCA GCA GAT
                                                                     30
         Gly-Trp-Glu-Gly-Met-Ile-Asp-Gly-Trp-Tyr-Gly-Phe-Arg-His-Gln-Asn-Ser-Glu-Gly-Thr-Gly-Gln-Ala-Ala-Asp-

         Gly-Trp-Glu-Gly-Met-Ile-Asp-Gly-Trp-Tyr-Gly-Phe-Arg-His-Gln-Asn-Ser-Glu-Gly-Thr-Gly-Gln-Ala-Ala-Asp-

         Gly-Trp-Glu-Gly-Leu-Val-Asp-Gly-Trp-Tyr-Gly-Phe-Arg-His-Gln-Asn-Ala-Gln-Gly-Gln-Gly-Thr-Ala-Ala-Asp-


         CTT AAA AGC ACT CAA GCA GCC ATC GAC CAA ATC AAT GGG AAA CTG AAT AGG GTA ATC GAG AAG ACG AAC GAG AAA
            40                                      50                                      60
         Leu-Lys-Ser-Thr-Gln-Ala-Ala-Ile-Asp-Gln-Ile-Asn-Gly-Lys-Leu-Asn-Arg-Val-Ile-Glu-Lys-Thr-Asn-Glu-Lys-

         Leu-Lys-Ser-Thr-Gln-Ala-Ala-Ile-Asp-Gln-Ile-Asp-Gly-Lys-Leu-Asn-Arg-Val-Ile-Glu-Lys-Thr-Asn-Glu-Lys-

         Tyr-Lys-Ser-Thr-Gln-Ser-Ala-Ile-Asp-Gln-Ile-Thr-Gly-Lys-Leu-Asn-Arg-Leu-Ile-Glu-Lys-Thr-Asn-Gln-Gln-


         TTC CAT CAA ATC GAA AAG GAA TTC TCA GAA GTA GAA GGG AGA ATT CAG GAC CTC GAG AAA TAC GTT GAA GAC ACT
                                      70                                      80
         Phe-His-Gln-Ile-Glu-Lys-Glu-Phe-Ser-Glu-Val-Glu-Gly-Arg-Ile-Gln-Asp-Leu-Glu-Lys-Tyr-Val-Glu-Asp-Thr-

         Phe-His-Gln-Ile-Glu-Lys-Glu-Phe-Ser-Glu-Val-Glu-Gly-Arg-Ile-Gln-Asp-Leu-Glu-Lys-Tyr-Val-Glu-Asp-Thr-

         Phe-Glu-Leu-Ile-Asp-Asn-Glu-Phe-Thr-Glu-Val-Glu-Lys-Gln-Ile-Gly-Asn-Leu-Ile-Asn-Trp-Thr-Lys-Asp-Phe-


         AAA ATA GAT CTC TGG TCT TAC AAT GCG GAG CTT CTT GTC GCT CTG GAG AAC CAA CAT ACA ATT GAT CTG ACT GAC
             90                                     100                                     110
         Lys-Ile-Asp-Leu-Trp-Ser-Tyr-Asn-Ala-Glu-Leu-Leu-Val-Ala-Leu-Glu-Asn-Gln-His-Thr-Ile-Asp-Leu-Thr-Asp-

         Lys-Ile-Asp-Leu-Trp-Ser-Tyr-Asn-Ala-Glu-Leu-Leu-Val-Ala-Leu-Glu-Asn-Gln-His-Thr-Ile-Asp-Leu-Thr-Asp-

         Ile-Thr-Glu-Val-Trp-Ser-Tyr-Asn-Ala-Glu-Leu-Leu-Val-Ala-Met-Glu-Asn-Gln-His-Thr-Ile-Asp-Leu-Ala-Asp-


         TCG GAA ATG AAC AAA CTG TTT GAA AAA ACA AGG AGG CAA CTG AGG GAA AAT GCT GAG GAC ATG GGC AAT GGT TGC
                                      120                                     130
         Ser-Glu-Met-Asn-Lys-Leu-Phe-Glu-Lys-Thr-Arg-Arg-Gln-Leu-Arg-Glu-Asn-Ala-Glu-Asp-Met-Gly-Asn-Gly-Cys-

         Ser-Glu-Met-Asn-Lys-Leu-Phe-Glu-Lys-Thr-Arg-Arg-Gln-Leu-Arg-Glu-Asn-Ala-Glu-Asp-Met-Gly-Asn-Gly-Cys-

         Ser-Glu-Met-Asn-Lys-Leu-Tyr-Glu-Arg-Val-Arg-Lys-Gln-Leu-Arg-Glu-Asn-Ala-Glu-Glu-Asp-Gly-Thr-Gly-Cys-


         TTC AAA ATA TAC CAC AAA TGT GAC AAT GCT TGC ATA GGG TCA ATC AGA AAT GGG ACT TAT GAC CAT GAT GTA TAC
             140                                     150                                     160
         Phe-Lys-Ile-Tyr-His-Lys-Cys-Asp-Asn-Ala-Cys-Ile-Gly-Ser-Ile-Arg-Asn-Gly-Thr-Tyr-Asp-His-Asp-Val-Tyr-

         Phe-Lys-Phe-Gln-Ile-Lys-Cys-Asp-Asn-Ala-Cys-Ile-Gly-Ser-Ile-Arg... end of known A/Mem sequence

         Phe-Glu-Ile-Phe-His-Lys-Cys-Asp-Asp-Asp-Cys-Met-Ala-Ser-Ile-Arg-Asn-Asn-Thr-Tyr-Asp-His-Ser-Lys-Tyr-


A/Vic    AGA GAC GAA GCA TTA AAC AAC CGG TTT CAG ATC AAA GGT GTT GAA CTG AAG TCA GGA TAC AAA GAC TGG
                                      170                                     180
A/Vic    Arg-Asp-Glu-Ala-Leu-Asn-Asn-Arg-Phe-Gln-Ile-Lys-Gly-Val-Glu-Leu-Lys-Ser-Gly-Tyr-Lys-Asp-Trp-

A/FPV    Arg-Glu-Glu-Ala-Met-Gln-Asn-Arg-Ile-Gln-Ile-Asp-Pro-Val-Lys-Leu-Ser-Ser-Gly-Tyr-Lys-Asp-Val-


         ATC CTG TGG ATT TCC TTT GCC ATA TCA TGC TTT TTG CTT TGT GTT GTT TTG CTG GGG TTC ATC ATG TGG GCC TGC
                         190                                     200                                     210
         Ile-Leu-Trp-Ile-Ser-Phe-Ala-Ile-Ser-Cys-Phe-Leu-Leu-Cys-Val-Val-Leu-Leu-Gly-Phe-Ile-Met-Trp-Ala-Cys-

         Ile-Leu-Trp-Phe-Ser-Phe-Gly-Ala-Ser-Cys-Phe-Leu-Leu-Leu-Ala-Ile-Ala-Val-Gly-Leu-Val-Phe-Ile-Cys-Val-


                                      End of cloned DNA↓
         CAA AAA GGC AAC ATT AGG TGC AAC ATT TGC ATT TGA GTGTATTAGTAATTAAAAACACCCTTGTTTCTA(CT) 3'
                                      220
         Gln-Lys-Gly-Asn-Ile-Arg-Cys-Asn-Ile-Cys-Ile.

         Lys-Asn-Gly-Asn-Met-Arg-Cys-Thr-Ile-Cys-Ile.
```

Fig. 4. Nucleotide sequence of the HA_2 region of the A/Victoria/3/75 haemag-glutinin gene. Included are the end of the HA_1 region and its junction with HA_2, and the untranslated region corresponding to the 5' end of the viral RNA. The predicted amino acid sequence is compared with that of A/FPV and the known sequence of A/Memphis/102/72.

58

the viral RNA. A knowledge of the complete sequence of the 3' terminus of gene
4 allows the model shown in Figure 5 to be proposed for this mechanism
involving the maximum degree of intramolecular base pairing possible in this
region (Figure 5) permitting a relatively stable structure[18] to be formed at
which transcription might initiate.

A. Nucleotide sequence at 3' end of gene 4.

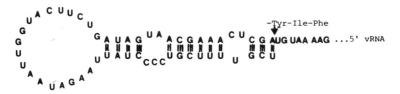

B. Intra-molecular base pairing at 3' end of gene 4.

Fig. 5. Fig. 5A shows the nucleotide sequence at the 3' end of gene 4, indicating the start of the coding region. Fig. 5B shows the possible conformation
adopted by this sequence to account for its property of self-priming for DNA
synthesis. Arrows indicate the point at which cDNA synthesis begins.

Amino acid sequence of the HA_2 protein

The HA_2 protein of A/Victoria, shown in Figure 4, consists of a sequence of
221 amino acids containing two strongly hydrophobic regions. It is the same
length as the HA_2 of Fowl Plague Virus, with which it shares only 65% amino
acid sequence homology. Comparison with the sequence of 153 amino acids
starting at the NH_2- terminus of the HA_2 of A/Memphis/102/72, another variant
of A/Hong Kong/68 (H3N2), reveals a much greater degree of homology, 97%. In
this sequence there is a difference in only 1 amino acid, this being at position
2 where Leu in A/Memphis becomes Ile in A/Victoria.

The sequence of 24 amino acids at the NH_2- terminus constitutes one region
of hydrophobicity in the HA_2 molecule. This region is highly conserved in
several subtypes including A/Memphis (H3)[8], A/FPV (Havl)[9] and A/Japan (H2)[19].
A/Victoria differs from A/Memphis by only one amino acid of this sequence. It
has been suggested that this region may be functionally important for the

interaction of haemagglutinin with the cell membrane prior to the onset of infection[19].

The other hydrophobic region of HA$_2$ is near the -COOH terminus, which is thought to contain the sequence necessary to secure the haemagglutinin to the viral membrane[19]. This sequence comprises the 26 amino acids from positions 185 to 210 and has a counterpart in exactly the same region of FPV which contains predominantly non-polar amino acids. Interestingly, though there is only 40% sequence homology with FPV in this region, the similarity of amino acid composition is 80%.

The positions of the cysteine residues are highly conserved between strains as might be expected since at least some are involved in the production and maintenance of secondary structure. Of a total of 8 cysteine residues in the HA$_2$ of A/Victoria, 3 are clustered at positions 137, 144 and 148, these being exactly conserved in A/Memphis, A/Japan and FPV. Of the remainder, 3 are within the -COOH terminal hydrophobic region and the other 2 are at positions 217 and 220, the latter 2 being identically placed in FPV.

There is one potential site for glycosylation of an asparagine residue[20] in the HA$_2$ molecule, this being at position 154 where the sequence is Asn-Gly-Thr. This corresponds exactly with the position of a potential site for carbohydrate attachment in FPV.

Cleavage of the HA molecule into the HA$_1$ and HA$_2$ chains is necessary for infectivity[2]; it is carried out by host cell proteolytic activity which can be mimicked in vitro by trypsin[1,2]. In A/Victoria, the sequence at the cleavage site is -Thr-Arg-Gly-, where the Arg residue is excised to produce HA$_1$ and HA$_2$. In A/Japan also, a single Arg is removed during this process (M.J. Gething, pers. comm.) but in FPV the corresponding excised region contains 5 amino acids, -Lys-Arg-Glu-Lys-Arg-[9].

CONCLUSIONS

Comparison of the amino acid sequence of the A/Victoria HA$_2$ protein with the known sequence of the A/Memphis HA$_2$ reveals a high degree of conservation between these H3N2 strains. This sequence together with that of the A/Victoria HA$_1$ chain (see W. Min Jou, these proceedings), when compared with that of other H3N2 strains especially in the region known to contain the antigenic sites[21], will give a more complete picture of the changes that arise in primary structure during antigenic drift.

ACKNOWLEDGEMENTS

We thank Bridget Lister for typing the manuscript, John Hobbs for photographic assistance, Andrew Threlfall for help in checking sequence data and Dr. A.J. Hale for providing excellent research facilities. We thank Graham Catlin and Brian Jenkins for valuable technical assistance.

All cloning experiments described here were carried out under Category III conditions in a laboratory approved by GMAG.

REFERENCES

1. Klenk, H.D., Rott, R., Orlich, M. and Blödorn, J. (1975) Virology, 68, 426-439.
2. Lazarowitz, S.G. and Choppin, P.W. (1975) Virology, 68, 440-454.
3. Drzeniek, R., Seto, J.T. and Rott, R. (1966) Biochim. Biophys. Acta, 128, 547-558.
4. Laver, W.G. and Kilbourne, E.D. (1966) Virology, 30, 493-501.
5. Webster, R.G. and Laver, W.G. (1975) in The Influenza Virus and Influenza, Kilbourne, E.D. ed., Academic Press, New York, pp. 269-314.
6. Laver, W.G., Air, G.M., Webster, R.G., Gerhard, W., Ward, C.W. and Dopheide, T.A. (1979) Virology, 98, 226-237.
7. Choppin, P.W., Lazarowitz, S.G. and Goldberg, A.R. (1975) in Negative Strand Viruses, Mahy, B.W.J. ed., Academic Press, London, pp. 105-119.
8. Ward, C.W. and Dopheide, T.A. (1979) Brit. Med. Bull., 35, 51-56.
9. Porter, A.G., Barber, C., Carey, N.H., Hallewell, R.A., Threlfall, G. and Emtage, J.S. (1979) Nature, 282, 471-477.
10. Vogt, V.M. (1973) Eur. J. Biochem., 33, 192-200.
11. Emtage, J.S., Catlin, G.H. and Carey, N.H. (1979) Nucleic Acids Res., 6, 1221-1240.
12. Roychoudhury, R., Jay, E. and Wu, R. (1976) Nucleic Acids Res., 3, 863-877.
13. Grunstein, M. and Hogness, D.S. (1975) Proc. Nat. Acad. Sci. USA, 72, 3961-3965.
14. Sutcliffe, J.G. (1978) Cold Spring Harbor Symp. Quant. Biol., 42, 77-90.
15. Maxam, A.M. and Gilbert, W. (1977) Proc. Nat. Acad. Sci. USA 74, 560-564.
16. Sanger, F. and Coulson, A.R. (1978) FEBS Letters, 87, 107-110.
17. Sleigh, M.J., Both, G.W. and Brownlee, G.G. (1979) Nucleic Acids Res., 7, 879-893.
18. Tinoco, I., Uhlenbeck, O.C. and Levine, M.D. (1971) Nature, 230, 362-367.
19. Waterfield, M.D., Espelie, K., Elder, K. and Skehel, J.J. (1979) Brit. Med. Bull., 35, 57-63.
20. Neuberger, A., Gottschalk, A., Marshall, R.D. and Spiro, R.G. (1972) in The Glycoproteins; their Composition, Structure and Function, Gottschalk, A. ed., Elsevier, Amsterdam, pp. 450-490.
21. Jackson, D.C., Dopheide, T.A., Russell, R.J., White, D.O. and Ward, C.W. (1979) Virology, 93, 458-465.

EDITOR'S COMMENTS

There is probably only one difference in the amino acid sequence of HA2 between Mem/102/72 and Vic/3/75 (at position 2). The sequence of Mem/102/72 HA2 derived by protein methods has been revised at positions 140-142 (Dopheide and Ward, this volume, Fig. 2) and is the same as Vic/3/75 at these residues. The Asp instead of Asn at position 49 is almost certainly the result of deamidation, since two forms of this peptide (neutral and acidic) were present in tryptic digests of Mem/102/72 HA2 (Laver et al., Nature, in press).

DISCUSSION

Salser: Self-priming by a loop for the reverse transcription reaction would lead to a product where cDNA is linked to the RNA. Is the sizing consistent with that?

Threlfall: Since we alkali-treat the product before sizing, we don't know.

Brownlee: Were there any errors in the clones?

Threlfall: Not as far as we know.

Gething: In the H2 clone there were no errors. This was using Pol 1 for second strand synthesis, and perhaps there is a difference between Pol 1 and reverse transcriptase.

Threlfall: We use reverse transcriptase for the second strand, and the terminal fragment from the clone gave an identical sequence to the sequence we already had.

Cummings: In the globin clones, using Pol 1 for second strand, we find two cases with errors in the middle - one an insertion, one a deletion.

CLONING AND DNA NUCLEOTIDE SEQUENCE ANALYSIS OF THE HEMAGGLUTININ AND
NEURAMINIDASE GENES OF INFLUENZA A STRAINS

WILLY MIN JOU, MARTINE VERHOEYEN, RENE DEVOS, ERIC SAMAN, DANNY HUYLEBROECK,
LUDO VAN ROMPUY, RONG XIANG FANG AND WALTER FIERS
Laboratory of Molecular Biology, State University of Ghent,
Ledeganckstraat 35, B-9000 Ghent, Belgium

INTRODUCTION

Influenza A virus infections continue to be a major cause of illness in
man because of the ability of the virus to change its antigenic properties.
These changes[1] in the surface proteins may be drastic (antigenic shift, leading
to the appearance of a new viral subtype) or relatively minor within a certain
subtype (antigenic drift). The two surface antigens, hemagglutinin and neuraminidase, are glycoproteins coded for by RNAs 4 and 5 (or 6, depending on the
strain).

In order to try to understand this antigenic variation, our approach has
been to polyadenylate these genes in vitro[2], to make synthetic DNA copies and
to clone them in a bacterial plasmid. In this way one can easily obtain sufficient amounts of material for rapid DNA sequencing[3]. Sofar, recombinant plasmids of the hemagglutinin and neuraminidase of two strains from the H3N2 subtype have been obtained and the complete sequence of one of the hemagglutinins
(from A/Victoria/3/75) has been determined.

MATERIALS AND METHODS

Bacterial strains, Plasmids, Enzymes and Viruses

Escherichia coli K12 strain HB101 and HB101 carrying the plasmid pBR322 were
kindly made available by Dr. H. Boyer. Avian myeloblastosis virus reverse transcriptase was a gift from Dr. J.W. Beard. The restriction enzymes used were from
New England Biolabs (Beverly, Mass.). Other enzymes and reagents were from
the suppliers described by Devos et al.[4] Two high yield recombinant viruses
were used. X47 (obtained from Evans Medical Co, Liverpool, England) is a recombinant between A/Victoria/3/75 (H3N2) and A/PR/8/34 (HON1) with both surface
antigens from the Victoria strain. X-31 (X-31 RNA was kindly made available
by Dr. J. Skehel) is a recombinant between A/Hong Kong/1/68 (H3N2) and A/PR/8/
34, carrying the H3N2 determinants from Hong Kong.

Construction of recombinant plasmids

Polyadenylation, reverse transcription, RNase treatment, E.coli DNA Polymerase I and SI nuclease reaction were as described[4] using the mixture of eight viral RNAs. The dsDNA mixture was sized on a 1.5% agarose gel and bands corresponding to gene 4, gene 5 and 6 (moving as one band), gene 7 and gene 8 were recovered from the gel. The DNA copies were tailed with polynucleotide phosphorylase and TTP and cloned in the Pst I site of the plasmid pBR322 tailed with ATP. The transformation mixture was plated out on tetracycline containing Luria agar plates. The colonies were transferred to nitrocellulose filters and colony hybridized according to a simplified version of Grunstein and Hogness[5] using ^{32}P-kinated RNA fragments[6] of the individual RNAs previously separated on a 3% acrylamide-urea gel. The length of the insert was determined on small scale DNA preparations separated on agarose gels.

Labeling procedures and DNA sequencing

5'- and 3'-labeling procedures[3,7] and DNA-sequencing[3] was according to established procedures.

RESULTS

Transformation

Between 10 and 70 ng of poly(dT)-tailed dsDNA was annealed to a 1.5 to 3 times molar excess of poly(dA)-tailed pBR322 DNA. The length of the tails varied from forty to two-hundred nucleotides according to the radioactivity incorporated. Using the dsDNA copies from genes 4, the mixture of 5 and 6, 7 and 8 from strain X-47, and 4, the mixture of 5 and 6, and 7 from X-31 between seventeen and hundred twenty five tetracycline-resistant colonies were obtained. Of these a fraction between 0 and 60% showed positive hybridisation[5] with the appropriate RNA probe. Hybridisation with RNAs 5 and 6 respectively, was also used to discriminate between colonies having incorporated neuraminidase and nucleoprotein information.

Physical characterization of the inserts

Estimation of the size of the inserts of the first series of clones from the Victoria hemagglutinin on agarose gel revealed that no full-size gene 4 copy had been obtained. The longest inserts were 720 base pairs (pVHA55; pVHA stands for plasmid-Victoria-Hemagglutinin) and 600 base pairs (pVHA57 and pVHA101). Further characterization showed that the information in pVHA55 was an extension of that in pVHA57, while pVHA55 and pVHA101 were non-overlapping.

Further cloning experiments yielded presumes full-size inserts for the hemagglutinin gene of Victoria and Hong Kong (approx. 1860 base pairs including the tails), for the neuraminidase of Victoria and Hong Kong (approx. 1570 base pairs) and for the Matrix protein of X47 (approx. 1030 nucleotides), which is derived from the PR8 strain (P. Palese, personal communication). Colonies from the other genes have not been physically characterized so far.

Sequence of the Victoria hemagglutinin gene

A restriction map of pVHA55 and pVHA101 and (later on) of pVHA14 (the latter containing the presumed full-size insert) was constructed using the Smith and Birnstiel method[8], and 5'- or 3'-terminally labeled fragments were prepared and sequenced[3]. To increase the accuracy most of the sequence was read from both strands and overlapping sequence data were collected in all cases.

The total hemagglutinin information in PVHA14 is 1744 nucleotides with a continuously open reading frame coding for 567 amino acids. The presence of the sequence 5'-AGCAAAAGCAGG proves that the complete information starting from the 3' end of the viral RNA has been cloned[9-11]. It follows from direct sequencing of a cDNA copy from the 5'-end of the RNA (G. Threlfall, personal communication) that 24 nucleotides are missing at the other end, thus bringing the length of the viral RNA to 1768. This is very similar to the FPV hemagglutinin gene[12] (1742 nucleotides) and the presumed full-size insertion of the strain 29C hemagglutinin gene[13] ($\pm$ 1760 nucleotides). There is only limited genetic information not coding for protein : 29 nucleotides at the 5'-end of the coding strand and 38 at the 3'-end. This seems to be a general feature of influenza RNAs[10,12,14-16]. The termination codon both in Victoria and Hong Kong is UGA, whereas a UAA is found in the FPV hemagglutinin[12].

Amino acid sequence of the Victoria hemagglutinin

The precursor Victoria HA consists of 567 amino acids (Figure 1) : most likely the signal peptide[17] is 16 amino acids long (by comparison with other signal peptides and the fact that the HA1 chain of H3 hemagglutinins is blocked, probably as a pyroglutamic acid residue[18]). This leaves 329 amino acids in the HA1, one arginine residue in the connecting region between HA1 and HA2, and 221 amino acids in the HA2 chain, as follows unambiguously from comparison with both the known carboxyl-terminal amino acid sequence of the HA1 and the amino-terminal sequence of the HA2 from another H3 strain A/Memphis/102/72[18]. The signal peptide shows almost no sequence conservation

Met-Lys-Thr-Ile-Ile-Ala-Leu-Ser-Tyr-Ile-Phe-Cys-Leu-Val-Phe-Ala-Gln-Asp-Leu-Pro
4

Gly-Asn-Asp-Asn-Asn-Ser-Thr-Ala-Thr-Leu-Cys-Leu-Gly-His-His-Ala-Val-Pro-Asn-
23

Gly-Thr-Leu-Val-Lys-Thr-Ile-Thr-Asn-Asp-Gln-Ile-Glu-Val-Thr-Asn-Ala-Thr-Glu-
42

Leu-Val-Gln-Ser-Ser-Ser-Thr-Gly-Lys-Ile-Cys-Asn-Asn-Pro-His-Arg-Ile-Leu-Asp-
61

Gly-Ile-Asn-Cys-Thr-Leu-Ile-Asp-Ala-Leu-Leu-Gly-Asp-Pro-His-Cys-Asp-Gly-Phe-
80

Gln-Asn-Glu-Lys-Trp-Asp-Leu-Phe-Val-Glu-Arg-Ser-Lys-Ala-Phe-Ser-Asn-Cys-Tyr-
99

Pro-Tyr-Asp-Val-Pro-Asp-Tyr-Ala-Ser-Leu-Arg-Ser-Leu-Val-Ala-Ser-Ser-Gly-Thr-
118

Leu-Glu-Phe-Ile-Asn-Glu-Gly-Phe-Asn-Trp-Thr-Gly-Val-Thr-Gln-Asn-Gly-Gly-Ser-
137

Ser-Ala-Cys-Lys-Arg-Gly-Pro-Asp-Ser-Gly-Phe-Phe-Ser-Arg-Leu-Asn-Trp-Leu-Tyr-
156

Lys-Ser-Gly-Ser-Thr-Tyr-Pro-Val-Gln-Asn-Val-Thr-Met-Pro-Asn-Asn-Asp-Asn-Ser-
175

Asp-Lys-Leu-Tyr-Ile-Trp-Gly-Val-His-His-Pro-Ser-Thr-Asp-Lys-Glu-Gln-Thr-Asn-
194

Leu-Tyr-Val-Gln-Ala-Ser-Gly-Lys-Val-Thr-Val-Ser-Thr-Lys-Arg-Ser-Gln-Gln-Thr-
213

Ile-Ile-Pro-Asn-Val-Gly-Ser-Arg-Pro-Trp-Val-Arg-Gly-Leu-Ser-Ser-Arg-Ile-Ser-
232

Ile-Tyr-Trp-Thr-Ile-Val-Lys-Pro-Gly-Asp-Ile-Leu-Val-Ile-Asn-Ser-Asn-Gly-Asn-
251

Leu-Ile-Ala-Pro-Arg-Gly-Tyr-Phe-Lys-Met-Arg-Thr-Gly-Lys-Ser-Ser-Ile-Met-Arg-
270

Ser-Asp-Ala-Pro-Ile-Gly-Thr-Cys-Ser-Ser-Glu-Cys-Ile-Thr-Pro-Asn-Gly-Ser-Ile-
289

Pro-Asn-Asp-Lys-Pro-Phe-Gln-Asn-Val-Asn-Lys-Ile-Thr-Tyr-Gly-Ala-Cys-Pro-Lys-
308

Tyr-Val-Lys-Gln-Asn-Thr-Leu-Lys-Leu-Ala-Thr-Gly-Met-Arg-Asn-Val-Pro-Glu-Lys-
327

Gln-Thr-Arg
330

Gly-Ile-Phe-Gly-Ala-Ile-Ala-Gly-Phe-Ile-Glu-Asn-Gly-Trp-Glu-Gly-Met-Ile-Asp-
19

Gly-Trp-Tyr-Gly-Phe-Arg-His-Gln-Asn-Ser-Glu-Gly-Thr-Gly-Gln-Ala-Ala-Asp-Leu-
38

Lys-Ser-Thr-Gln-Ala-Ala-Ile-Asp-Gln-Ile-Asn-Gly-Lys-Leu-Asn-Arg-Val-Ile-Glu-
57

Lys-Thr-Asn-Glu-Lys-Phe-His-Gln-Ile-Glu-Lys-Glu-Phe-Ser-Glu-Val-Glu-Gly-Arg-
76

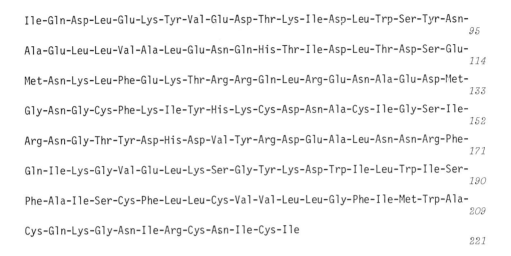

Ile-Gln-Asp-Leu-Glu-Lys-Tyr-Val-Glu-Asp-Thr-Lys-Ile-Asp-Leu-Trp-Ser-Tyr-Asn-
95

Ala-Glu-Leu-Leu-Val-Ala-Leu-Glu-Asn-Gln-His-Thr-Ile-Asp-Leu-Thr-Asp-Ser-Glu-
114

Met-Asn-Lys-Leu-Phe-Glu-Lys-Thr-Arg-Arg-Gln-Leu-Arg-Glu-Asn-Ala-Glu-Asp-Met-
133

Gly-Asn-Gly-Cys-Phe-Lys-Ile-Tyr-His-Lys-Cys-Asp-Asn-Ala-Cys-Ile-Gly-Ser-Ile-
152

Arg-Asn-Gly-Thr-Tyr-Asp-His-Asp-Val-Tyr-Arg-Asp-Glu-Ala-Leu-Asn-Asn-Arg-Phe-
171

Gln-Ile-Lys-Gly-Val-Glu-Leu-Lys-Ser-Gly-Tyr-Lys-Asp-Trp-Ile-Leu-Trp-Ile-Ser-
190

Phe-Ala-Ile-Ser-Cys-Phe-Leu-Leu-Cys-Val-Val-Leu-Leu-Gly-Phe-Ile-Met-Trp-Ala-
209

Cys-Gln-Lys-Gly-Asn-Ile-Arg-Cys-Asn-Ile-Cys-Ile
221

Fig. 1. Amino acid sequence of the precursor Victoria HA as derived from the DNA sequence. The HA1 and HA2 chains are numbered separately.

except for its hydrophobic character when compared with FPV[18] and with the sequence at the 5'-end of an Asian subtype[15,16].

There is sufficient amino acid sequence homology with FPV[12] to line up the two sequences all over the chain by the introduction of two insertions (of nine amino acids and one amino acid respectively) and three deletions (of one amino acid in two different positions and four amino acids in another one) into the HA1 part of the Victoria sequence. Both most extensive insertions are found at the ends of HA1, one leading to an extension of the amino terminal sequence and the second one occurring in the connecting region between HA1 and HA2. The positions of cysteines are highly conserved in these two strains and also when the partial amino acid sequence data of another member of the H3 subtype[18] and of an H2 strain[19] are considered. Both observations indicate a similar general folding of the hemagglutinin molecule even in the more variable HA1 chain between different subtypes. Of 320 corresponding amino acids in HA1 116 amino acids have been conserved in FPV (36.2%), the conservation being higher towards both ends. The amino acid conservation between Victoria and the Memphis strain[18] is 93% in the carboxylterminal part of the HA1.

The connecting region between HA1 and HA2 consists only of a single arginine residue in Victoria whereas in FPV five residues are removed.

The HA2 chain contains 221 amino acids both in Victoria and FPV and the amino acid sequence homology amounts to 65.6%. Again, the conservation between Victoria and Memphis is very high (only 5 differences in the 153 amino-terminal amino acids). The hydrophobic region associated with the membrane can clearly be recognized near the carboxyl-terminus from amino acid residues 185 to 208. This sequence is exactly conserved in the Hong Kong strain. A similar hydrophobic region is found at the same position in FPV.

REFERENCES

1. Pereira, M.S. (1979) British Med. Bull., 35, 9.
2. Devos, R., Gillis, E. and Fiers, W. (1976) Eur. J. Biochem., 62, 401.
3. Maxam, A. and Gilbert, W. (1977) Proc. Natl. Acad. Sci. USA, 74, 560.
4. Devos, R., van Emmelo, J., Contreras, R. and Fiers, W. (1979) J. Mol. Biol., 128, 595.
5. Grunstein, M. and Hogness, D.S. (1975) Proc. Natl. Acad. Sci. USA, 72, 3961.
6. Coffin, J.M. and Billeter, M.A. (1976) J. Mol. Biol., 100, 293.
7. Soeda, E., Kimura, G. and Miura, K.-L. (1978) Proc. Natl. Acad. Sci. USA, 75, 162.
8. Smith, H.O. and Birnstiel, M.L. (1976) Nucl. Acids Res., 3, 3287.
9. Skehel, J.J. and Hay, A.J. (1978) Nucl. Acids Res., 5, 1207.
10. Robertson, J.S. (1979) Nucl. Acids Res., 6, 3745.
11. Desselberger, U., Racaniello, V.R., Zazra, J.R. and Palese, P. (1979) Gene, in press.
12. Porter, A.G., Barber, C., Carey, N.H., Hallewell, R.A., Threlfall, G. and Emtage, J.S. (1979) Nature, in press.
13. Sleigh, M.J., Both, G.W. and Brownlee, G.G. (1979) Nucl. Acids Res., 7, 879.
14. Both, G.W. and Air, G.M. (1979) Eur. J. Biochem., 96, 363.
15. Air, G.M. (1979) Virology, 97, 468.
16. Mc Cauley, J., Bye, J., Elder, K., Gething, M.J., Skehel, J.J., Smith, A. and Waterfield, M.D. (1979) FEBS Letters, in press.
17. Elder, K.T., Bye, J.M., Skehel, J.J., Waterfield, M.D. and Smith, A.E. (1979) Virology, 95, 343.
18. Ward, C.W. and Dopheide, T.A. (1979) Brit. Med. Bull, 35, 51.
19. Waterfield, M.D., Espelie, E., Elder, K. and Skehel, J.J. (1979) Brit. Med. Bull., 35, 57.

DISCUSSION

Gibbs: You have an extra amino acid compared to the other H3 sequences. It is hard to imagine how 3 nucleotides can be added, how do you explain that?

Min Jou: We really don't know. Already the H3 sequence is 10-11 amino acids longer at the N-terminus compared to H2. I just saw last night at 11 o'clock that we had one amino acid more than the other H3's (residue 9 of HA1)!

THE HAEMAGGLUTININ GENE OF INFLUENZA A VIRUS: NUCLEOTIDE SEQUENCE
ANALYSIS OF CLONED DNA COPIES

M.J. SLEIGH[+], G.W. BOTH[+], G.G. BROWNLEE[++], V.J. BENDER[+] AND B.A MOSS[+]
+CSIRO Molecular and Cellular Biology Unit, P.O. Box 184, North Ryde, N.S.W.,
2113, Australia; ++MRC Molecular Biology Laboratory, Cambridge, CB2 2QH, U.K.

INTRODUCTION

Within a particular subtype, the influenza virus undergoes a continual
process of evolution, characterised by frequent small changes in the properties
of its surface antigens (antigenic drift). Such changes occurring in the viral
haemagglutinin (HA) can be studied by comparing and analysing the peptide maps
of proteins from different strains (for example, references 1,2). However, with
the development of rapid nucleotide sequencing methods, it is now often easier
to analyse a gene than the protein for which it codes.

As a prelude to an investigation at the nucleic acid level of the variation
between haemagglutinins from different influenza strains of the Hong Kong (H3N2)
subtype, we have prepared double stranded DNA copies of their HA genes (the
fourth largest of the viral RNA genome segments). The gene copies were
amplified in E. coli after insertion into the plasmid pBR322. By nucleotide
sequence analysis of these cloned copies, we have determined the structure of
the HA gene, and have compared the amino acid sequence it predicts with the
data available for the amino acid sequence of the HA from the Hong Kong
influenza strain A/Mem/102/72 [2,3].

MATERIALS AND METHODS

Growth and Purification of Virus and RNA. The influenza strain 29C is a
mutant derived in the laboratory from the field strain A/NT/60/68 grown in the
presence of the most avid fraction of homologous antibody [4] in embryonated
chicken eggs [5]. The virus was kindly supplied by Dr. C. Hannoun and purified
as previously described [6]. Influenza A/Mem/102/72 was supplied by Dr. W.G.
Laver as a recombinant with A/PR/8/34. The preparation of viral RNA has been
described [6].

Preparation of Cloned HA gene copies for A/NT/60/68 and A/NT/60/68/29C.
The preparation of a double stranded DNA copy of the 29C HA gene, its insertion
into the plasmid pBR322 and amplification in E. coli RRI have been described
previously [7]. The cloned gene copy for A/NT/60/68 was obtained in the same way
but without separation of full length gene copies from lower molecular weight

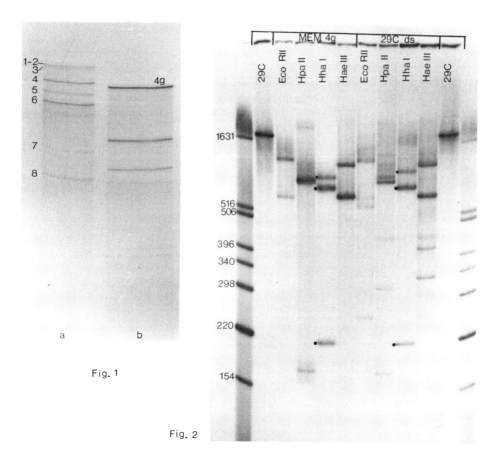

Fig. 1

Fig. 2

Fig. 1. Polyacrylamide gel electrophoresis of single stranded cDNA synthesised
from adenylated and non-adenylated influenza genome RNA. The cDNA species were
separated on a 2.6% polyacrylamide gel containing 7M urea. cDNA segments 1-8
correspond in size to the influenza RNA gene segments [6] (a) single stranded
DNA copied from polyadenylated RNA from strain A/NT/60/68/29C using reverse
transcriptase and p(dT)$_{12-18}$ as primer [6] (b) cDNA synthesised by reverse
transcriptase under the same conditions but with no added primer, and
unadenylated RNA from A/Mem/102/72 as template.

Fig. 2. Comparison of restriction enzyme digests of ds 4g DNA from
A/Mem/102/72 with those of ds DNA synthesised using polyadenylated RNA from
A/NT/60/68/29C. The outside slots show Hinf I digestion fragments from pBR322,
with sizes in base pairs, and the slots next to them S$_1$ nuclease-digested
ds DNA from strain 29C. Markers on the HhaI digests demonstrate that all but
one of the fragments obtained are of a similar size for the two DNA species.

species at the double stranded DNA stage [7]. The hybrid plasmid containing the NT/60/68 HA gene copy was initially isolated by transformation of E. coli χ1776, but was later transferred to E. coli RRI.

All recombinant DNA experiments were carried out under CII and EK1 and EK2 conditions, as prescribed by the Australian Academy of Science Recombinant DNA Committee.

Preparation of a Cloned HA gene copy for A/Mem/102/72. Total genome RNA from influenza A/Mem/102/72 was incubated with reverse transcriptase [7] in the absence of added primer, and without prior adenylation. Several discrete cDNA products were separated by polyacrylamide gel electrophoresis (Fig. 1), the largest (band 4g) being slightly smaller than the cDNA transcribed from the HA gene (band 4) [6]. Band 4g DNA was extracted from the gel and converted to the double stranded form [7]. Subsequent treatment of the double stranded DNA for insertion into pBR322 and cloning in E. coli RRI were as described previously [7].

That the double stranded DNA prepared in this way was a slightly shortened copy of the HA gene was demonstrated by comparing restriction enzyme digests of ^{32}P- labelled double stranded band 4g DNA from A/Mem/102/72 with digests of DNA prepared from polyadenylated gene 4 RNA (A/NT/60/68/29C) [7], previously confirmed as a copy of the HA gene by cloning and sequencing [7]. This comparison is shown in Figure 2.

Restriction Enzyme Analysis and Nucleotide Sequencing of cloned HA Gene copies. Restriction enzyme cleavage maps were prepared for each of the three cloned gene copies using enzymes obtained from New England Biolabs and the reaction conditions described previously [6]. DNA fragments, ^{32}P- labelled using reverse transcriptase [6] were sequenced by the method of Maxam and Gilbert [8]. Some sequence information was also obtained directly by copying viral RNA, using the chain termination method of Sanger [9]. In these experiments, restriction fragments from the cloned gene copies were used to prime cDNA synthesis by reverse transcriptase, using total polyadenylated genome RNA as template [10].

Nucleotide sequence data was stored and analysed using computer programmes devised by Staden [11,12].

RESULTS

Characterisation of cloned HA gene copies. Analysis of cloned HA gene copies for influenza A/NT/60/68/29C demonstrated that in clone C89, the DNA inserted into pBR322 was approximately 1730 bases in length, 30 bases shorter than the estimated size of the HA gene [6,7]. For A/NT/60/68, where there was no size

selection of material after double stranded DNA synthesis, only partial copies
of the HA gene were found inserted into pBR322. The largest insert (clone N327)
was approximately 1300 bases long, and corresponded to the 5' end of the gene,
(i.e. that region coding for the C-terminal area of the HA protein).

For A/Mem/102/72, a double stranded copy of the HA gene was synthesised using
self-priming by influenza RNA genome segments for cDNA synthesis by reverse
transcriptase. In the absence of added primer, the synthesis of band 4g DNA
(Fig. 1) was probably initiated at a site within the 3' terminal region of the
HA gene RNA, as a result of complementarity between a base sequence in this area
and the 3' terminal sequence common to all influenza gene segments [13,14]. This
mechanism of cDNA synthesis implies that the nucleotides on the 3' side of the
priming site will be missing from the cDNA copy. Restriction enzyme mapping
confirmed that the HA gene copy obtained in this way for A/Mem/102/72
(clone MX29) was approximately 60 bases shorter in this region than the full
length gene copy in C89.

Detailed restriction enzyme cleavage maps for the HA gene copies from the 3
influenza strains are summarised in Fig. 3. The patterns for NT/60/68 and its
descendant, 29C, were identical for all enzymes tested, but differed at some
sites from the pattern for the A/Mem/102/72 gene copy.

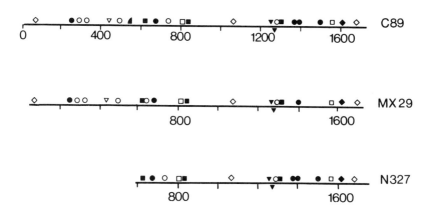

Fig. 3. Restriction enzyme cleavage maps of HA gene copies. The maps show
sites for cleavage by various restriction enzymes in the copied HA gene
sequences cloned in pBR322. Numbering (in base pairs) is from the start
(3' end) of the HA gene. MX29 - A/Mem/102/72; N327 - A/NT/60/68;
C89 - A/NT/60/68/29C; (●) Hinf I; (◆) Bam HI; (v) Hind III; (◀) Hind II;
(▼) Eco RI; (■) Ava I; (O) Ava II; (◇) Hae III; (□) Hpa II.

Nucleotide Sequence Analysis of Inserted HA Gene Copies. The strategy used
for the sequencing of MX29 [8] is shown in Fig. 4. Sequences for MX29 and N327
were obtained largely from one DNA strand only, using as a reference amino acid
sequence data for the HA from A/Mem/102/72 [2,3] and the sequence for clone C89,
75% of which was obtained for both DNA strands (unpublished results). All of
the HA gene copies studied were inserted into pBR322 in a similar orientation,
i.e. with the 5' end of the gene (coding for the C-terminal region of the
protein) at the end closest to the Eco RI site of the plasmid.

At a position 107 nucleotides from the 3' end of the gene a single base
which was present in the Mem/102/72 gene copy was missing in clone C89. Direct
sequencing of genome RNA [10], demonstrated that the missing nucleotide was also
present in the A/NT/60/68 gene. The sequence in this region for A/Mem/102/72
(marked ● in Fig. 4) was also confirmed by sequencing the RNA, since band
patterns on sequencing gels between bases 95 and 105 were difficult to interpret. Some peculiarity of secondary structure in this region may account for
the difficulty, and perhaps for the apparent deletion of a base in C89.

A composite plan of the HA gene, compiled from the three HA gene copies
sequenced, is shown in Fig. 5. Terminal sequences are shown both for the
negative strand (the gene) and the positive strand, which has the same sense as
the mRNA. Coding sequences are shown only for the positive strand.

Twenty nine nucleotides precede the codon for the N-terminal methionine and
at least the first 12 of these are identical with the 3' terminal sequence
found for the HA genes from fowl plague virus and the H3N2 strain X31 [13,14].

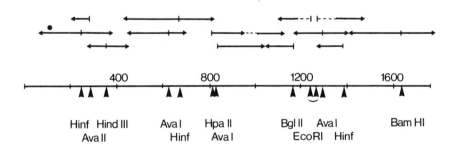

Fig.4. Strategy for obtaining the nucleotide sequence of the HA gene copy from
A/Mem/102/72 (clone MX29). Nucleotides are numbered from the start of the gene
as in Fig. 3. The arrows show the area of the insert over which sequence was
obtained and the direction of sequencing, and begin from the ^{32}P-labelled
restriction enzyme cleavage site. (●) Marks a region of 10 nucleotides whose
sequence was confirmed directly from viral RNA (see text).

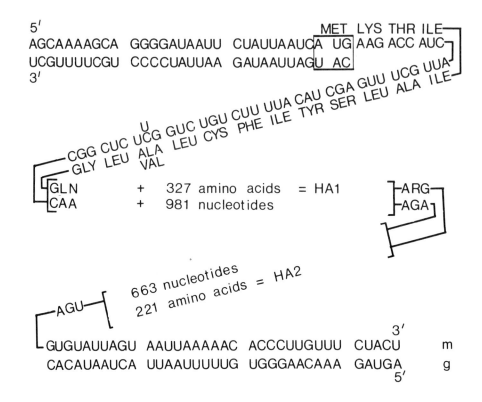

Fig. 5. Composite plan of the HA gene for Hong Kong subtype influenza viruses. The diagram shows the negative (genome) strand (labelled g) as well as the positive messenger-sense strand (m). There is at least one amino acid change in the signal peptide between A/Mem/102/72 (val) and A/NT/60/68/29C (ala). The 3' terminal gene sequence is from 29C and the 5' terminal sequence is from A/NT/60/68.

The gene then provides information for a signal peptide of 16 amino acids (with at least one amino acid difference between Mem/102/72 and NT/60/68/29C) followed by the HA protein of which glutamine is the N-terminal amino acid [15].

The gene copies for Mem/102/72 and 29C were missing 25-30 nucleotides at the 5' end of the gene (these were lost during S_1 nuclease treatment to remove the terminal hairpin loop which primes double stranded DNA synthesis by reverse transcriptase). However, we obtained the missing sequences from the cloned gene for A/NT/60/68 because of a peculiarity of the HA insert in clone N327. This contained 35 nucleotides between the translation termination codon UGA

3' end of the messenger-sense strand   base no. of the gene - 137

```
CAA GAC UUU CCA GGA AAU GAC AAC AGC ACA GCA ACG CUG UGC CUG GGA CAU CAU GCG GUG
gln asp phe pro gly asn asp asn ser thr ala thr leu cys leu gly his his ala val
N-terminal amino acid of HA1
```

```
                                                                            197
CCA AAC GGA ACA CUA GUG AAA ACA AUC ACA AAU GAU CAG AUU GAA GUG ACU AAU GCU ACU
pro asn gly thr leu val lys thr ile thr asn asp gln ile glu val thr asn ala thr
```

```
                                                                            257
GAG CUG GUU CAG AGU UCC UCA ACG GGG AAA AUA UGC AAC AAU CCU CAU CGA AUC CUU GAU
glu leu val gln ser ser ser thr gly lys ile cys asn asn pro his arg ile leu asp
```

```
                                                                            317
GGA AUA GAC UGC ACA CUG AUA GAU GCU CUA UUG GGG GAC CCU CAU UGU GAU GGC UUU CAA
gly ile asp cys thr leu ile asp ala leu leu gly asp pro his cys asp gly phe gln
```

```
                                                                            377
AAU GAG ACA UGG GAC CUU UUC GUU GAA CGC AGC AAA GCU UUC AGC AAC UGU UAC CCU UAU
asn glu thr trp asp leu phe val glu arg ser lys ala phe ser asn cys tyr pro tyr
```

```
                                                                            437
GAU GUG CCA GAU UAU GCC UCC CUU AGG UUA CUA GUU GCC UCG UCA GGC ACU UUG GAG UUU
asp val pro asp tyr ala ser leu arg leu leu val ala ser ser gly thr leu glu phe
```

```
                                                                            497
AUC AAU GAA GGC UUC ACU UUG ACU GGG GUC ACU CAG AAU GGG GGA AGC AAU GCU UGC AAA
ile asn glu gly phe thr leu thr gly val thr gln asn gly gly ser asn ala cys lys
```

```
                                                                            557
AGG GGA CCU GAU AGC GGU UUU UUC AGU AGA CUG AAC UGG UUG UAC AAA UCA GGA AGC ACA
arg gly pro asp ser gly phe phe ser arg leu asn trp leu tyr lys ser gly ser thr
```

```
                                                                            617
UAU CCA GUG CUG AAU GUG ACU AUG CCA AAC AAU GAC AAU UUU GAC AAA CUA UAC AUU UGG
tyr pro val leu asn val thr met pro asn asn asp asn phe asp lys leu tyr ile trp
```

```
                                                                            677
GGG GUU CAC CAC CCG AGC ACG GAC CAA GAA CAA ACC AGC CUA UAU GUU CAA GCA UCA GGG
gly val his his pro ser thr asp gln glu gln thr ser leu tyr val gln ala ser gly
```

```
                                                                            737
AGA GUC ACA GUC UCU ACC AAG AGA AGC CAG CAA ACU AUA AUC CCG AAU AUC GGG UCU AGA
arg val thr val ser thr lys arg ser gln gln thr ile ile pro asn ile gly ser arg
```

```
                                                                            797
CCC UGG GUA AGG GGU CAG UCU AGU AGA AUA AGC AUC UAU UGG ACA AUA GUU AAA CCG GGA
pro trp val arg gly gln ser ser arg ile ser ile tyr trp thr ile val lys pro gly
                        leu
```

```
                                                                            857
GAC AUA CUG GUA AUU AAU AGU AAU GGG AAC CUA AUU GCU CCU CGG GGU UAU UUC AAA AUG
asp ile leu val ile asn ser asn gly asn leu ile ala pro arg gly tyr phe lys met
```

```
                                                                            917
CGC ACU GGG AAA AGC UCA AUA AUG AGG UCA GAU GCA CCU AUU GGC ACC UGC AUU UCU GAA
arg thr gly lys ser ser ile met arg ser asp ala pro ile gly thr cys ile ser glu
```

```
                                                                            977
UGC AUC ACU CCA AAU GGA AGC AUU CCC AAU GAC AAG CCC UUU CAA AAC GUA AAC AAG AUC
cys ile thr pro asn gly ser ile pro asn asp lys pro phe gln asn val asn lys ile
                                           lys pro asp asp
```

```
                                                                           1037
ACA UAU GGG GCA UGU CCC AAG UAU GUU AAG CAA AAC ACC CUG AAG UUG GCA ACA GGG AUG
thr tyr gly ala cys pro lys tyr val lys gln asn thr leu lys leu ala thr gly met
```

```
                 end of HA1 | start of HA2              1097
CGG AAU GUA CCA GAG AAA CGA ACU AGA GGC CUA UUC GGC GCA AUA GCA GGU UUC AUA GAA
arg asn val pro glu lys arg thr arg gly leu phe gly ala ile ala gly phe ile glu
                            gln
```

(continued)

```
AAU GGU UGG GAG GGA AUG AUA GAC GGU UGG UAC GGU UUC AGG CAU CAA AAU UCU GAG GGC
asn gly trp glu gly met ile asp gly trp tyr gly phe arg his gln asn ser glu gly

                                                                              1217
ACA GGA CAA GCA GCA GAU CUU AAA AGC ACU CAA GCA GCC AUC GAC CAA AUC AAU GGG AAA
thr gly gln ala ala asp leu lys ser thr gln ala ala ile asp gln ile asn gly lys

                                                                              1277
CUG AAU AGG GUA AUC GAG AAG ACG AAC GAG AAA UUC CAU CAA AUC GAA AAG GAA UUC UCA
leu asn arg val ile glu lys thr asn glu lys phe his gln ile glu lys glu phe ser

                                                                              1337
GAA GUA GAA GGG AGA AUU CAG GAC CUC GAG AAA UAC GUU GAA GAC ACU AAA AUA GAU CUC
glu val glu gly arg ile gln asp leu glu lys tyr val glu asp thr lys ile asp leu

                                                                              1397
UGG UCU UAC AAU GCG GAG CUU CUU GUC GCU CUG GGG AAC CAA CAU ACA AUU GAU CUG ACU
trp ser tyr asn ala glu leu leu val ala leu gly asn gln his thr ile asp leu thr
                                                  glu

                                                                              1457
GAC UCG GAA AUG AAC AAA CUG UUU GAA AAA ACA AGG AGG CAA CUG AGG GAA AAU GCU GAG
asp ser glu met asn lys leu phe glu lys thr arg arg gln leu arg glu asn ala glu

                                                                              1517
GAC AUG GGC AAU GGU UGC UUC AAA AUA UAC CAC AAA UGU GAC AAU GCU UGC AUA GGG UCA
asp met gly asn gly cys phe lys ile tyr his lys cys asp asn ala cys ile gly ser
                                tyr his ile

                                                                              1577
AUC AGA AAU GGG ACU UAU GAC CAU GAU GUA UAC AGA GAC GAA GCA UUA AAC AAC CGG UUU
ile arg asn gly thr tyr asp his asp val tyr arg asp glu ala leu asn asn arg phe

                                                                              1637
CAG AUC AAA GGU GUU GAA CUG AAG UCA GGA UAC AAA GAC UGG AUC CUG UGG AUU UCC UUU
gln ile lys gly val glu leu lys ser gly tyr lys asp trp ile leu trp ile ser phe

                                                                              1697
GCC AUA UCA UGC UUU UUG CUU UGU GUA GUU UUG CUG GGG UUC AUC AUG UGG GCC UGC CAG
ala ile ser cys phe leu leu cys val val leu leu gly phe ile met trp ala cys gln

AAA GGC AAC AUU AGG UGC AAC AUU UGC AUU UGA    5' end of messenger-sense strand.
lys gly asn ile arg cys asn ile cys ile ***   C-terminus of HA2
```

Fig. 6. Sequence coding for the mature HA protein from A/Mem/102/72 (clone MX29). Sequence is shown for the positive (messenger-sense) strand only, with the predicted amino acid sequence. Areas of the HA protein sequenced by Ward and Dopheide [2,3,16] are underlined, and a second row of amino acids is included where there is a discrepancy between the sequence predicted and found.

(on the positive strand) and the end of the HA gene (identified as base 1765). The last 21 nucleotides were identical to the 5' terminal sequence for the HA gene from fowl plague virus described by Robertson [14]. The insert then continued for approximately 150 nucleotides (apparently derived neither from HA gene nor from plasmid) before the poly(dG)-poly(dC) tails marking the site of insertion into the plasmid.

Fig. 6 shows the complete sequence of that region of the HA gene from A/Mem/102/72 (PR8 recombinant) coding for the mature HA protein. The amino acid sequence predicted from this is compared in the same figure with published data on the sequence of the HA protein from a Bel recombinant of

A/Mem/102/72 [2,3,16].

DISCUSSION

Double stranded DNA copies of the HA gene from three different influenza strains of the Hong Kong (H3N2) subtype, inserted into the plasmid pBR322 and amplified in E. coli, have enabled us to determine a general structure for the HA gene of this subtype. The ability of Hong Kong influenza genome RNA to initiate cDNA synthesis without added primer provides a useful shortcut to the synthesis of slightly shortened double stranded HA gene copies, without the losses normally incurred during polyadenylation of RNA. Band 4g DNA synthesis seems to be a property of all of the strains from the Hong Kong subtype so far tested (A/Mem/102/72, A/Eng/42/72, A/Qu/7/70 and A/NT/60/68) although it is not always the major product of the reaction. Band 4g dDNA also provides a highly specific and pure probe, useful for identifying E. coli transformants containing HA gene sequences [7].

Several differences are apparent between HA gene structures for H3N2 viruses, and for fowl plague virus and A/Japan/305/37, an H2N2 strain [16,17]. Most noticeable is that the N-terminal amino acid for HA from A/Mem/102/72, glutamine [15], precedes the N-terminal amino acid for FPV and Japan HAs by 10 residues, resulting in a longer HA1 for Mem/102/72 (328 amino acids) than for FPV (319 amino acids). The HA gene for FPV has shorter 3' and 5' terminal sequences, and a peptide connecting HA1 and HA2 of five amino acids (a single arginine in Mem/102/72). The amino acid sequence predicted for the HA from A/Mem/102/72 (Fig. 6) shows 27% homology with HA1 from FPV [16] and 63% homology in HA2. The regions where sequence is conserved also generally coincide with regions of similarity between FPV and A/Japan/305/57 (H2N2) genes [16,17].

A comparison of the amino acid sequence predicted from the A/Mem/102/72 HA gene sequence with that determined by Ward and Dopheide [2,3,16] is in agreement for all but 10 amino acids out of the 377 (67% of the molecule) so far published. Of these differences, 6 appear to be due to incorrect ordering of amino acids within peptides (beginning at bases 946 and 1482 on the gene sequence). The remaining changes from the amino acid data are leu→gln at base 753, asp→asn at base 946, gln→arg at 1056 and glu→gly at 1371.

Two possibilities could account for these discrepancies. The HA for amino acid sequencing was derived from an A/Mem/102/72 recombinant with A/Bel/42, while the virus used for nucleic acid studies was a Memphis-A/PR/8/34 recombinant. Some antigenic and peptide differences have been detected between the two recombinants (P.A. Underwood, B.A. Moss, personal communication and this volume) including the leu→gln difference at base 753.

On the other hand, the cloned gene sequences for A/NT/60/68 and 29C, as well as for fowl plague virus [16] contained anomalies possibly due to copying errors during HA gene DNA synthesis or replication. For this reason, and because of the risk during cloning of selecting a variant from what appear to be mixed viral populations, we intend to check the discrepancies between the predicted and determined amino acid sequences by sequencing the viral RNA directly. It is apparent that when comparing nucleic acid sequences of genes from antigenically different virus strains, it will be important to examine sequences representing the average for the viral population, in the same way that antigenic reactivity is measured for the whole population rather than for its individual members.

ACKNOWLEDGEMENTS

We thank Elizabeth Hamilton for competent technical assistance, CSIRO Division of Plant Industry for the provision of biological containment facilities, and Dr. A. Reisner and Ms. C. Bucholtz for their invaluable assistance in establishing and adapting computer programmes. χ1776 was kindly provided by Dr. R. Curtiss, University of Alabama, Birmingham, and pBR322 by the Plasmid Reference Centre, Stanford University.

REFERENCES

1. Moss, B.A. and Underwood, P.A. (1978) in The Influenza Virus Haemagglutinin Laver, W.G., Bachmayer, H. and Weil, R. ed., Springer-Verlag, Vienna, pp. 145-166.
2. Laver, W.G., Air, G.M., Dopheide, T.A. and Ward, C.W. Nature, in press.
3. Ward, C.W. and Dopheide, T.A. (1979) Br. Med. Bull, 35, 51-56.
4. Fazekas de St. Groth, S. (1967) Cold Spring Harb. Symp. Quant. Biol. 32, 525-536.
5. Fazekas de St. Groth, S. and Hannoun, C. (1973) C.R. Acad. Sci. Paris Ser. 276, 1917-1920.
6. Sleigh, M.J., Both, G.W. and Brownlee, G.G. (1979) Nucl. Acids Res. 6, 1309-1321.
7. Sleigh, M.J., Both, G.W. and Brownlee, G.G. (1979) Nucl. Acids Res. 7, 879-893.
8. Maxam, A. and Gilbert, W. (1977) Proc. Natl. Acad. Sci. USA 74, 560-564.
9. Sanger, F., Nicklen, S. and Coulson, A.R. (1977) Proc. Natl. Acad. Sci. USA 74, 5463-5467.
10. Both, G.W., Sleigh, M.J., Bender, V.A. and Moss, B.A. This volume.
11. Staden, R. (1977) Nucl. Acids Res. 4, 4037-4051.
12. Staden, R. (1979) Nucl. Acids Res. 6, 2601-2611.
13. Skehel, J.J. and Hay, A.J. (1978) Nucl. Acids Res. 5, 1207-1219.
14. Robertson, J.S. (1979) Nucl. Acids Res. 6, 3745-3757.
15. Ward, C.W. and Dopheide, T.A. This volume.
16. Porter, A.G., Barber, C., Carey, N., Hallewell, R.A., Threlfall, G. and Emtage, J.S. Nature, in press.
17. Waterfield, M.D., Espelie, K., Elder, K. and Skehel, J.J. (1979) Br. Med. Bull. 35, 57-63.

DISCUSSION

Laver: In the variants we selected with monoclonal antibodies only one can be distinguished with heterogeneous antibody. This is the one which shows a change at position 144 in HA1 of Gly → Asp, so this seems to be a key change.

Palese: When we passage WSN virus 10 times we see mutations in the oligonucleotide maps. We should be careful in attaching significance to differences seen in laboratory strains.

Both: In the laboratory mutants we see only 2-4 differences, so we don't seem to get many unselected changes in sequences.

Palese: In PR8 we get a low level of self-priming but we find that the self-priming starts exactly at the 3' end and therefore cannot involve a loop.

Brownlee: Ours definitely does not start at the 3' end, and if the 3' end of the RNA is blocked, the self-priming does not occur. With PR8 we get no self-priming.

A COMPARISON OF ANTIGENIC VARIATION IN HONG KONG INFLUENZA VIRUS HAEMAGGLUTININS AT THE NUCLEIC ACID LEVEL

G.W. BOTH, M.J. SLEIGH, V.J. BENDER AND B.A. MOSS,
CSIRO Molecular and Cellular Biology Unit, P.O. Box 184,
North Ryde, N.S.W. 2113, Australia.

INTRODUCTION

Influenza virus is distinguished by its ability to vary the antigenic character of its surface proteins. These alterations in structure of the viral haemagglutinin (HA) and, less importantly, the neuraminindase, are known as antigenic shift (radical antigenic changes leading to the appearance of a new subtype) and antigenic drift (progressive changes within a subtype)[1]. As described in the previous article in this volume [2], we are studying antigenic drift at the molecular level by comparing the nucleotide sequences of the HA genes from different influenza A strains of the Hong Kong (H3N2) subtype. Double stranded (ds) DNA copies of the HA RNA gene have been inserted in the plasmid pBR322 and amplified in E. coli RR1 [2,3]. Using these cloned gene copies, we have obtained complete nucleotide sequences for the coding regions of the HA genes from three influenza strains, including the field strains A/NT/60/68 and A/Mem/102/72 (ref. 2 and unpublished data).

The nucleotide sequences reveal a considerable number of base changes resulting in amino acid differences in the HA of the two field strains, but give no indication as to which of these affect viral antigenicity. Recently we have begun to examine a field strain more closely related to NT/60/68 and a series of antigenically distinct mutants derived from the latter strain under selective pressure in the presence of antibody [4,5]. We expect that the number of base and amino acid changes between these strains will be less, enabling us to pin-point regions of the HA which are antigenically important.

In this work we are comparing the HA gene sequences directly from the RNA of the viral population, rather than from a single, cloned DNA copy of the gene. In this way, the sequence of the major population is obtained; cloning the HA gene runs the risk that a minor variant in the population could be selected for analysis. DNA restriction fragments derived from a cloned HA gene copy are used as primers for reverse transcriptase which copies a portion of the HA RNA gene segment. The DNA primer is chosen such that one of its strands will hybridize to the RNA gene near the region of interest and because the restriction fragment is sufficiently large (> 30 bases), its complement is

unique to the HA gene. This eliminates the necessity to separate the gene
from the influenza genome RNA mixture. Total polyadenylated RNA is used as a
template since this abolishes self-priming [2] and ensures that only the DNA
restriction fragment will prime cDNA synthesis on the RNA gene. The Sanger
chain termination method [6] is then used to generate sequence data. In this
way, equivalent regions of HA genes from different viruses of the same subtype
can be compared at the nucleic acid level.

This paper presents a preliminary account of the comparison of HA from the
field strains A/Mem/102/72, A/Qu/7/70, A/NT/60/68 and three laboratory strains
derived from the latter virus.

MATERIALS AND METHODS

Procedures for the growth and purification of virus and extraction of the
RNA have been described [3,7]. The virus A/Mem/102/72 used was a strain obtained
by recombination with A/PR/8/34 and supplied by Dr. W.G. Laver.

Cloning of the Influenza HA Gene. Procedures for the synthesis of a ds DNA
copy of the HA RNA gene and its subsequent cloning using the plasmid pBR322
amplified in E. coli RR1 have been described [3,7]. The analysis of cloned HA
genes from the strains A/NT/60/68, A/Mem/102/72 and A/NT/60/68/29C is described
in the preceding paper [2].

Preparation of Restriction Fragments. Restriction fragments used as primers
for reverse transcriptase were prepared by digestion of the cloned plasmids,
C89 and MX29 which contained HA gene inserts from A/NT/60/68/29C and
A/Mem/102/72, respectively [2]. Procedures for digestion of the DNA with
restriction enzymes and for separation and isolation of DNA fragments by
polyacrylamide gel electrophoresis are published [3]. In order to obtain
cleavage within the hybrid plasmid at sites subject to methylation by the host
E. coli RR1, MX29 was also grown in the non-methylating strain, E. coli χ2230.

DNA Sequencing.
(a) Sequence analysis of cloned HA gene copies by the method of Maxam
    and Gilbert. The cloned DNA copies of the HA gene from the strains
A/Mem/102/72, A/NT/60/68 and A/NT/60/68/29C were sequenced by published
procedures [8].
(b) Direct sequencing of the viral RNA using the Sanger chain termination
    method. The appropriate ds DNA restriction fragment ($\sim$.5 pmols) was mixed
with 5μl of total polyadenylated influenza virion RNA [7] (4.5 pmols) in 5μl of
buffer containing Tris. HCl pH8.0 (20mM), KCl (13mM) and EDTA (0.2mM). The
mixture was sealed in a glass capillary, heated at 90-100°C for 1 min.,

annealed at 65°C for 30 min. and diluted into 5μl of H_2O. This primer/template solution (2.5μl) was used for each dideoxynucleoside triphosphate reaction [6]. Standard conditions for these incubations were used [9], except that the minimum concentration of each deoxynucleoside triphosphate was raised to 10μM and the chase with unlabelled deoxynucleoside triphosphates was omitted. After incubation at 37° for 25 min. the mixtures were dried under vacuum, dissolved in 2-5μl of formamide/dye mix, boiled for 2-3 min. and loaded onto a polyacrylamide gel [9]. Conditions for electrophoresis and autoradiography of the wet gel were as described [3,10]. Nucleotide sequence data was stored and edited in a PDP 11/10 Digital Computer using Staden's programmes [11,12].

RESULTS AND DISCUSSION

Comparison of HA gene sequences from A/NT/60/68 and A/Mem/102/72. Using the sequencing strategy outlined in the previous paper [2] and in Fig. 1 we determined the nucleotide sequence of the HA gene from the field strains A/Mem/102/72 (bases 63-1730) and A/NT/60/68 (bases 78-1765).

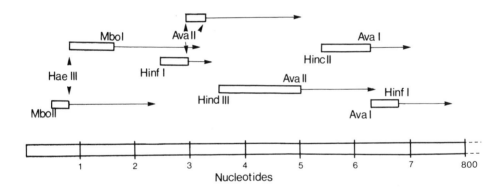

Fig. 1. Strategy for sequencing the HA1 region of the HA RNA gene from A/NT/60/68. The boxes represent restriction fragments, used to prime cDNA synthesis on the RNA and these were prepared by digestion of plasmids C89 and MX29 as described [2,3]. The Hae 111/Mbol primer was prepared from MX29 plasmid DNA grown in a non-methylating host, E. coli 2230. The line and arrowhead extending from each box represents the amount of sequence information obtained with each primer. Since the nucleotide sequence of strain 29C is known in this region, some of the overlaps across priming sites are not extensive.

The differences between the strains are shown in Fig. 2a (top and bottom lines) and Fig. 2b. The sequences compared include the triplet CAA coding for the

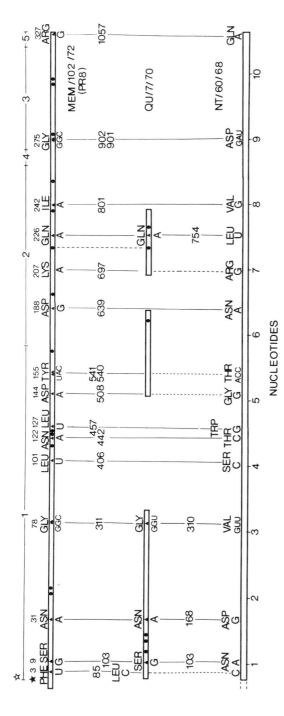

NUCLEOTIDES

Fig. 2a. Comparison of the amino acid and base changes in HA1 between A/NT/60/68, A/Ou/7/70 and A/Mem/102/72. The base sequences of NT/60/68 (bases 684-1765) and Mem/102/72 were determined by sequencing a cloned dsDNA copy of the gene. NT/60/68 (bases 78-775) and Qu/7/70 sequences were determined by priming cDNA synthesis on the RNA difference is indicated in Fig. 1 and Methods. The number and the identity of the base and the resulting amino acid difference is indicated for each amino acid change (▲). Silent base changes are indicated (●). ☆ Numbers in this line correspond to the cyanogen bromide fragments of HA1 18. ★ Numbers refer to the amino acid residues of HA1 beginning with the N-terminal Gln 13. Codons in which a double base change occurs are located at residues 78, 155 and 275.

N-terminal Gln [13] (bases 78-80) and the translation termination codon, UGA (bases 1728-1730). While extensive regions of the base and amino acid sequences are conserved between the two strains, there are nevertheless 42 base changes of which 18 result in amino acid differences. Fifteen of these occur in HA1 and three in HA2 (Fig. 2a,b). Eight of the changes in HA1 occur in peptides not analysed in other field strains [17]. Three amino acid changes, all in HA1, are the result of double base changes within a codon, but most result from single mutations. Thus, the number of differences between these field strains makes it difficult to assess the antigenic importance of individual amino acid changes. Therefore we began an examination of three strains of influenza selected in the laboratory and a field strain (A/Qu/7/70) more closely related to A/NT/60/68, in the belief that the pattern of amino acid changes might be less complex.

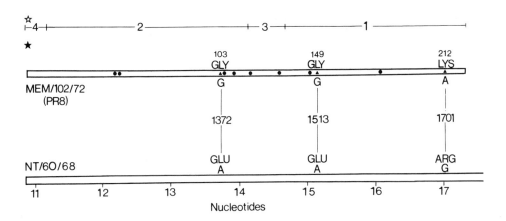

Fig. 2b. Comparison of the amino acid and base changes in HA2 between A/NT/60/68 and A/Mem/102/72. Notation for this figure is described in the legend to Figure 2a. Amino acids are numbered from the beginning of HA2.

Comparison of a partial HA gene sequence for A/Qu/7/70 with A/NT/60/68. As described earlier, a restriction fragment can be used to prime cDNA synthesis such that the sequence of RNA genes in a given region can be compared. In this way, some of the restriction fragments prepared for sequencing the first ∿770 bases of A/NT/60/68 (Fig. 1) were used to generate sequence data for A/Qu/7/70. The differences found between this strain and A/NT/60/68 are summarised in Fig. 2a (middle and bottom lines). Although the sequence is not complete, the data available shows that in the regions sequenced there are fewer amino acid differences between NT/60/68 and Qu/7/70 than between NT/60/68 and Mem/102/72 (Fig. 2). All the amino acid changes found in Qu/7/70 so far are conserved in Mem/102/72. In addition Mem/102/72 differs from Ou/7/70, by changes of Leu→Phe at amino acid residue 3, Gly→Asp at 144 and Arg→Lys at 207. The latter was also seen in other field strains isolated between 1970-72 [17]. There are at least four amino acid changes between NT/60/68 and Ou/7/70 and it is likely that more differences will be detected when the base sequence of Ou/7/70 is completed; eight changes were detected between NT/60/68 and Mem/102/72 in areas of the HA not yet completed in Qu/7/70. Although a previous study showed that strains isolated soon after the emergence of the Hong Kong subtype differed by only one amino acid in the regions analysed [17], the situation described here for strains with similar chronology is more complex. Therefore it may be difficult to relate amino acid changes to antigenicity simply by examining relationships between field strains, even if they are very closely related. With this point in mind, it is interesting to examine our results obtained with the laboratory selected mutants.

Comparison of HA gene sequences from Influenza strains selected in the laboratory. Using A/NT/60/68 as a parent, a series of strains of influenza was selected in the laboratory in the present of the most avid fraction of homologous antibody [4,5]. Titration of these strains against whole rabbit antisera and against a panel of monoclonal antibodies raised against A/Mem/1/71 [15] reveals that these mutants are antigenically distinct (P. Ann Underwood, unpublished results). Selection of these strains under controlled conditions means they are likely to represent a series of mutants which have undergone relatively simple antigenic changes. Thus, they may be useful to identify regions of antigenic importance in the HA molecule, particularly if similar antigenic and amino acid changes also occur in the field.

Of the laboratory strains, 29C has been sequenced as a cloned DNA copy of the HA gene (unpublished results). Partial sequence data has been obtained for 30D and 34C by the method of priming cDNA synthesis on the RNA gene. Of the three amino acid changes observed in 29C (Fig. 3), the Leu→Gln change has been confirmed by peptide mapping [16] and by priming on the RNA gene and peptide mapping data [16] supports the presence of Asp and Arg at the positions shown in Fig. 3. The Gln→Arg change may represent a variant selected in the NT/60/68 clone, since many other field strains have Arg in this position [17]. Thus, the Gly→Asp change at base 508 and the Leu→Gln change at position 754 may be the most significant differences between NT/60/68 and 29C.

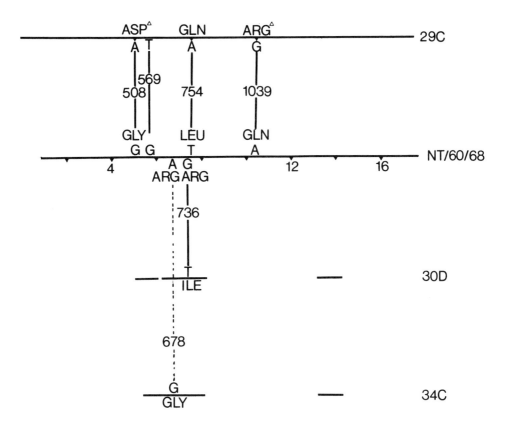

Fig. 3. A comparison of the base and amino acid changes between A/NT/60/68 and the strains derived from it in the laboratory. The majority of sequence obtained for 29C was determined by analysis of a cloned ds DNA copy of the HA gene. Some amino acid changes have not yet been confirmed by sequencing the RNA (Δ). The number and identity of a base and the resulting amino acid difference is indicated for each amino acid change. The G→T change at base 569 in 29C is silent.

It is noteworthy that the Leu→Gln change also occurs in Qu/7/70 and is conserved in the Mem/102/72-PR/8/34 recombinant strain while the Gly→Asp change (base 508) between 29C and NT/60/68 is observed in a variety of other field strains [17]. Peptide mapping data is not completely consistent with Gly being present in NT/60/68 at base 508, rather a mixture of Gly and Asp is seen with the latter apparently predominant [16]. Since the HA protein and the viral RNA were prepared from the same stock virus grown in separate batches of eggs, this

88

suggests that this site in the HA gene mutates easily and may be one of the first changes in antigenic drift. This is being examined further. In summary, the pattern of amino acid changes between A/NT/60/68 and 29C is relatively simple and two of them seem likely to contribute to the antigenic differences between the strains.

For the other laboratory strains, 30D and 34C, interpretation of the results is more difficult at this stage. Although only one amino acid difference (Arg→Ile) has been found between 30D and NT/60/68 (Fig. 3) and only one other is expected based on peptide mapping data [16], neither change corresponds to any seen among field strains so far. Similarly, the single amino acid difference (Arg→Gly) detected in 34C (Fig. 3) does not appear to correspond precisely to any change seen in the field [17]. However, for both these strains, amino acid changes occur 16 residues apart in the same large tryptic peptide. Since a complete analysis of this peptide for different field strains is not complete [17], there may yet be changes found which correspond to those observed here in 30D and 34C. Because this region of the HA does undergo mutation in the field [17], it may also contribute to the antigenicity of HA.

In summary, we have determined (1) the complete sequence of the coding portion of the HA genes from A/NT/60/68 and A/Mem/102/72 beginning at the N-terminal Gln (base 78), (2) the complete sequence of the laboratory strain 29C derived from NT/60/68, except for the last 23 bases (unpublished results) and, (3) partial sequence data from various regions of A/Qu/7/70 and the laboratory strains 34C and 30D. The picture emerging is quite encouraging. While there are many differences between the field strains, there are very few changes between A/NT/60/68 and the strains derived from it in the laboratory. 29C differs from NT/60/68 by only 3 amino acids and two of these changes have been observed in the field. Similarly, although in these cases the data is not complete, strains 30D and 34C show a simple pattern of amino acid changes so far, and when the analysis of field strains is completed in this area, the significance of the changes we have observed may be clearer.

Acknowledgements

We thank Elizabeth Hamilton for competent technical assistance and Caroline Bucholtz and Dr. Alex Reisner for establishing the computer technology for sequence analysis.

References

1 Stuart-Harris, C.H. and Schild, G.C. (1976). Influenza. The Viruses and the Disease. pp. 57-68, Edward Arnold, London.

2 Sleigh, M.J., Both, G.W., Brownlee, G.G., Bender, V.J. and Moss, B.A. This volume.

3 Sleigh, M.J., Both, G.W. and Brownlee, G.G. (1979). Nucl. Acids Res. 7, 879-893.

4 Fazekas de St. Groth, S. (1967). Cold Spring Harb. Symp. Quant. Biol. 32, 525-535.

5 Fazekas de St. Groth, S. and Hannoun, C. (1973). C.R. Acad. Sci. Paris Ser. D. 276, 1917-1920.

6 Sanger, F., Nicklen, S. and Coulson, A.R. (1977). Proc. Natl. Acad. Sci., USA 74, 5463-5467.

7 Sleigh, M.J., Both, G.W. and Brownlee, G.G. (1979). Nucl. Acids Res. 6, 1309-1321.

8 Maxam, A. and Gilbert, W. (1977). Proc. Natl. Acad. Sci. USA 74, 560-564.

9 Both, G.W. and Air, G.M. (1979). Eur. J. Biochem. 96, 363-372.

10 Sanger, F. and Coulson, A.R. (1978). FEBS Letters. 87, 107-110.

11 Staden, R. (1977). Nucl. Acids Res. 4, 4037-4051.

12 Staden, R. (1979). Nucl. Acids Res. 6, 2601-2610.

13 Ward, C.W. and Dopheide, T.A. This volume.

14 Fazekas de St. Groth, S. (1978). In "The Influenza Virus Haemagglutinin", Laver, W.G., Bachmayer, H. and Weil, R. eds. Springer-Verlag, Wien. pp 25.

15 Koprowski, H., Gerhard, W. and Croce, C.M. (1977). Proc. Nat. Acad. Sci. USA 74, 2985-2988.

16 Moss, B.A., Underwood, P.A., Bender, V.J. and Whitakker, R.G. This volume.

17 Laver, W.G., Air, G.M., Dopheide, T. and Ward, C.W. (1979). Nature (Lond.) In press.

18 Ward, C.W. and Dopheide, T.A. (1979). Brit. Med. Bull. 35, 51-56.

RNA SEGMENT 8 OF THE INFLUENZA VIRUS GENOME CONTAINS TWO OVERLAPPING GENES:
MAPPING THE GENES FOR POLYPEPTIDES NS_1 AND NS_2.

ROBERT A. LAMB,*§ PURNELL W. CHOPPIN,* ROBERT M. CHANOCK[†] and CHING-JUH LAI[†]
*The Rockefeller University, New York, New York 10021 and [†]Laboratory of
Infectious Diseases, National Institute of Allergy and Infectious Diseases,
National Institutes of Health, Bethesda, Maryland 20205

INTRODUCTION

In addition to the eight well characterized influenza virus polypeptides
(see this volume) we have investigated in some detail the synthesis of a ninth
polypeptide (M_r 11,000) now designated NS_2.[1-4] This polypeptide is not synthesized from primary transcripts of viral genome RNA and early protein synthesis
is required for its synthesis. NS_2 was shown to be a unique ninth influenza
virus polypeptide on the basis of its peptide composition, its synthesis in
vitro using mRNAs from infected cells, the isolation of a separate mRNA for it,
and strain-specific differences in its migration in gels.[1-4] Because of the
evidence for nine virus-coded polypeptides and the existence of only eight
influenza virus RNA segments, we postulated that one RNA segment must code for
two polypeptides.[2] Subsequently we[3] and others[5] showed that virus RNA segment
8 coded for both NS_1 and NS_2 in studies with recombinant viruses in which NS_1
and NS_2 reassorted together and, in addition, hybridization of segment 8 to
total viral mRNAs specifically prevented the synthesis of both NS_1 and NS_2
in vitro. We describe here the results of experiments using cloned DNA segments of the NS gene,[6,8] to map the mRNAs on RNA segment 8 and have distinguished between overlapping or contiguous genes for NS_1 and NS_2 within RNA
segment 8. A detailed report of these results is described elsewhere.[7]

MATERIALS AND METHODS
These have been published previously[2,3,6,7] and the cloning procedures are
described in this volume.[8]

RESULTS AND DISCUSSION
A restriction endonuclease cleavage map of the cloned DNA derived from RNA
segment 8 (NS DNA) was obtained,[6,7] and is partially shown in Figs 1 & 2.

§To whom correspondence should be addressed

92

To determine the size and genomic positions of the NS_1 and NS_2 mRNAs we used
the method of Berk and Sharp[9] in which ^{32}P-labeled NS DNA fragments, in 5-10
fold molar excess, were hybridized under conditions in which the DNA was kept
dissociated, to poly(A) containing mRNA from influenza virus infected HeLa
cells, and then digested with nuclease S_1 and the ssDNA analyzed on alkaline
agarose gels. As shown in Fig. 1 hybridization with unit length NS DNA and
S_1 nuclease digestion revealed two ssDNA bands of ∿860 nucleotides and ∿340
nucleotides, indicating indirectly that two NS specific mRNA species are present
in the cell, with the larger mRNA coding for NS_1 and the smaller mRNA for NS_2.
Hybridization with smaller NS DNA fragments, as shown in Fig. 1, permitted
the location of the NS_1 and NS_2 mRNAs to be deduced. When the Hae III A
fragment (0.34-1.0 units) was used as probe, a band of ∿615 nucleotides was
produced, corresponding to the reduced large mRNA, and another band of ∿340
nucleotides, corresponding to the intact small mRNA (lane b, both panels).
When the Hae III B probe (0-0.34 units) was used, a single band of ∿300 nucleo-

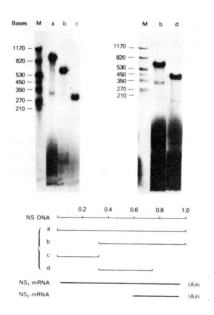

Fig. 1. Nuclease S_1 analysis of the
NS_1 and NS_2 mRNAs. Poly(A)- containing mRNAs from influenza virus-infected HeLa cells were denatured and
allowed to hybridize in 80% formamide
at 48°C for 3hr with ^{32}P-labeled NS
DNA cleaved with restriction endonucleases, and the hybridization mixtures were treated with nuclease S_1.
The digests were analyzed by electrophoresis on 1.4% alkaline agarose gels
to determine the size of the S_1-resis-
tant DNA segments. Lane M: Marker
SV40 DNA digested with Hind II and III
endonucleases. Lane a: mRNAs hybridized with total NS DNA. Lane b:
mRNAs hybridized with the Hae III A
fragment of NS DNA (0.34-1.00 units).
Lane c: mRNAs hybridized with the Hae
III B fragment of NS DNA (0-0.34
units). Lane d: mRNAs hybridized with
the Hae III-Alu I fragment of NS DNA
(0.34-0.77 units). The schematic diagram shows the positions of the DNA
fragments used in hybridization and
the mapping of the NS_1 and NS_2 mRNAs
on the cloned NS DNA.

From Lamb et al.[7]

tides was found, corresponding to the 5' end of the NS_1 mRNA, and no other discrete DNA segment was observed. Hybridization using the Hae III A-Alu I fragment (0.34-0.77 units) produced a DNA band of ∿410 nucleotides and another band of ∿160 nucleotides (lane d). The large DNA segment was derived from protection with the NS_1 mRNA, and the small segment was derived from protection with the NS_2 mRNA. Thus, the map position of the body of the NS_1 mRNA is located between 0.05-0.95 units, and the body of the NS_2 mRNA between 0.59-0.95 units, which suggests that the two mRNAs have the same 3'-terminus to which poly(A) is added.

To confirm the above results of the mapping of the NS_1 and NS_2 mRNAs and to obtain information concerning the extent of translation of the NS_1 mRNA, we used the hybrid-arrested translation method of Paterson and coworkers.[10] Hybridization of a restriction fragment of NS DNA to a mRNA would be expected to stop translation proceeding downstream from the 5'-terminus of the mRNA at the region of the boundary of the hybrid, and this was found to be the case. The results shown in Fig. 2 are consistent with the NS_2 mRNA extending from 0.59-0.95 map units, as the Hinf I B and Hae III - Hpa II A fragments inhibit the translation of NS_2. Using the restriction fragments indicated in Fig. 2 premature termination products of NS_1 were produced. By using the size of these products (determined from gels and calibrated with markers of known size) and the location of the restriction endonuclease sites, it can be estimated that termination of translation of NS_1 (M_r ∿25,000) is at ∿0.76 map units. The M_r of NS_2 is ∿11,000 and its mRNA contains ∿340 nucleotides, therefore nearly all the NS_2 mRNA must be used for translation. Thus, from these data the coding regions of the NS_1 and NS_2 mRNAs overlap by ∿144-159 nucleotides, the equivalent of ∿48-53 amino acids. As the methionine- and leucine-labeled tryptic peptides of NS_1 and NS_2 do not contain any similar peptides, and as the leucine-labeled chymotryptic peptides of NS_1 and NS_2 contain at most one or two similar peptides, which is probably fortuitous, it would appear that these polypeptides are completely distinct. Therefore, these findings together with the above evidence that the coding regions overlap, indicate that the translation of the NS_2 mRNA is in a reading frame different from that used for NS_1.

It has yet to be demonstrated how the mRNA for NS_2 arises. It could occur by RNA processing of the NS_1 mRNA to produce NS_2 mRNA, or a second site for the initiation of transcription of the NS_2 mRNA might be revealed on the virion RNA segment 8 with early protein synthesis being required in each case. It would be interesting to obtain the 5' end sequence arrangement of the NS_2 mRNA, to compare it with that of the mRNAs made early in infection, and to investigate whether any part of the 5' end of the NS_2 mRNA is the same as that of the NS_1

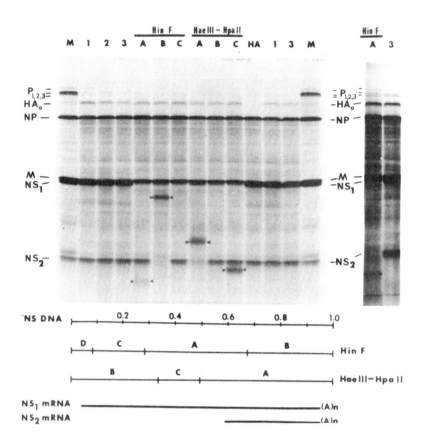

Fig. 2. Hybrid-arrested translation of the NS_1 and NS_2 mRNAs with NS DNA restriction endonuclease fragments.

LEFT PANEL. Lanes M: Influenza virus marker polypeptides synthesized in influenza virus infected HeLa cells mixed with a wheat germ extract which had been incubated with no exogenous RNA. The dark band comigrating with the 3 P polypeptides is glycosylated HA synthesized in vivo, which migrates more slowly than HA_0 synthesized in vitro. Lanes 1: mRNA in H_2O frozen at $-20°C$ for 2hr and then treated for translation as described.[7] Lane 2: mRNA incubated at $44°C$ for 2hr in buffer with H_2O instead of formamide. Lanes 3: mRNA incubated at $44°C$ for 2hr in buffer and 80% formamide. Lanes Hinf A,B,C: hybridization done under conditions given for 3 but with Hinf I A,B, or C fragments added. Lanes Hae III-Hpa II, A,B,C: hybridization as above but with Hae III-Hpa II A,B,C fragments added. Lane HA: hybridization as above but with cloned DNA of the hemagglutinin (HA) gene (PFV 88/HA) added. RIGHT PANEL. Lane Hinf A: mRNA and Hinf l A fragment hybridization at $44°C$ for 5hr in buffer and 80% formamide. Lane 3: mRNA incubated at $44°C$ for 5 hr in buffer and 80% formamide without DNA.

A schematic representation of the fragments used is shown below.

From Lamb et al.[7]

mRNA. If a region of the NS_2 mRNA was the same as that of the NS_1 mRNA, it would presumably be less than 50 nucleotides, because a band larger than that would have been observed in the nuclease S_1 analysis of the mRNAs (Fig. 1 Lane C). In addition, in the hybrid arrested translation experiments, the Hae III B fragment (0-0.34 units) did not inhibit the synthesis of NS_2 under stringent conditions in which a hybrid of ∿80 nucleotides using the Hinf A fragment (0.28-0.67 units) did inhibit translation of NS_2 (Fig. 2 right panel). These results suggest that the mRNAs do not share 5' regions, but the existence of a small common region has not been completely excluded.

ACKNOWLEDGMENTS

We thank Miss Mary-Louise Scully, Mrs Jo Ann Berndt and Ms Bronna Cohen for excellent technical assistance. Supported by research grants AI-056000 from the National Institute of Allergy and Infectious Diseases and PCM 78-09091 from the National Science Foundation. R.A.L. is an Irma T. Hirschl Career Scientist Awardee.

REFERENCES

1. Lamb, R.A. and Choppin, P.W. (1978) in Negative Strand Viruses and the Host Cell. Mahy, B.W.J. and Barry, R.D. eds. Academic Press. London pp. 229-238.
2. Lamb, R.A., Etkind, P.R. and Choppin, P.W. (1978) Virology 91, 60-78.
3. Lamb, R.A. and Choppin, P.W. (1979) Proc.Natl.Acad. Sci.USA 76, 4908-4912.
4. Lamb, R.A. and Choppin, P.W. (1980) Phil. Trans. R. Soc. Lond. B (in press).
5. Inglis, S.C., Barrett, T., Brown, C.M. and Almond, J.W. (1979) Proc.Natl. Acad. Sci. USA 76, 3790-3794.
6. Lai, C-J., Markoff, L.J., Zimmerman, S., Cohen, B., Berndt, J.A. and Chanock, R.M. (1980) Proc. Natl. Acad. Sci. USA 77 (in press).
7. Lamb, R.A., Choppin, P.W., Chanock, R.M. and Lai, C-J. (1980) Proc. Natl. Acad. Sci. USA 77 (in press).
8. Lai, C-J., Markoff, L.J., Zveda, M., Dhar, R. and Chanock, R.M. This volume.
9. Berk, A.J. and Sharp, P.A. (1978) Proc. Natl. Acad. Sci. USA 75, 1274-1278.
10. Patterson, B.M., Roberts, B.E. and Kuff, E.L. (1977) Proc. Natl. Acad. Sci. USA 74, 4370-4374.

(See DISCUSSION on following page)

DISCUSSION

Porter: How do you solubilize these peptides?

Choppin: They are not very soluble and the concentrations I gave
   are what we added, so the concentration in solution is much
   lower than that.   The carboberzoxy group makes them even less
   soluble.

Laver: Why should D-Phe be more active than L-Phe?

Choppin: With the L form we may be getting inactivation by
   chymotrypsin-like activity, but I think it is more likely to be
   a steric effect.

Carey: There is a similar effect in enkephalins, where D forms
   stimulate activity.

Rott: Have you tried fatty acids, i.e. completely unrelated, but
   hydrophobic molecules?

Choppin: No, but the sequence is certainly important, so it is
   not a non-specific, hydrophobic effect.   The effect is on
   penetration, but not adsorption.

Rott: Then you conclude that there are two virus-specific receptors on the cell surface, one for adsorption and one for fusion?

Choppin: Yes.

HAEMAGGLUTININ BIOSYNTHESIS

J. McCAULEY AND J. SKEHEL
Division of Virology, National Institute for Medical Research, Mill Hill,
London, NW7 1AA.
K. ELDER, M.-J. GETHING, A. SMITH AND M. WATERFIELD
Imperial Cancer Research Fund, Lincoln's Inn Fields, London, WC2.

In influenza virus infected cells the haemagglutinin is exclusively
associated with membranes. It is initially detected in the rough endoplasmic reticulum as a glycosylated precursor of approximate molecular weight
75000 and subsequently as a component of the plasma membrane where
processing of the precursor by an undefined protease leads to the production
of HA_1 and HA_2. Haemagglutinin biosynthesis has also been investigated in
cell-free translation systems with or without added membrane vesicles such
as those described by Blobel and Dobberstein (1975) and Rothman and Lodish
(1977) and a comparison of the structure of the products of these systems
and of the haemagglutinin polypeptides detected in infected cells is of some
value in determining the steps in biosynthesis and the mechanisms of membrane
association.

The products of in vivo and in vitro translation of influenza virus
messenger RNAs are shown in Figure 1. The 63000 and 75000 dalton polypeptides
indicated have been identified as haemagglutinin precursors by precipitation
with specific antibodies and by analyses of the tryptic peptides obtained
following digestion of the eluted polypeptides (Elder et al., 1979). The
75000 dalton components produced either in vivo or in vitro in the presence
of membranes are glycosylated as judged by their affinity for lentil lectin;
the 63000 dalton polypeptide is not. In addition in vitro synthesis in the
presence of membranes leads to the transfer of the precursor into the
membrane vesicles as judged by the differential sensitivity of the product
to proteolysis (Elder et al., 1979).

The rate of synthesis of the haemagglutinin polypeptide in vitro can be
estimated following inhibition of the initiation of translation by
7-Methylguanosine 3' monophosphate as described in Figure 2. From the results
of such experiments 50% of the haemagglutinin produced was completed by
about 32 minutes of incubation and since the polypeptide contains 562 amino
acid residues the rate of synthesis was approximately 18 residues per minute.

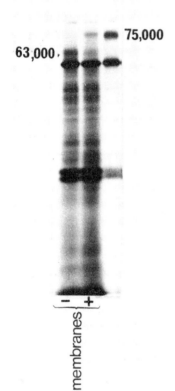

in vitro | in vivo

75,000

63,000

— +

membranes

Fig. 1. Synthesis of influenza viral proteins in wheat germ extracts. For details see Elder et al., 1979.

In a similar fashion by initiating synthesis in the absence of membranes, blocking further initiation and then adding membranes at different times, estimates can be obtained of the extent of synthesis required before membrane insertion. The data shown in Figure 3 indicate that membrane insertion and subsequent glycosylation is obtained only when membranes are added within 5 minutes of initiation, i.e. before polymerization of more than 90 amino

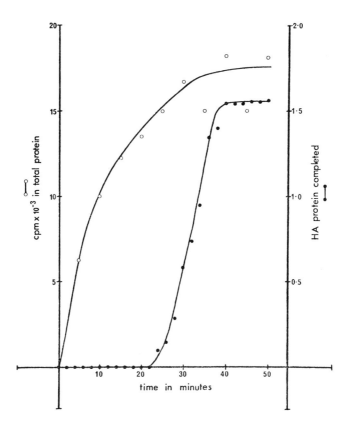

Fig. 2. Wheat germ extract was incubated in the presence of 5 µg of cellular
RNA for two minutes; 1 µl of 10 mg/ml 7meGp was then added, and incubation
continued for 90 mins. At two minute intervals, aliquots were removed from
the incubation mixture for determination of TCA precipitable counts, and for
analysis by PAGE. The amount of HA synthesised was determined from densi-
tometer scans of an autoradiograph of the dried gel, and by cutting the bands
out of the PPO-impregnated dried gel for scintillation counting.
o -- o, TCA-precipitable counts in total protein (5 µl aliquots)
o -- o, amount of HA polypeptide completed.

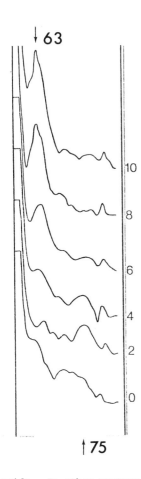

↓ 63

10

8

6

4

2

0

↑ 75

Fig. 3.   Addition of membranes after initiation of protein synthesis. A wheat germ protein synthesis reaction was synchronised as in figure 2;   at two minute intervals, 15 µl aliquots were added to 1 µl of membranes, and incubation continued in the presence of membranes for 90 minutes.   Aliquots of these incubations were analysed by PAGE on 7.5% gels, and autoradiographs of the dried gels were scanned with a Joyce-Loebl microdensitometer.   The figure shows scans of proteins in the 50,000–80,000 molecular weight range made when membranes were added at 0, 2, 4, 6, 8 and 10 minutes.

acids. In other systems (e.g. Rothman and Lodish, 1977; Blobel and Dobberstein, 1975; Lingappa et al., 1978) information such as this has been taken to indicate the presence of 'signal' sequences at the NH_2-termini of the precursors of secreted and membrane proteins which are proposed to be involved in the association of the nascent polypeptides with the membranes of the endoplasmic reticulum and their transfer across the membranes, and which are subsequently removed from the completed chain. The results of comparitive NH_2-terminal sequence analysis of the 75,000 and 63,000 dalton polypeptides are compatible with these proposals for the haemagglutinin since the sequence of the 75,000 polypeptide produced in the presence of membranes

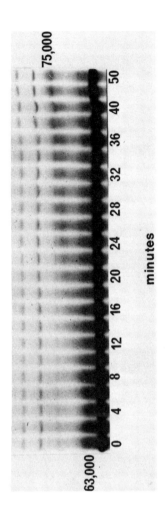
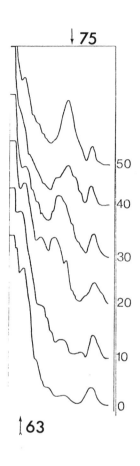

Fig. 4. Synthesis of intermediate precursors to glycosylated HA. Protein synthesis was synchronised in wheat germ extracts as in Figure 2, in the presence of microsomal membranes. At two-minute intervals, 1% Triton X-100 was added to 15 μl aliquots of the reaction, and incubation continued for 50 minutes. Aliquots of each tube were analysed by PAGE. The figures show the 50,000-80,000 molecular weight area of the gel.

is identical to that of the HA_1 component of completed haemagglutinin and the 63000 polypeptide produced in the absence of membranes contains an additional NH_2-terminal peptide. The sequences deduced from these experiments (McCauley et al., 1979) were completed and extended by the results of nucleotide sequence analyses of the virion RNA complementary in sequence to haemagglutinin messenger RNA. Table 1.

Finally similar kinetic analyses to those described in Figures 2 and 3 can be made to estimate the rate of glycosylation of the nascent polypeptide. By initiating in the presence of membranes and by adding detergent to dissociate them at different times after initiation it can be seen, Figure 4A and B, that glycosylation is first detected at about 10 minutes after initiation and appears to continue stepwise until completion of the 75000 precursor after about 45 minutes.

The mechanisms of biosynthesis and membrane insertion of the haemagglutinin, therefore, appear to comply with those proposed in the signal hypothesis. It is certainly apparent that in vivo haemagglutinin is synthesized by membrane associated polysomes and that in vitro only nascent haemagglutinin can interact with and be subsequently transferred into membrane vesicles. At the same time, since the products of translation in vitro in the presence or absence of membranes, interact specifically with anti haemagglutinin immunoglobulin, it would also appear unlikely that there are large conformational differences between them. As a consequence of all these observations the "trigger" hypothesis (e.g. Wickner, 1979) would at present seem less appropriate.

Table 1. The 3' terminal nucleotide sequence of the haemagglutinin gene, its component and the amino-
terminal sequence of the haemagglutinin.

Position						
	5	10	15	20	25	30
vRNA	U C G U U U	U U C C A C	C U G G U A	U G G U A U	C C U U U G	G
Complementary RNA	A G C A A A	A A G G U G	G A C C A U	A C C A U A	G G A A A C	C
Protein sequence	Ile Leu	Leu Phe	Thr Met	Val Ile	Ile Tyr	Leu Asp

Position						
	35	40	50	55		60
vRNA	G U U C U	U U C U G G	U A C C U C	G G, G C C U	U C A A A U	A G
Complementary RNA	C A A G A	A A G A C C	A U G G A G	C C, C G G A	A G U U U A	U C
Protein sequence	Ala	Ile	Ala	Tyr	Ile Tyr	Leu

Position						
	65	70	80	85		90
vRNA	G U A A G	G A C A A C	U C U G U C	A C C U U	C C C C U	U
Complementary RNA	C, A U U C, C	U G U U G	A G A C A, G	U G G A A	G G G G, G	A
Protein sequence	Ile Leu	Phe	Thr	Ala	Val Arg	Gly Asp

Position						
	95	100	110	115		120
vRNA	G G U C U	A C G U A A	C U A U G G	A U U A C G	C A A U U C	U
Complementary RNA	C, C A G A	U G C A U U	G A U A C C	U A A U G C	G U U A A G	A
Protein sequence	Ile	Cys	Ile	Gly Tyr	Ala His	Ala Asn

Position						
	125	130	140	145		150
vRNA	A A G G U C	U U C C U U	C C A C G U	G U U G U A	C A A A C U	U
Complementary RNA	U, U C, A C A G	A A G G, A A	G G U G C A	C A, A C A U	G U U U G, A	A
Protein sequence	Ser Thr	Glu Lys	Val	Asp Thr	Ile Leu	Glu

Position						
	155	160	170	175		180
vRNA	C G C C C U	U G A C A G	C U G U A C	A U G G A C	C G G C C C	G
Complementary RNA	G, C G G, A A	A C U, A G U C	G A, C A U G	U A C C U, G	G C C, G G G	G
Protein sequence	Arg	Asn Val	Thr Val	His	His Gly	Arg

REFERENCES

Blobel, G. and Dobberstein, B. (1975) J. Cell. Biol., 67, 835-851

Rothman, J.E. and Lodish, H.F. (1977) Nature, 269, 775-780

Elder, K.T., Bye, J.M., Skehel, J.J., Waterfield, M.D. and Smith, A.E.
    (1979) Virology, 95, 343-351

Lingappa, V.R., Katz, F.N., Lodish, H.F. and Blobel, G. (1978)
    J. Biol. Chem., 253, 8667-8670

McCauley, J., Bye, J., Elder, K., Gething, M.-J., Skehel, J.J., Smith, A.
    and Waterfield, M.D. (1979) Febs. Lett. in the press.

Wickner, W. (1979) Annual Rev. Biochem., 48, 23-45

NATURALLY OCCURRING RECOMBINANTS OF HUMAN INFLUENZA A VIRUSES

WILLIAM J. BEAN, JR.*, NANCY J. COX,†, AND ALAN P. KENDAL†
*Division of Virology, St. Jude Children's Research Hospital, Memphis, Tennessee 38101, U.S.A.; †WHO Collaboration Center for Influenza, Virology Division, Center for Disease Control, Atlanta, Georgia 30333, U.S.A.

INTRODUCTION

The appearance in 1977 of an influenza A (H1N1) virus similar to a virus from 1950, led to the co-circulation of both H1N1 and H3N2 strains throughout the world.[1-7] Laboratory surveillance indicated that on occasion, individuals were mixedly infected[8,9] raising the possibility that recombination between the two strains might affect the future epidemiologic behavior of influenza. Serological analysis of virus isolates from influenza outbreaks during the winter of 1978-1979, however, failed to detect any antigenic hybrids (H3N1 or H1N2). Therefore, the investigation described in this report was undertaken to detect recombinants among recent isolates of the H1N1 and H3N2 serotypes involving genes coding for other than the surface proteins by RNA-RNA hybridization.

MATERIALS AND METHODS

Preparation of viral genome RNA segments

The growth and purification of virus and the extraction of viral RNA has been described recently.[10] Virion RNA (10-15 ug) was resolved into its constituent gene segments by electrophoresis on 7 M urea-acrylamide slab gels, containing 3% acrylamide cross-linked with 0.37% bis-acrylylcystamine.[10] This cross-linking agent allows the gel to be solubilized by reduction.[11] Following electrophoresis, gels were stained with ethidium bromide and the RNA bands were visualized with an ultraviolet light and cut from the gel. These gel fragments were then dissolved in 2 ml EDTA 0.05 M containing 10% 2-mercaptoethanol and 20 ug poly uridylic acid (Miles Laboratories). (The poly-U acts as a carrier RNA during subsequent steps, but does not interefere with iodination[10]). The RNA and acrylamide were then ethanol-precipitated, washed once with 70% ethanol, and resuspended in 2.5 ml sodium acetate buffer (pH 5.0) and the RNA was separated from the acrylamide by electrophoresis in an Isco electrophoretic concentrator cell, operated at 50V for 2 hr. The RNA was recovered and ethanol-precipitated.

Iodination

The isolated RNA segments were iodinated using the method described by Commerford.[12] Each RNA pellet was dissolved in 13 ul 0.2 M sodium acetate (pH 5.0) and to this was added 8 ul (800 uCi) [125]I and 5 ul of TlCl$_3$ (6 mg/ml). The mixture was incubated at 60° for 15 min and the reaction was stopped by the addition of 5 ul of 2 mercaptoethanol and 0.6 ml STE (0.1 M NaCl, 0.05 M Tris, 0.05 M EDTA, pH 7.4) containing 20 ug yeast RNA and 10% glycerol. The mixture was then reincubated at 60° for 30 min. Unreacted iodine was removed by passage through a 10 ml column of Sephadex G-25 and ethanol was added to a final concentration of 35%. The RNA was then adsorbed onto a column of CF 11 cellulose[13] and eluted with STE-15% ethanol and finally ethanol-precipitated.

Preparation of viral complementary RNA

Viral complementary RNA (cRNA) was obtained from infected monolayer cultures of Maden-Darby canine kidney cells. Cells were infected at high multiplicity and incubated at 37° for 90 min. Cyclohexmide (100 ug/ml) was then added to block further viral RNA synthesis, while cRNA synthesis continued.[14] Total RNA extracted from these cells contained an excess of cRNA and was used for hybridization with labeled v-RNA segments as described below.

Direct RNA-RNA Hybridization

Quantitative RNA-RNA hybridization was carried out using ^{32}P-labeled virion RNA extracted from virus grown in primary chick embryo kidney cells in the presence of [32]P. Virion RNA was resolved into its constituent segments by electrophoresis on acrylamide slab gels as described previously[15] and recovered from the gel by phenol extraction. The ^{32}P-labeled segments were used in quantitation hybridization assays as described by Scholtissek et al.,[16] except that the cRNA was obtained from chick embryo fibroblast cells infected in the presence of cycloheximide with the homologous or with the heterologous strains. This procedure, outlined by Stephenson et al.[17] minimizes replication of RNA with virion polarity. Hybrids were heated to 75° in the presence of 1% formaldehyde prior to digestion with ribonuclease.

The Comparison of Genome Homologies by Competitive RNA:RNA Reassociation

The genomes of the various influenza isolates were compared for homology with the individual RNA segments of selected reference strains using a competitive reassociation assay. For this assay, a double-strand RNA probe is prepared by annealing an ^{125}I-labeled individual RNA segment to its homologous unlabeled cRNA. To determine if a particular virus isolate contains an RNA segment related to that of the reference RNA segment, the double-strand RNA is melted and allowed to reanneal in the presence of increasing amounts of RNA from the virus isolate being tested. If the unlabeled viral RNA being tested against the probe contains an RNA sequence identical to that of the ^{125}I-labeled segment, the unlabeled RNA will then compete for annealing sites on the complementary RNA and prevent the reannealing of the labeled RNA. If, however, the unknown virus RNA does not contain a homologous segment or contains one that is only partially homologous, then the RNA either would not compete for annealing sites on the cRNA or it would compete less efficiently and the labeled RNA would reanneal (either completely or partially) with the cRNA.

Competitive reassociation reactions were carried out in 15 ul of 2.3 x SSC, 50% formamide.[18] Mixtures of double-strand probe RNA and unlabeled viral RNA were melted at 90° for 90 seconds, cooled to 70° and held at this temperature for 40 hours. This annealing temperature is approximately 10° below the Tm of the homologous double-strand. Following annealing, the amount of labeled double-strand RNA was determined by incubating with ribonuclease A and T1.[18]

RESULTS

Initial RNA comparisons were made using probes prepared with RNA segments isolated from an H3N2 virus of the "Victoria" serotype (A/Memphis/110/76) and an H1N1 strain, A/FW/1/50, previously shown to be nearly identical to the "USSR" virus.[3-5] Figure 1 shows results of competitive reassociation assays of various virus strains with the H3N2 probes and two representatives of the H1N1 probes. RNA extracted from the homologous strain or closely related strains gave essentially complete competition of the labeled probes. The heterologous RNAs competed to varying levels with the different RNA segments. There was, for example, little cross-competition with the genes coding for the surface proteins of the prototype strains (genes 4 and 6), while genes 5 and 7 (nucleoprotein and matrix) showed much more cross-competition indicating a greater conservation of the base sequence coding for these internal proteins.[4] In all cases, however, competition with RNA derived from the heterologous prototype strain was clearly distinguishable from the homologous competition.

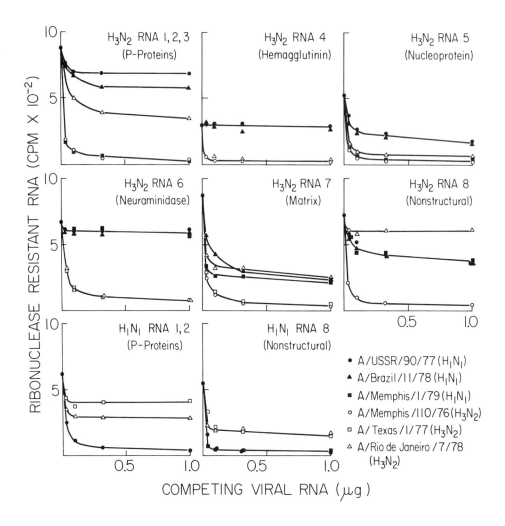

Fig. 1.   Comparison of the RNA segments of recent influenza isolates
with those of previous H3N2 and H1N1 strains by competitive
hybridization.

Virion RNA segments were isolated from A/Memphis/110/76
(H3N2) and A/FW/1/50 (H1N1) and ^{125}I-labeled double-strand probes
were prepared as described in Materials and Methods. These were
melted and allowed to reanneal in the presence of unlabeled virion
RNA extracted from the virus strains listed.

One strain shown in Figure 1, A/Memphis/1/79 (a recent H1N1 isolate), is clearly a recombinant, since four genes (1, 2, 3 and 5) coding for the three 90,000 dalton "P" polypeptides and for the nucleoprotein are homologous with those of the H3N2 strain, while those coding for the surface proteins and genes 7 and 8, coding for the matrix and non-structural proteins, are homologous with those of the H1N1 strain. Comparable results (Table 1) were obtained by directly hybridizing ^{32}P-labeled gene segments

TABLE 1

HOMOLOGY BETWEEN RNAs OF REFERENCE INFLUENZA VIRUS AND ISOLATES, DETECTED BY QUANTITATIVE RNA-RNA HYBRIDIZATION*

	% homology of cRNA with ^{32}P vRNA-labeled segments of A/Texas/1/77					
cRNA of	1	2	3	5	7	8
Reference Virus		P		NP	M	NS
A/Texas/1/77(H3N2)	100	100	100	100	100	100
A/USSR/90/77(H1N1)	66	44	54	62	76	78
Recent Isolates						
A/Shanghai/9/79(H3N2)	97	(105)		94	99	100
A/Singapore/333/79(H3N2)	110	(102)		98	101	97
A/Brazil/11/78(H1N1)	59	27	53	55	82	77
A/California/10/78(H1N1)	93	103	107	74†	84	73
A/Texas/8/78(H1N1)	92	97	98	79†	74	75
A/Texas/10/78(H1N1)	100	91	108	74†	78	80

*^{32}P-labeled RNA segments of A/Texas/1/77 and cRNA of the strains listed were isolated and hybridized as described in Materials and Methods. Values are expressed as the % of counts protected in the homologous reaction. Standard error of the procedure determined by repetitive tests of different RNA segments is ± 5%.
†Value > 100% probably due to cross-contamination of NP RNA (segment 5) with RNA of N2 neuraminidase (segment 6).

isolated from A/ Texas/1/77 (H3N2) with complementary RNA isolated from cells infected with A/California/10/78 (H1N1) and other isolates from early outbreaks of influenza during the winter of 1978-79 in the U.S. (A/Texas/8/78 and A/Texas/10/78). Three other H1N1 isolates obtained during the winter of 1978-79 (A/California/ 10/78; A/Berkeley/40/78; A/Georgia/64 /78) were also tested by competitive hybridization and shown to be identical recombinants (Table 2). These results are in agreement with the findings of Young and Palese[19] who analyzed the genetic composition of these recent H1N1 virus strains by oligonucleotide and peptide mapping.

TABLE 2

SUMMARY OF GENE DERIVATION OF RECENT H1N1 AND H3N2 VIRUS ISOLATES ANALYZED
IN THIS STUDY

H1N1 Strains	RNA Segments							
	1	2	3	4	5	6	7	8
		P		HA	NP	NA	M	NS
A/Brazil/11/78 8 May 78	H1	H1	H1	H1	H1	H1	H1	H1
A/Berkley/40/78 29 Nov 78								
A/Calif/10/78 10 Dec 78								
A/Texas/8/78 28 Nov 78	H3	H3	H3	H1	H3	H1	H1	H1
A/Texas/10/78 12 Dec 78								
A/Memphis/1/79 2 Feb 79								
A/Ga/64/79 19 Feb 79								
H3N2 Strains								
A/Rio de Janeiro/7/78 8 May 78	?	?	?	H3	?	H3	?	?
A/Singapore/333/79 7 April 79	H3	H3	H3	H3	H3	H3	H3	H3
A/Shanghai/9/7 16 April 79								

H1 = RNA segment homologous with corresponding gene of A/USSR/90/77 (H1N1).

H3 = RNA segment homologous with corresponding gene of recent H3N2 isolates of the "Victoria" or "Texas" serotypes.

? = RNA segment not closely related to H1N1 or H3N2 strains or any other influenza strain yet tested.

Many of the recent H1N1 strains mentioned above which were shown to be recombinants between previous H1N1 and H3N2 viruses, are antigenically indistinguishable, when tested with ferret sera or monoclonal antibodies (unpublished data), from A/Brazil/11/78 which is the prototype for a minor

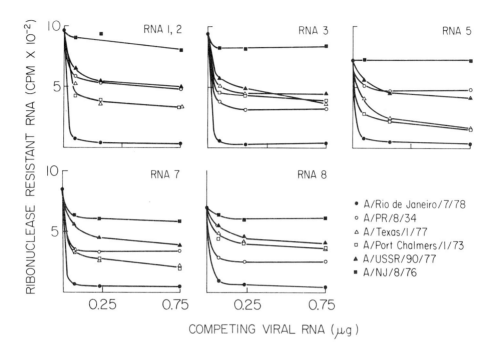

Fig. 2.   Comparison of the RNAs of various influenza strains with segments isolated from A/Rio de Janeiro/7/78 (H3N2) by competitive
reassociation.

Virion RNA segments were isolated from influenza strain A/Rio
de Janeiro/7/78 and labeled ds RNA probes prepared as described in
Materials and Methods. Unlabeled virion RNA extracted from 20
virus strains was used in competitive reassociation assays with
these probes. Six of these are shown in the figure. The other
strains tested were, A/USSR/90/77 (H1N1); A/Memphis/110/76 (H3N2);
A/FM/1/47 (H1N1); A/Jap/305/57 (H2N2); A/Ned/64/68 (H2N2);
A/Aichi/2/68 (H3N2); A/Eng/42/72 (H3N2); A/Port Chalmers/1/73
(H3N2); A/Scotland/ 840/74 (H3N2); A/Fukushima/103/78 (H1N1);
A/Texas/1/77 (H3N2); A/Victoria/3/75 (H3N2); A/Wash/1/79 (H3N2);
A/Swine/Tn/1/75 (Hsw1N1); A/duck/Alberta/35/76 (Hsw1N1);
A/Swine/Iowa/15/30 (Hsw1N1); and B/Hong Kong/8/73.

variant of the USSR strain predominant in South America during 1978.[20] Analysis of the RNAs of this prototype variant (Fig. 1, Table 1) indicated, however, that all of its gene segments were derived from an H1N1 strain.

To determine if the recent circulation of recombinant influenza viruses was limited to the above described H1N1 strains, the genetic composition of some recent H3N2 isolates[21] was also analyzed. No evidence was found for the presence of genes of H1N1 origin in H3N2 strains isolated in S.E. Asia in 1979 (Table 1). A South American H3N2 virus isolate (A/Rio de Janeiro/7/78), however, proved to have a different genetic composition. When RNA from this strain was tested in competitive reassociation assays (Fig. 1), only genes 4 and 6, coding for the surface proteins, of the H3N2 strain were shown to have homologous counterparts in this virus. The RNA did not contain sequences homologous to the other genes of either the H1N1 or H3N2 prototypes, although gene 5 (nucleoprotein) appeared to be more closely related to the corresponding H3N2 gene than to that of H1N1.

In an effort to determine the origin of the genes coding for the non-surface proteins of this virus, ^{125}I-labeled probes were prepared from its RNA segments and these were used in competitive reassociation assays with RNA from a series of 20 viruses. These included representatives of the major human influenza A viruses and selected strains from lower animals, as well as an influenza B virus, and are listed in the legend of Figure 2. Mixtures of H3N2 and H1N1 RNA were also tested to rule out the possibility that this virus might actually be a mixture with two copies of each gene. The results are shown in Figure 2. With each segment only the homologous RNA from A/Rio de Janeiro/7/78 was effective in competition assays. None of the other strains tested appeared to be closely related and no consistent pattern of relationships could be seen. For example, segments 3 and 8 were most effectively competed with RNA from the A/PR/8/34 strain, while the other segments were more effectively competed with the recent H3N2 isolates.

DISCUSSION

The prevalence of an H1N1 virus during the winter of 1978-79, containing genes from an H3N2 virus indicates that this recombinant must have had a distinct selective advantage over the parental stains. Possibly, the immune status of the population favored the surface protein of the H1N1 variant, while the replication complex of the H3N2 strain was better adapted for infection and transmission. The earliest examples of these recombinant viruses were obtained in November and December of 1978. Since these viruses were are antigenically identical to the prototype of this H1N1 variant, A/Brazil/11/78, which was isolated about six months earlier and contained all genes from the USSR strain, it is apparent that the change in antigenic characteristics was not directly related to the recombinational event with the H3N2 strain.

The significance of the finding that the H3N2 virus A/Rio de Janeiro/7/78, which contains genes coding for surface proteins identical to those of other recent H3N2 isolates, but derives all other genes from an unknown source remains uncertain. This isolate was chosen for study primarily because it came from an outbreak in the same country and in the same week as A/Brazil/ 11/78, and therefore was of interest to us as a potential recombinant with H1N1 genes. This virus and others from the outbreak also have the unusual property of cross-reacting equally with both the "Texas" and "Victoria" serotypes, as found for a small number of other H3N2 isolates in recent years.[7] The unknown genes of A/Rio de Janeiro/7/78 may have been derived from a previously unrecognized human influenza virus or from some animal influenza that was not tested in the experiments described here. In either case, the identity of only the hemagglutinin and neuraminidase genes of A/Rio de Janeiro/7/ 78 with those of recent H3N2 strains suggests that this unusual virus may be a further example of a recombinant virus infecting man.

This work was supported, in part, by Grant AI 14293 from the National Institute of Allergy and Infectious Disease, by Cancer Center Support (CORE) Grant CA 21765 from the National Cancer Institute and by ALSAC.

We thank Mr. Raymond Wilson for excellent technical assistance and Dr. Peter Palese for prepublication information.

REFERENCES
1. WHO Wkly Epidem. Rec., No. 4, pp 25-28 (1979).
2. Zhdanov, V.M., Lvov, D.K., Reznik, V.I., et al., Lancet I, 294-295 (1978).
3. Kendal, A.P., Noble, G.R., Skehel, J.J. & Dowdle, W.R., Virology 89, 632-636 (1978).
4. Scholtissek, C., von Hoynigen, V. & Rott, R., Virology 89, 613-617 (1978).
5. Nakajima, K., Desselberger, U. & Palese, P., Nature 274, 334-339 (1978).
6. Morbidity and Mortality Weekly Report, U.S. Department of Health, Education, and Welfare 28, 166-167 (1979).
7. Kendal, A.P., Joseph, J.M., Kobyashi, G., Nelson, D., Reyes, C.R., Ross, M.R., Sarandea, J.Z., White, R., Woodall, D.S., Noble, G.R. & Dowdle, W.R., Am. J. Epidemiol. 110, 449-461 (1979).

8. Kendal, A.P., Lee, D.T., Parish, H.S., et al., Am. J. Epidemiol. 110, 462-468 (1979).
9. Kendal, A.P., Beare, A.S., Cox, N.J., et al., Abst. Ann. Mtng. Amer. Soc. Microbiol., pp 304 (1979).
10. Bean, W.J., Sriram, G. & Webster, R.G., Anal. Biochem. (1979) (in the press).
11. Hansen, J.N., Anal. Biochem. 76, 37-44 (1976).
12. Commerford, S.L., Biochemistry 10, 1943-1999 (1971).
13. Franklin, R.M., Proc. Natl. Acad. Sci. USA 55, 1504-1511 (1966).
14. Etkind, P.R. & Krug, R.M., J. Virol. 16, 1464-1475 (1975).
15. Kendal, A.P., Cox, N.J., Galphin, J.C. & Maassab, H.F., J. Gen. Virol. 44, 443-452 (1979).
16. Scholtissek, C., Harms, E., Rohde, W., Orlich, M. & Rott, R., Virology 74, 332-344 (1976).
17. Stephenson, J.R., Hay, A.J. & Skehel, J.J., J. Gen. Virol. 36, 237-248 (1977).
18. Bean, W.J., Jr. & Simpson, R.W., J. Virol. 18, 365-369 (1976).
19. Young, J.F. & Palese, P., Proc. Natl. Acad. Sci. USA (1979 (in the press).
20. Webster, R.G., Kendal, A.P. & Gerhard, W., Virology 96, 258-264 (1979).
21. Morbidity and Mortality Weekly Report, U.S. Department of Health, Education, and Welfare 28, pp 348 (1979).

DISCUSSION

Scholtissek: Most data shown was of highly conserved genes. What happens when the homology is not so high? On some of your curves you did not reach a plateau. If you compare unrelated HA genes do you get zero?

Bean: This happens with some strains - we don't know why, and without sequence data we cannot quantitate any of this data. We normally do reach a plateau. If the temperature is high enough we do get zero.

Sambrook: Have you ever run the products out on a gel after RNAse digestion to look for the size of the pieces?

Bean: No.

Krug: Have you assayed to see if the transcriptase is more active in the H3N2 than in the H1N1, thus giving a selective advantage to a recombinant virus?

Bean: No.

Skehel: How do these findings fit with Dr. Palese's results?

Palese: Very well - European strains have the A/California/10/78 prototype, but very recent strains have also M and NS genes derived from Texas-like virus.

DNA SEQUENCES DERIVED FROM GENOMIC AND mRNA SPECIES THAT CODE FOR THE
HEMAGGLUTININ AND THE NEURAMINIDASE OF INFLUENZA A VIRUS

CHING-JUH LAI, LEWIS J. MARKOFF, MICHAEL SVEDA, RAVI DHAR[+] AND
ROBERT M. CHANOCK
Laboratory of Infectious Diseases, National Institute of Allergy and Infectious
Diseases, and [+]Laboratory of Molecular Virology, Nantional Cancer Institute,
National Institutes of Health, Bethesda, Maryland USA

INTRODUCTION

Human influenza A viruses recovered from pandemics always differ from
previous strains in their antigenic properties. Smaller but discernable
differences often characterize strains responsible for epidemics that occur
during interpandemic intervals. Analysis of successive pandemic or epidemic
variants indicates that antigenic alteration affects the viral surface
antigens, i.e., hemagglutinin (HA) and neuraminidase (NA) which are involved in
immunity and resistance. Substitution of corrsponding gene segments during
coinfection has been proposed to account for alterations involving major
changes of the surface glycoproteins (antigenic shift) while point-mutation
appears to be responsible for minor changes of the surface glycoproteins
(antigenic drift) (reviewed in ref. 14). Recent re-emergence of the H1N1
subtype indiates that transfer of a previous human influenza A virus from its
ecologic niche in nature back to man represents another mechanism for antigenic
shift.[37] These diverse pathways for alteration or substitution of influenza
viral genes attest to the variability of this virus. The recombinant DNA
approach offers new opportunities to further understand the mechanisms of
variations and other important properties of influenza virus. We describe
procedures used to obtain complementary DNA copies from virion RNA (vRNA) and
mRNA segments that code for the hemagglutinin and neuraminidase of influenza
virus (A/Udorn/72[H3N2]). The DNA sequences cloned in pBR 322 were
characterized by mapping with restriction enzymes and by sequence analysis.

RESULTS

(1) Influenza viral RNA segments and cloning design

The genome of influenza A virus consists of eight separate single stranded
RNA segments ranging from 900 to 2400 nucleotides.[5-9] These vRNA segments are
transcribed and the transcripts are polyadenylated to generate the

corresponding positive-strand mRNA species.[10,11] Sequence analysis of vRNA from virus strains of diverse antigenic subtype indicates that there is a common sequence of 12 nucleotides at the 3'-terminus and another common sequence of 13 nucleotides at the 5'-terminus.[12,13] The conserved sequence at the 3'-terminus provides a convenient way to generate cDNA copies by reverse transcription using a specific DNA primer. The procedure used to obtain double-stranded DNA molecules from bacteriophage Qβ RNA was adapted for cloning influenza viral RNA segments.[14] As illustrated in Figure 1, positive strands of complementary DNA[(+)cDNA] were synthesized by reverse-transcription of vRNA using a deoxyribonucleotide dodecamer primer, d(AGCAAAAGCAGG), complementary to the conserved 3'-terminus. Negative strands of cDNA were derived from reverse-transcription of poly(A)-containing cytoplasmic viral mRNA primed by oligo(dT). Corresponding cDNA strands were hybridized and the hybrids selected by chromatography on a hydroxyapatite column. The purified DNA duplexes were inserted into the Pst I site of plasmid pBR322 using dC/dG joining sequences.[15,16] The recombinant DNA was then used for transformation of E. coli K-12.

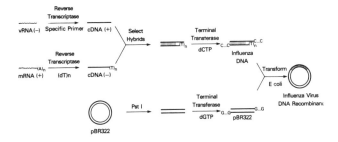

Fig. 1. Scheme for construction and cloning of influenza virus DNA (reproduced from Lai, et al[20]).

(2) Reverse-transcription of genomic RNA and mRNA segments

Both cDNA products were analyzed by electrophoresis on alkaline agarose gel (Fig. 2). There were 7 prominent bands and one faint band of (+)cDNA. Estimation of molecular size of the (+) cDNAs in this gel analysis and a comparison with the values obtained by others[17-19] suggests that these (+) cDNA species may be complete or almost complete transcripts of all eight separate viral RNA segments. Also shown in Fig. 2 were (+)cDNA products reverse-transcribed by the specific priming of vRNA's from other major subtypes of human influenza A viruses including FM-1/47 (H1N1) and Taiwan/62 (H2N2). The (-)cDNA products of reverse transcription of cytoplasmic mRNA also exhibited the expected size for complete or nearly complete transcripts. Eight bands were observed, although the largest 3 bands in Fig. 2 were only faintly visible.

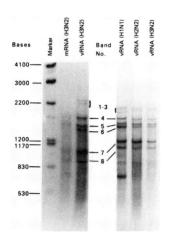

Fig. 2. Reverse-transcription of vRNA and mRNA segments. Influenza virus A/Udorn/72 (H3N2) was used to prepare vRNA and cytoplasmic viral mRNA segments for reverse-transcription with specific docecamer DNA primer and oligo(dT) primer, respectively. Conditions for the reverse transcriptase reaction were detailed by Meyer et al[35]. The ^{32}p-labelled cDNA products were analyzed on a 1.4% alkaline agarose gel and autoradiographed. Markers are SV40 DNA fragments used as size standards.

(3) Cloning DNA sequences coding for the hemagglutinin and the neuraminidase

After annealing the (+) and (-) cDNA strands, DNA duplexes were purified by chromatography on a hydroxyapatite column and separated according to size by polyacrylamide gel electrophoresis. DNA segments corresponding respectively in molecular size to the genes of the hemagglutinin and the neuraminidase were inserted into the Pst I site of pBR 322 (for details see ref 20). The constructed recombinant DNA molecules were used to transform E. coli K-12.

118

Tetracycline resistant transformants were analyzed for the presence of
influenza viral sequences by in situ hybridization with a labelled (+)cDNA
probe containing either the hemagglutinin gene sequences (band 4 of Fig. 2) or
the neuraminidase gene sequences (band 6 of Fig. 2).[21,22] Two independent
isolates (pFV88 and pFV92) that hybridized with the cDNA probe from band 4 were
examined for the inserted sequences released by Pst I digestion (Fig. 3).
Recombinant DNA from both isolates which contained the hemagglutinin gene
yielded a segment of 1950 base pairs (bp).

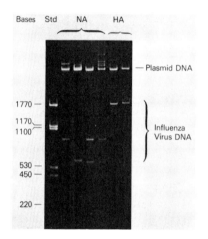

Fig. 3. Restriction enzyme analysis
of influenza virus recombinant DNA.
Plasmid DNA form I from E. coli
transformants containing influenza
virus gene segments coding for the
hemagglutinin and the neuraminidase
was prepared according to the
procedure described by Clewell[36] and
the DNA digested with restriction
enzyme Pst I. The digests were
separated by electrophoresis on 1.4%
agarose gels and visualized by
staining with ethidium bromide[27].
Sample order (from the right):
HA(pFV 88, pFV 92), NA(pFV 101, pFV
102, pFV 103, pFV 104).

Fig. 3 also shows the result of Pst I digestion on four recombinant DNA's
which contained the putative neuraminidase gene. Two recombinants (pFV101 and
pFV102) each yielded two Pst I fragments of 630 and 980 base pairs. Therefore,
the total size of the inserted neuraminidase DNA sequences was 1610 bp. The
other two cloned neuraminidase DNA plasmids, pFV103 and pFV104, yielded one or
the other Pst I fragment but not both. Apparently, these isolates generated
only one of the flanking Pst I sites. Recombinant neuraminidase plasmids
(pFV101 and pFV102) containing both Pst I segments were selected for further
analysis.(Markoff et al., manuscript in preparation) It should be noted that
each of the cloned influenza DNA segments contained linker G/C sequences at

both termini. If the linker sequences are about 30 bp in length at each end of the inserted influenza DNA sequences, then these inserts may be complete or nearly complete copies of the respective influenza genes.

(4) Verification of the cloned influenza virus DNA

Plasmid DNA from pFV88, 101, and 102 was prepared and digested with Eco RI to yield linear DNA molecules. This DNA was denatured and bound to nitrocellulose filters and hybridized in the presence of an excess of all eight vRNA segments. Bound vRNA was subsequently eluted and analyzed on a 2.6% polyacrylamide gel containing 6M urea. Under these partially denaturing conditions, Palese and his collaborators[23] and Markoff et al.[24] have shown the hemagglutinin gene is RNA 4 and the neuraminidase gene is RNA 5 for H3N2 influenza A viruses. Fig. 4 shows that filters bearing pFV88 bound predominantly vRNA 4 and the filters bearing pFV101 bound predominantly vRNA 5 (as did the filters bearing pFV102 DNA, not shown). These experiments confirmed that the influenza DNA sequences of pFV88 were those of the HA gene and that the influenza DNA sequences of pFV 101 and 102 were those of the NA gene.

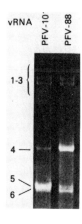

Fig. 4. Identification of cloned influenza virus DNA segments. Recombinant DNA from pFV 88 and pFV 101 was denatured and immobilized on nitrocellulose filters for hybridization with total vRNA. Influenza virus RNA segments hybridized to the cloned DNA were eluted from the filters and analyzed by polyacrylamide gel electrophoresis as described in the text.

(5) Strand orientation and restriction enzyme maps

The influenza virus-specific sequences isolated after digestion of recombinant plasmids with Pst I were characterized further by cleavage with other restriction enzymes. The localization of the restriction enzyme sites on DNA segments coding for the hemagglutinin and for the neuraminidase is summarized in Fig. 5.

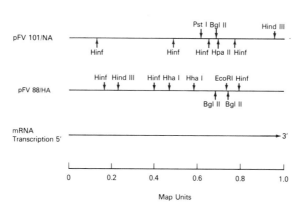

Fig. 5. Restriction enzyme cleavage map and strand orientation of influenza virus DNA segments. The restriction enzyme cleavage sites on the cloned influenza virus DNA segments were determined by analysis of the cleaved DNA fragments. One map unit is the total length of a cloned gene including the linker dG/dC sequences. The direction of mRNA transcription defines the strand orientation of a cloned DNA segment.

The orientation of the cloned DNA (corresponding to synthesis of mRNA during infection) was established as follows. HA DNA duplexes were labelled at both 3'-termini and cleaved by Eco RI (at 0.26 map units) yielding two fragments. Hybridization of vRNA occurred with the 3'labelled strand of the dissociated 0.26 unit fragment. In the case of NA, DNA duplexes formed between linear denatured plasmid 101 and 102 DNA and the 3'-^{32}P-labelled (+)cDNA strand representing the NA vRNA were digested with Pst I. Analysis of the digest on an alkaline agarose gel showed that the 630 bp unit fragment carried the sequences complementary to the 3' end of (+)cDNA. Mapping by restriction enzymes was performed to determine the orientation of influenza virus DNA with respect to the pBR322 DNA sequences. Plasmids pBR322, pFV101 and 102 were digested with Hinf I and the DNA fragments that were unique to the recombinant plasmids were isolated. Pst I cleavage of the largest influenza specific Hinf fragment from pFV101 yielded two fragments: one identical in length (240 base pairs) to the pBR322 moiety[15], and the second identical in size to the fragment produced by Hinf I digestion of the small (630 bp) Pst I fragment from pFV101 representing the 3"-terminus of (+) strand NA DNA. Similar analysis indicated the orientation of NA DNA in pFV102 was the reverse of that in pFV101 (data not shown) with respect to the pBR 322 sequences.

(6) DNA sequences corresponding to the 5'-terminus of in vivo mRNA

Recent evidence indicates that in vitro transcription of influenza vRNA is efficiently primed by mRNA's of β globin and reovirus.[25,26] In this system, the influenza polymerase complex appears to utilize the 5' "cap" structure and the adjacent 10-15 nucleotides of mRNA forming a donor RNA molecule. This sequence initiates the transcription of new influenza mRNA to which it becomes covalently linked. However, initiation of viral mRNA synthesis in influenza virus infected cells and therefore the 5'-structure of the in vivo mRNA remain to be determined. To approach this problem we sequenced DNA fragments that included the portion of the sequences corresponding to the 5'-terminus of the in vivo mRNA from two independently cloned hemagglutinin DNA containing plasmids, pFV88 and pFV 92.[29,30], Dhar and Lai, manuscript in preparation) The sequences are shown in Fig. 6. The dodecamer DNA that was used to initiate the reverse-transcription of vRNA was present intact in both isolates, indicating that the cloned DNA contained the complete 3'-end sequence of the genomic RNA. Each of the cloned DNAs contained 30-35 residues of dG/dC linker at the sequenced end. Between the primer and the linker there were additional sequences which correspond in position to the 5'-terminus of the in vivo mRNA molecules. There were 14-15 nucleotides in pFV88 and 9-10 nucleotides in pFV92. These additional sequences appeared to be different in base composition. The apparent heterogeneity corresponding to the 5'-terminus of the in vivo mRNA suggests that these sequences were derived from cellular RNA molecules consistent with the observations of Krug et al.[28] Our results provide direct evidence indicating that a short RNA segment of cellular origin may be used to prime transcription of influenza viral mRNA in infected cells.

```
pFV 92    5'(+) ┌──────┬─────┬──────────┬─────────────┐
          3'(-) │ 30±5 │ (G) │ AGTGTTCGC │ AGCAAAAGCAGG │ ...
                │      │ (C) │ TCACAAGCG │ TCGTTTTCGTCC │ ...
                └──────┴─────┴──────────┴─────────────┘

pFV 88    5'(+) ┌──────┬─────┬──────────────────┬─────────────┐
          3'(-) │ 30±5 │ (G) │ ACCGGAGGGAGCAA   │ AGCAAAAGCAGG │ ...
                │      │ (C) │ TGGCCTCCCTCGTT   │ TCGTTTTCGTCC │ ...
                └──────┴─────┴──────────────────┴─────────────┘
                       Linker                      Primer
```

Fig. 6. DNA sequences corresponding to the 5'-terminus of _in vivo_ mRNA coding for the hemagglutinin. Two independently derived clones, pFV 92 and pFV 88, were analyzed.

DISCUSSION

A scheme was described for cloning DNA sequences that corresponded to the gene segments of influenza A viruses. Since we were interested in retaining complete sequences from the cDNA transcripts, this approach did not employ S1 nuclease treatment normally used to obtain an open gene after the self-primed synthesis of the second strand DNA.[31] As shown in Fig. 2, a DNA dodecamer complementary to the 3'-terminus of vRNA efficiently primed the reverse-transcription of vRNA segments from all three subtypes of human influenza A virus. The size of these (+) cDNA transcripts as estimated by gel electrophoresis suggests that they represent full-length or almost full-length genomic sequences of 8 viral genes.

On the other hand, (-) cDNA strands used for forming duplexes were derived by reverse-transcription of cytoplasmic viral mRNA segments using oligo(dT) primer. It has been shown that the mRNA transcripts are shorter at their 3'-terminus than vRNA template molecules by 20-30 nucleotides, and in addition, a short stretch of additional sequences derived from host cell mRNA may be present at the 5'-terminus.[32-34] Thus, the cDNA duplexes formed between the (+) and (-) cDNA strands contain mismatched and unpaired regions at each end. After transfection of _E. coli_ such mismatched and unpaired region in the DNA molecules should be corrected by the cellular DNA repair enzymes. This appeared to be the case, since many of the recombinant plasmids recovered from E. coli transformants had two Pst I sites that were generated _in vivo_.

Analysis of DNA sequences from two isolates coding for the hemagglutinin demonstrates a complete representation of the 3'-terminus of genomic RNA. It will be necessary to determine nucleotide sequences at the other terminus in order to identify which, if any, of the cloned plasmids contain complete genomic information.

In regard to gene expression at the transcriptional level the cloned DNA molecules provide a convenient way to probe various forms of RNA transcripts present in the infected cells. For example cloning influenza viral recombinant DNA and analyzing nucleotide sequences provided evidence illustrating the presence of a population of mRNA containing diverse sequences at their 5'-termini.

ACKNOWLEDGEMENTS

We thank Ms. Jo Ann Berndt and Bronna Cohen for their technical assistance.

REFERENCES

1. Webster, R.G. and Laver, W.G. (1975) The Influenza Viruses and Influenza, E.D. Kilbourne, ed., Academic Press, New York, pp. 269-314.
2. Burnett, F.M. (1959) The Virus, F.M. Burnett and W.M. Stanley, eds., Academic Press, New York, Vol III, pp. 275-306.
3. Schulman, J.L. (1975) The Infuenza Viruses and Influenza, E.D. Kilbourne, ed., Academic Press, New York, pp. 373-379.
4. Kilbourne, E.D. (1975) The Influenza Viruses and Influenza, E.D. Kilbourne, ed., Academic Press, New York, pp. 483-538.
5. Young, J.F., Desselberger, U. and Palese, P. (1979) Cell 18, 73-83.
6. Pons, M.W. and Hirst, G.K. (1968) Virology 34, 385-388.
7. McGeoch, D., Felner, P. and Newton, C. (1976) Proc. Natl. Acad. Sci. USA 73, 3045-3049.
8. Desselberger, U. and Palese, P. (1978) Virology 88, 394-399.
9. Scholtissek, C., Harms, E., Rohde, W., Orlich, M., and Rott, R. (1976) Virology 74, 332-344.
10. Etkind, P.R., Buckhagen, D.L., Herz, C., Broni, B. and Krug, R.M. (1977) J. Virol. 22, 346-342.
11. Hay, A.J., Lomniczi, B., Bellamy, A.R., and Skehel, .J. (1977) Virology 83, 337-355.
12. Robertson, J.S. (1979) Nucleic Acids Res. 6, 3745-3757.
13. Skenhel, J.J. and Hay, A.J. (1978) Nucleic Acids Res. 5, 1207-1219.
14. Taniguchi, T., Palmieri, M. and Weissman, C. (1978) Nature (London) 274, 223-228.
15. Sutcliffe, J.G. (1979) Cold Spring Harbor Symposia on Quantitative Biology, Vol 43, pp. 77-90.
16. Boyer, H.W., Betlach, M., Boliver, F., Rodriguez, R.L., Heyneker, H.L., Shine, J. and Goodman, H.M. (1977) Impact on Science and Society, Proceedings of the 10th Miles International Symposium, R.F. Beers, Jr. and E.G. Bassett, E.G., Raven, New York, pp, 9-20.

17. Emtage, J.S., Catlin, G.H. and Carey, N.H. (1979) Nucleic Acids Res. 6, 1221-1239.

18. Sleigh, M.J., Both, G.W., and Brownlee, G.G. (1979) Nucleic Acids Res. 6, 1309-1321.

19. Porter, A.G., Barber, C., Carey, N.H., Hallewell, R.A., Threlfall, G. and Emtage, J.S. (1979) Nature (London) 282, 471-477.

20. Lai, C.-J., Markoff, L.J., Zimmerman, S., Cohen, B., Berndt, J.A., and Chanock, R.M. (1980) Proc. Natl. Acad. Sci. 77,

21. Enea, V., Voris, G.F. and Zinder, N.D. (1975) J. Mol. Biol. 96, 495-509.

22. Grunstein, M. nd Hogness, D.S. (1975) Proc. Natl. Acad. Sci. USA 72, 3961-3965.

23. Palese, P. and Ritchey, M.B. (1977) Virology 78, 183-191.

24. Markoff, L.W., Thierry, F., Murphy, B.R. and Chanock, R.M. (1979) Infect. Immun. 26, 280-286.

25. Bouloy, M., Plotch, S.J. and Krug, R.M. (1978) Proc. Natl. Acad. Sci. USA 75, 4886-4890.

26. Bouloy, M., Morgan, M.A., Shatkin, A.J. and Krug, R.M. (1979) J. Virol. 32, 895-904.

27. Sharp. P.A., Sugden, B. and Sambrook, J. (1973) Biochemistry 12,3055-3963.

28. Krug, R.M., Broni, B.A., and Bouloy, M. (1979) Cell 18, 329-334.

29. Seif, I., Khoury, G. and Dhai, R. (1980) Manuscript in preparation.

30. Maxam, A.M. and Gilbert, W. (1971) Proc. Natl. Acad. Sci. USA 74, 560-564.

31. Efstratiadis, A., Kafatos, F.C., Maxam, A.M. and Maniatis, T. (1976) Cell 7, 279-288.

32. Plotch, S.J., and Krug, R.M. (1977) J. Virol. 21, 24-34.

33. Skehel, J.J. and Hay, A.J. (1978) Nucleic Acids Res. 4, 1207-1209.

34. Plotch, S.J., Tomasz, J. and Krug, R.M. (1978) J. Virol. 28, 75-83.

35. Meyer, J.C., Spiegelman, S. and Kacian, D.L. (1977) Proc. Natl. Acad. Sci. USA 74, 2840-2843.

36. Clewell, D.B. (1972) J. Bacteriol. 110, 667-676.

37. Kendal, A.P., Noble, G.R., Skenhel, J.J., and Dowdle, W.R. (1978) Virology 89, 632-636.

SEQUENCE VARIATIONS OBSERVED IN THE NEURAMINIDASES OF SEVERAL STRAINS OF
INFLUENZA VIRUS

J. BLOK AND G.M. AIR
John Curtin School of Medical Research, Australian National University,
P.O. Box 334, Canberra City, A.C.T. 2601, Australia

INTRODUCTION

There are two forms of antigenic variation which occur in the surface
glycoproteins of influenza A viruses. These are antigenic drift which is a
series of minor changes arising from point mutations, and antigenic shift
which is a major change possibly arising by gene reassortment from a mixed
infection of one host cell (for reviews see 1,2).

The antigenic drift and shift found in neuraminidase can be studied by
several methods such as the neuraminidase inhibition tests[3], comparative
peptide maps or by comparing nucleotide and amino acid sequences. The latter
method is the most accurate for it reveals the precise changes at the
molecular level. By sequencing the neuraminidase gene of several field
strains using the dideoxy method, one can observe the point mutations which
occur during drift; and the totally different sequences which appeared in
the shift from N1 to N2 strains.

MATERIALS AND METHODS

Chemicals and enzymes

^{32}P and ^{3}H-labelled nucleoside triphosphates were obtained from the
Radiochemical Centre, Amersham, England. Dideoxynucleoside triphosphates and
p(dT)$_8$-dA were obtained from P.L.-Biochemicals, Milwaukee, Wisconsin, U.S.A.
The synthetic oligonucleotide d(A-G-C-A-A-A-A-G-C-A-G-G) was from Collaborative
Research and was a generous gift from Dr Ching-Juh Lai. Reverse transcriptase
was generously supplied by Dr J.W. Beard (Life Sciences, St. Petersberg,
Florida, U.S.A.) under NCI contract.

Viruses

Influenza viruses were grown in embryonated chicken eggs and purified by
adsorption to and elution from chicken red blood cells followed by sucrose
density centrifugation[4]. The virus strains used were A/NWS/33(H0N1),
A/PR/8/34(H0N1), A/Bellamy/42(H0N1), A/Loyang/4/57(H1N1), A/Memphis/10/78
(H1N1), and A/RI/5$^-$/57(H2N2). High growing recombinants between A/NWS/33(H0N1),

and A/Tokyo/67(H2N2), A/NWS/33(HON1) and A/Netherlands/68(H2N2), A/NWS/33(HON1)
and A/RI/5$^+$/57(H2N2))named X-7(FI)[5], and A/PR/8/34(HON1) and A/Memphis/102/72
(H3N2) were also used. In each case the neuraminidase gene came from the
latter virus in each pair. Virus stocks were kindly provided by Dr W.G. Laver.

Preparation of template for cDNA synthesis

Extraction of virion RNA, separation of the genome segments on polyacrylamide gels and their elution from gels were as previously described[6,7]. In
some experiments, where the primer p(dT)$_8$-dA was used, a poly A tail was
added to the 3' end of the viral RNA *in vitro* using *E.Coli* adenyltransferase
either before or after gel separation of segments.

Sequencing procedures

Sequences of segment 6, which is the gene coding for neuraminidase, were
obtained from the 3' end of the viral RNA using the dideoxy method[8] as
previously described[6,7]. Thin polyacrylamide gels (200 x 400 x 0.4mm)[9]
were used to separate the sequencing products. In some experiments the
oligonucleotide d(A-G-C-A-A-A-A-G-C-A-G-G) was used as a primer instead of
p(dT)$_8$-dA, thus avoiding the necessity to polyadenylate the viral RNA. In
these experiments double labelling, with ^{32}P dATP and ^{32}P dGTP, was used to
obtain short products.

RESULTS AND DISCUSSION

The 3' nucleotide of each RNA segment from several influenza A strains has
been determined as uracil[10]. The oligonucleotide p(dT)$_8$-dA can therefore be
used as a phased primer to synthesize cDNA from polyadenylated influenza RNA
segments using reverse transcriptase. This has been the basis of the dideoxy
sequencing procedure used to sequence segments 8[11], 7[6], 4[7] and 6.

The results of this sequencing procedure on segment 6 of A/NWS/33 can be
seen in Fig. 1. The numbering of nucleotides starts nine nucleotides from
the 5' end of the cDNA where the dA of the primer, which is complementary
to the 3' nucleotide U of the viral RNA, is the first nucleotide. The first
12 nucleotides at the 3' end of all RNA segments of the influenza A strains
are conserved and have been determined by Skehel and Hay[12]. Some of these
first nucleotides can be seen with the dideoxy sequencing method and the
numbering is consistent with the published sequence. Fig. 1 shows the
nucleotides 9 to 128 of the A/NWS/33 neuraminidase gene.

Extra bands can sometimes be seen but these are usually not consistent between experiments so that one can deduce the sequence from several experiments if necessary. In some cases the artefact bands are weak but occasionally there are high intensity bands at the same position, making nucleotide assignment difficult. The extra bands are probably due to secondary structure in the template.

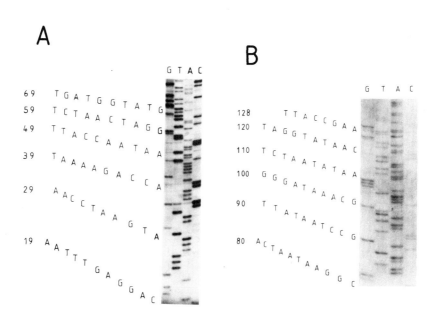

Fig. 1. The sequence of A/NWS/33 neuraminidase gene cDNA obtained by the dideoxy method. A is an autoradiograph of a 12% polyacrylamide gel showing nucleotides 9 to 70, while B is an 8% gel showing nucleotides 71 to 128.

The nucleotide sequence of A/NWS/33 and its predicted amino acid sequence are shown in Fig. 2. The first initiation codon is found 20-22 nucleotides from the 5' end of the cDNA(=mRNA) for this particular Nl strain. The other Nl strains sequenced have this initiation site at nucleotides 21-23 which agrees with the fowl plague virus work on segment 6[12,13]. Terminating codons in different reading frames can be found near this first AUG.

Common 5' sequence   A-G-C-A-A-A-A-G-C-A-G-G

(Skehel & Hay)

                                                                    20
cDNA   dT₈A — — — — — A-G-C-A-G-G-A-G-T-T-T-A-A-A-T-G-
predicted protein sequence   Met

                30   40   50   60
A-A-T-C-C-A-A-A-C-C-A-G-A-A-A-A-T-A-A-T-A-A-C-C-A-T-T-G-G-A-T-C-A-A-T-C-T-G-T-
Asn   Pro   Asn   Gln   Lys   Ile   Ile   Thr   Ile   Gly   Ser   Ile   Cys

                70   80   90   100
A-T-G-G-T-A-G-T-C-G-G-A-A-T-A-A-T-C-A-G-C-C-T-A-A-T-A-T-T-G-C-A-A-A-T-A-G-G-G-
Met   Val   Val   Gly   Ile   Ile   Ser   Leu   Ile   Leu   Gln   Ile   Gly

                110   120   128
A-A-T-A-T-A-A-T-C-T-C-A-A-T-A-T-G-G-A-T-A-A-G-C-C-A-T-T
Asn   Ile   Ile   Ser   Ile   Trp   Ile   Ser   His

Fig. 2. Nucleotide sequence complementary to the 3' end of segment 6 from
A/NWS/33(HON1), and the predicted amino acid sequence of the neuraminidase
for which it codes.

Neuraminidase genes of five N1 subtype influenza strains isolated in the
years 1933, 1934, 1942, 1957 and 1978 have so far been sequenced using the dideoxy method. The number of nucleotides obtained range from 128 to 230 which
corresponds to 37 to 70 predicted amino acids or about 6-12% of the protein
sequence. This is assuming that the first AUG downstream from the 5' end of
the viral mRNA initiates protein synthesis, as is found in several eukaryotic
mRNA's[14,15,16].

There are a few base changes between N1 neuraminidase genes as is predicted
by the small antigenic changes during drift. Some of these substitutions are
silent (third position nucleotides) while others (first or second position
nucleotides) result in amino acid differences. Table 1 shows the percentage
homology found in the predicted amino acid sequences of the five N1 strains
used. It reveals that there is a high degree of conservation between the
neuraminidase gene of the N1 subtype and that the drift observed may not be
linear, since segment 6 of A/NWS/33 is more closely related to A/Bellamy/42
than to A/PR/8/34. One can also observe that the A/Memphis/10/78 strain is
more closely related to the late N1 strains than to the very early ones.

TABLE 1

PERCENT HOMOLOGY OF PREDICTED AMINO ACID SEQUENCE WITHIN THE N1 SUBTYPE

	NWS	PR8	Bel	Loy	Mem
A/NWS/33	100	92	97	87	87
A/PR/8/34		100	95	88	87
A/Bellamy/42			100	90	92
A/Loyang/4/57				100	93
A/Memphis/10/78					100

These figures represent about 10% of the protein sequence.

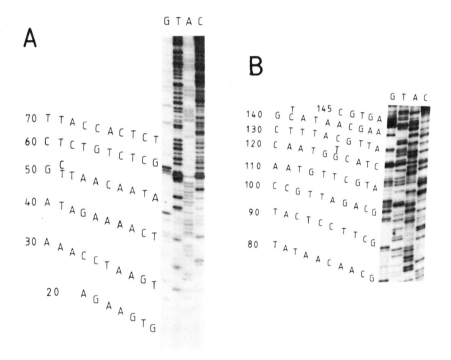

Fig. 3. The sequence of A/Memphis/102/72 neuraminidase gene cDNA obtained by the dideoxy method. A is an autoradiograph of a 12% polyacrylamide gel showing nucleotides 14 to 70. The synthetic primer d(A-G-C-A-A-A-A-G-C-A-G-G) was used in this experiment so that the first nucleotide one can see will be 14 from the 5' end of the cDNA. B is an 8% gel showing nucleotides 71 to 145.

130

Influenza neuraminidase has undergone one major antigenic change over the last 80 years. The Asian influenza epidemic was the beginning of the N2 subtype. Fig. 3 shows an autoradiograph of the neuraminidase gene sequencing gels of A/Memphis/102/72, an H3N2 strain. This sequence, shown in Fig. 4, was obtained as before except that the specific synthetic primer d(A-G-C-A-A-A-A-G-C-A-G-G) was used instead of p(dT)$_8$-dA, thus eliminating the step of adding a poly A tail to the 3' end of the viral RNA. The initiation site closest to the 5' end of the cDNA is 20-22 nucleotides away, as found in the N1 strain A/NWS/33. Again there are terminating codons in different reading frames around this first AUG triplet.

```
                                              12
Synthetic primer used:    A-G-C-A-A-A-A-G-C-A-G-G

(complementary to 3' common seq.)
                                         14        20
cDNA                              ----G-T-G-A-A-G-A-T-G-A-A-T-
predicted protein sequence                       Met   Asn

         30              40              50              60
C-C-A-A-A-T-C-A-A-A-A-G-A-T-A-A-T-A-A-C-A-A-T-T-G-G-C-T-C-T-G-T-C-T-C-T-C-T-C-
Pro   Asn   Gln   Lys   Ile   Ile   Thr   Ile   Gly   Ser   Val   Ser   Leu
                                              10


         70              80              90              100
A-C-C-A-T-T-G-C-A-A-C-A-A-T-A-T-G-C-T-T-C-C-T-C-A-T-G-C-A-G-A-T-T-G-C-C-A-T-G-
Thr   Ile   Ala   Thr   Ile   Cys   Phe   Leu   Met   Gln   Ile   Ala   Met
                        20


         110        G       120              130              140
C-T-T-G-T-A-A-C-T-A-C-T-G-T-A-A-C-A-T-T-G-C-A-T-T-T-C-A-A-G-C-A-A-T-A-T-G-A-G
Leu   Val   Thr   Thr   Val   Thr   Leu   His   Phe   Lys   Gln   Tyr   Glu
   30                                                               40
```

Fig. 4. Nucleotide sequence complementary to the 3' end of segment 6 from A/Memphis/102/72(H3N2), and the predicted amino acid sequence of the neuraminidase for which it codes.

Sequences have been obtained from other N2 field strains, ranging from 140 to 240 nucleotides in length and coding for 41 to 73 amino acids or about 9 - 13% of the protein sequence. A high degree of conservation is found in the neuraminidase gene within the N2 subtype as shown in Table 2. This is similar to the N1 subtype results and shows that antigenic drift occurs by point mutations in the nucleotide sequence.

TABLE 2

PERCENT HOMOLOGY OF PREDICTED AMINO ACID SEQUENCE WITHIN THE N2 SUBTYPE

	RI5⁻	RI5⁺	Tok	Ned	Mem
A/RI/5⁻/57	100	93	95	93	93
A/NWS$_{HA}$-RI/5⁺/57$_{NA}$		100	93	93	91
A/NWS$_{HA}$-Tokyo/67$_{NA}$			100	95	93
A/NWS$_{HA}$-Ned/68$_{NA}$				100	91
A/Memphis/102/72					100

These figures represent about 10% of the protein sequence.

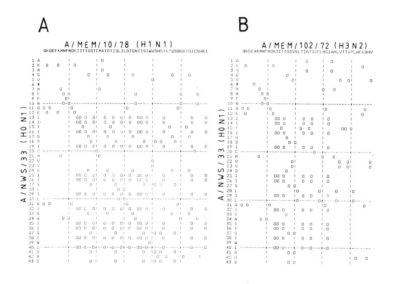

Fig. 5.   A - Computer matching of predicted N-terminal amino acid sequence
of NWS/33 (HON1) and Memphis/10/78 (H1N1); B - Comparison of predicted
N-terminal amino acid sequence of NWS/33 (HON1) and Memphis/102/72 (H3N2).

When one compares the predicted amino acid sequences of the neuraminidases of an Nl subtype with those of an N2, there is one striking feature which is illustrated in Fig. 5B. This figure shows that the only marked homology between the predicted N-terminal sequences of the two subtypes is in the first twelve of forty amino acids (including the initiating methionine) and 3-4 other amino acids scattered along the sequence. In contrast to this, Fig. 5A compares the predicted amino acid sequence of two Nl strains showing a few very small gaps in their homology.

The percentage homology between the two subtypes, Nl and N2, is less than 50% in the predicted N-terminal amino acid sequences obtained to date, compared to greater than 85% within each subtype. Comparisons have been made with the amino acid sequences coded by different reading frames in order to check for deletions or insertions which may have caused the vast difference in amino acid sequences without too much change in the nucleic acid sequences between subtypes. These comparisons revealed that the Nl and N2 subtype neuraminidases are not simply deletion or insertion mutations; they are very different, thus explaining the vast difference in antigenic properties between shift strains.

Neuraminidases of the influenza A strains examined show that the first twelve predicted amino acids are usually conserved. Following the first five of these amino acids, the sequences are relatively hydrophobic which could suggest a signal peptide usually found in membrane glycoproteins. There is no evidence for or against a longer *in vitro* translation product which would imply a leader sequence which is cleaved off during processing as is the case with the influenza hemagglutinin[17,6]. The influenza neuraminidase may of course have an internal signal peptide as is found in ovalbumin[18], but this has not yet been determined.

In order to be sure of the nucleotide sequence and whether the first AUG is the initiator, one needs some peptide data. Tryptic peptide maps have been prepared and the peptides eluted, hydrolysed, and analysed for amino acid composition. The predicted amino acid sequence of either an Nl or N2 strain contains no short tryptic peptides so far, except for one containing the first five amino acids. These may be cleaved off as part of a processing procedure and therefore not present in the mature protein isolated from the virions. The longer peptides which are predicted have been searched for unsuccessfully but these may be insoluble or glycosylated and thus not purified on peptide maps. No N-terminal amino acid can be detected by manual protein sequencing, suggesting that the N-terminus is blocked.

ACKNOWLEDGEMENTS

This work was supported in part by Grant AI 15343 from the National
Institute of Allergy and Infectious Diseases and the Australian Government
Poultry Industry Trust Fund. We thank Dr A. Gibbs for use of his computer
program, Dr W.G. Laver for preparing some of the peptide maps, and
Anne Mackenzie, Sally Campbell, and Bertrum Bubble for expert technical
assistance.

REFERENCES

1. Webster, R.G. and Laver, W.G. *in* The Influenza Viruses and Influenza,
    (Kilbourne, E.D. ed), pp. 270-314, Academic Press, New York (1975).
2. Schild, G.C. and Dowdle, W.R. *in* The Influenza Viruses and Influenza,
    (Kilbourne, E.D. ed), pp. 316-372, Academic Press, New York (1975).
3. Aymard-Henry, M., Coleman, M.T., Dowdle, W.R., Schild, G.C. and Webster,
    R.G. Bull. W.H.O. 48, 199-202 (1973).
4. Laver, W.G. *in* Fundamental Techniques in Virology (Habel, K. and
    Salzman, N.P. eds) pp. 82-86, Academic Press, New York (1969).
5. Kilbourne, E.D., Lief, F.S., Schulman, J.L., Jahiel, R.I. and Laver, W.G.
    Perspectives Virol. 5, 87-106 (1967).
6. Both, G.W. and Air, G.M. Eur. J. Biochem. 96, 363-372 (1979).
7. Air, G.M., Virology 97, 468-472 (1979).
8. Sanger, F., Nicklen, S. and Coulson, A.R. Proc. Nat. Acad. Sci. 74,
    5463-5467 (1977).
9. Sanger, F. and Coulson, A.R. FEBS Letters 87, 107-110 (1978).
10. Lewandowski, L.J., Content, J. and Leppla, S.H. J. Virol. 8, 701-707
    (1971).
11. Air, G.M. and Hackett, J.A., unpublished results.
12. Skehel, J.J. and Hay, A.J. Nucl. Acids Res. 5, 1207-1219 (1978).
13. Robertson, J.S., Nucl. Acids Res. 6, 3745-3757 (1979).
14. Kozak, M. and Shatkin, A.J. Cell 13, 201-212 (1978).
15. Filipowitz, W. and Haenni, A-L., Proc. Nat. Acad. Sci. 76, 3111-3115
    (1979).
16. Zain, S., Sambrook, J., Roberts, R.J., Keller, W., Fried, M. and Dunn,
    A.R. Cell 16, 851-861 (1979).
17. Waterfield, M.D., Skehel, J.J., Nakashima, Y., Gurnett, A. and Belham, T.
    in Topics of Infectious Diseases (Laver, W.G., Bachmayer, H., and Weil,
    R. eds), Vol. 3, pp. 167-180, Springer-Verlag, Wein (1977).
18. Lingappa, V.R., Lingappa, J.R. and Blobel, G. Nature 281, 117-121 (1979).

(See DISCUSSION on following page)

DISCUSSION

Ward: What does the sequence look like if you use other AUG's than the first to initiate?

Blok: In Nl the next AUG is in the same reading frame as the first. In N2 there is one AUG in a different reading frame but it is closely followed by a termination codon.

Ward: Can you line up the cysteines in Nl and N2 as in the HA?

Blok: No. They are in completely different environments.

Compans: Is there some data on the N-termini?

Blok: Using manual sequencing methods on N2, none is seen, so it may be blocked in this case.

Choppin: Is there any homology between the NA and HA? Somewhere in those molecules there is a region which recognises the same site, i.e., neuraminic acid linked to another sugar, so there may well be a region of homology.

Blok: We haven't looked.

Palese: There was no homology in the PR8 and WSN HA and NA sequences we have (150 nucleotides).

SEQUENCES FROM THE 3' ENDS OF INFLUENZA VIRUS RNA SEGMENTS

G.M. AIR
John Curtin School of Medical Research, Australian National University,
P.O. Box 334, Canberra City, A.C.T. 2601, Australia.

INTRODUCTION

Knowledge of the nucleotide sequences of influenza virus genes is necessary to understand the molecular basis of antigenic variation of the virus. Sequencing can show (i) how much variation occurs between different strains and subtypes, (ii) whether all genes of the virus change to the same extent, or whether variation is confined to genes coding for the surface antigens, and (iii) whether the nucleotide sequences of variable genes show evidence of high mutation, e.g. in altered codons where the amino acid sequences are conserved.

Influenza viruses have a segmented genome of single-stranded RNA molecules of negative polarity. Each has been found to contain the coding information for one of the known viral gene products, and from one segment there are two known products. As a first step in the sequence study, we have used primed synthesis of a complementary strand and the dideoxy sequencing method of Sanger et al.,[1] to obtain sequences 250-350 nucleotides long from the 3' ends of viral RNA segments. The sequence of each corresponds to the 5' end region of the messenger RNA, and therefore is expected to contain the coding information for the N-terminal region of the protein coded by that gene.

As in the other nucleotide sequencing methods currently in use, the dideoxy method depends on the introduction of a radioactive label, and RNA can be copied into cDNA using reverse transcriptase (usually from avian myeloblastosis virus) and incorporating a ^{32}P-deoxynucleoside triphosphate.

If the RNA template is polyadenylated at the 3' end, cDNA synthesis can be initiated from an oligo-dT primer. Since specific initiation is necessary for sequencing, primers of the type dT_8dN are used where N is complementary to the nucleotide preceding the poly A tail. If, as in the case of influenza virus gene segments, the RNA does not have a poly A tail, this can be added *in vitro* by the *E.coli* adenyltransferase[2]. All segments of several strains of influenza A viruses have U as the 3' nucleotide[3,4], therefore dT_8dA will prime on adenylated RNA. The basic principles of the dideoxy method as described by Sanger et al.,[1] for DNA sequencing apply when an RNA template is used, although there are several differences in the detailed protocol[5,6].

Gel methods to directly sequence RNA have also been described[7,8,9]. The RNA is end-labelled with ^{32}P, and while the technique is useful for comparing 5' or 3' ends of RNA molecules, the lack of enzymes equivalent to the DNA-specific restriction endonucleases to generate suitable fragments (100-200 nucleotides long), and the difficulty in working with RNA compared with the relative stability of DNA, indicate that it is not the method of choice for extensive sequence analysis. The best approach to sequencing influenza virus RNA segments would seem to be via the cDNA copy. If necessary, dsDNA can be prepared, cloned in a plasmid vector, and amplified in *E.coli* to provide internal primers for sequencing. Because sequence variation is one of the most obvious properties of influenza virus genes, we prefer not to sequence a cloned gene. The chance of such a cloned gene having a sequence which varies from the RNA sequence which codes for the major hemagglutinin molecule of the strain under study seems to us to be unacceptably high.

MATERIALS AND METHODS

Viruses

The influenza virus strains used were A/Mem/1/71(H3N2), A/Mem/10/78("USSR", H1N1), A/FW/1/50(H1N1), A/RI/5$^-$/57(H2N2), A/PR/8/34(H0N1), and B/Lee/40. All virus stocks were kindly provided by Dr. W.G. Laver. The viruses were grown in embryonated chicken eggs and purified by adsorption to and elution from red blood cells followed by sucrose density centrifugation[10].

Chemicals and enzymes

^{32}P-labelled deoxynucleoside triphosphates (350 Ci/mol or >2000 Ci/mol) were obtained from the Radiochemical Centre, Amersham, England. Dideoxynucleoside triphosphates and pd(T_8A) were from P-L Biochemicals, Milwaukee, Wis. U.S.A. Reverse transcriptase was generously supplied by Dr. J.W. Beard (Life Sci. Inc., St. Petersberg, Fla. U.S.A.) under NCI contract. The synthetic dodecanucleotide primer d(A-G-C-A-A-A-A-G-C-A-G-G) was from Collaborative Research, and was obtained from Dr. C-J Lai.

Preparation of template for cDNA synthesis

Extraction of virion RNA, *in vitro* addition of a 3' poly A sequence by *E.coli* adenyl transferase, separation of the RNA segments by polyacrylamide gel electrophoresis and elution of RNA segments from the gel were as previously described[5,6]. In some experiments the RNA segments were polyadenylated after the gel separation.

Nucleotide sequencing procedures

Sequences from the 3' end of the viral RNA were obtained by the dideoxy method[1] using thin polyacrylamide gels (200x400x0.4mm)[11] as previously described[6].

The polyadenylated RNA is used as template in the synthesis of cDNA with the primer d(pT$_8$A) and reverse transcriptase. More recently, a commercially available oligonucleotide which is complementary to the 12-nucleotide sequence at the 3' end common to all RNA segments of all influenza A strains[4] has been used to specifically prime cDNA synthesis on viral RNA without the need for polyadenylation.

RESULTS AND DISCUSSION

1. Sequences from the 3' end of RNA segment 7 (matrix gene)

Fig. 1 shows dideoxy sequencing gels with the sequence of cDNA from nucleotides 93 to 210 transcribed from the 3' ends of viral RNA segment 7 of strains

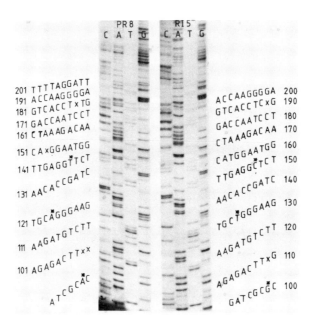

Fig. 1. Autoradiograph of an 8% polyacrylamide gel showing the sequences of cDNA transcribed from RNA segment 7 (matrix gene) from nucleotide 93 to 210 of influenza A strains PR8(HON1) and RI5⁻(H2N2). Nucleotides marked "X" cannot be identified from this gel, but were obtained from other experiments. Nucleotide differences are marked by an asterix. Nucleotide 1 is complementary to the 3' U of the RNA.

A/PR/8/34(HON1) and A/RI/5⁻/57(H2N2). As preliminary results[5] showed, this gene is highly conserved, only three nucleotide differences occuring in the first 200 of matrix gene sequences of PR8 and RI5⁻. These are at positions 99, 124 and 147, and are indicated in Fig. 1. The sequence of PR8 matrix protein predicted from the nucleotide sequence has been confirmed by tryptic and chymotryptic peptide compositions from nucleotide 29 to 55 and 95 to 210.

2. Sequences from the NS gene (RNA segment 8) of influenza A and B viruses.

Nucleotide sequences of cDNA transcribed from the 3' ends of RNA segment 8 of influenza strains A/PR/8/34, A/RI/5⁻/57 and B/Lee/40 have been obtained using the dideoxy method, with depurination analysis of specific dideoxy-terminated products used for partial confirmation of the sequences (Air and Hackett, unpublished results). In the first 80 nucleotides there are 3 differences when the sequences of segment 8 from PR8 (33T, 35C, 50T) and RI5⁻ (33C, 35T, 50C) are compared. The sequences are of the same sense as mRNA, but in the absence of protein data we cannot be certain where protein synthesis initiates. However, there is now considerable evidence that in eukaryotic mRNA's, the first AUG triplet downstream of the cap at the 5' end initiates

```
                                                                              T  C
A/PR/8/34                                    10            20           30   Ser
A/RI/5⁻/57            T₈A - - - - A A G C A G G G T G A C A A A G A C A T A A T G G A T C C T
                                                                            Met Asp Pro

               10            20           30            40           50
B/Lee/40   T₈A - - - - A A G C A G A G G A T T T A T T T A G T C A C T G G C A A A C G G A A A G A T G G C G G A
                                                                            Met Ala Asp


                       T
PR8              40          50            60            70           80
RI5⁻      A A C A C T G T G T C A A G C T T T C A G G T A G A T T G C T T C C T T T G G C A T G T C C G C A A
          Asn  Thr  Val  Ser  Ser  Phe  Gln  Val  Asp  Cys  Phe  Leu  Trp  His  Val  Arg  Lys

                     60            70           80            90          100
B/Lee     C A A C A T G A C C A C A A C A C A A A T T G A G G T G G G T C C G G G A G C A A C C A A T G C C A
          Asn  Met  Thr  Thr  Thr  Gln  Ile  Glu  Val  Gly  Pro  Gly  Ala  Thr  Asn  Ala


                  90          100           110           120          130
RI5⁻      A C A A G T T G C A G A C C A A G A A C T A G G T G A T G C C C C A T T C C T T G A T C G G
          Gln  Val  Ala  Asp  Gln  Glu  Leu  Gly  Asp  Ala  Pro  Phe  Leu  Asp  Arg

                    110           120          130           140          150
B/Lee     C T A T A A A C T T T G A A T C A G G A A T T C T G G A G T G C T A T A A A C G G T T T T C A T G G C
          Thr  Ile  Asn  Phe  Glu  Ser  Gly  Ile  Leu  Glu  Cys  Tyr  Lys  Gly  Phe  His  Gly
```

Fig. 2. Nucleotide and predicted amino acid sequences of cDNA transcribed from RNA segment 8 (NS gene) of influenza strains A/PR8, A/RI5⁻ and B/Lee. The sequences are aligned so that the presumed initiating codons correspond.

protein synthesis[12], and this is the case in other influenza genes[5,6,13]. The first AUG codons of gene 8 mRNA of A and B strains are therefore likely candidates for initiation codons, and the N-terminal protein sequences which can be predicted from the first AUG triplet are shown in Fig. 2.

RNA segment 8 has been shown to code for two polypeptides. One is the "non-structural" protein (NS1) which accumulates in infected cells, and the other, of which little is known except a MW estimate from gel electrophoresis is now called NS2[15]. No peptide analysis or sequences are yet available for the NS1 or NS2 polypeptides, and whether the protein sequence predicted is that of NS1 or NS2 (or neither) is not known. However, there is near identity in the nucleotide sequence in the 5' end region of the mRNA.

In influenza B viruses, RNA segment 8 also codes for the NS1 protein, and possibly also NS2[14,15]. In cDNA transcribed from RNA segments of influenza strain B/Lee/40, nucleotide 1 is A, as in the A strains, and nucleotides 6-11 are the same as the A strain common sequence. Nucleotide 12, however, is A instead of G in segments 4, 5, 6, 7 and 8 of B/Lee/40 cDNA (J. Blok & G. Air, unpublished results). Following the nucleotides 6-11 common to all A strains and B/Lee/40 the nucleotide sequence of B/Lee/40 cDNA complementary to RNA segment 8 shows no similarities to the highly conserved sequence of the A strains PR/8/34 and RI/5⁻/57 for at least 130 nucleotides. When the proposed N-terminal amino acid sequences are aligned (Fig. 2) there are still no apparent homologies.

3. Sequences from the hemagglutinin genes (RNA segment 4) of influenza A viruses.

Attempts to sequence from the 3' ends of adenylated RNA segment 4 priming with d(T$_8$A) were successful only for one strain (RI5⁻,H2N2), from which a sequence of 121 nucleotides was obtained[6]. Use of the synthetic dodecamer primer without the need to adenylate the RNA has enabled sequences from the hemagglutinin genes of this and other subtypes to be obtained consistently for 250 nucleotides and sometimes to 370 nucleotides. The strains used were A/PR/8/34(HON1), A/Mem/10/78(H1N1), and A/Mem/1/71(H3N2). Some of the sequences have been partially confirmed by amino acid sequence data[16,17] or peptide compositions[18].

Fig. 3 shows the sequence obtained of nucleotides 170 to 300 from RI5⁻(H2) hemagglutinin gene, and for comparison, the same region from the hemagglutinin gene of Mem/71(H3). There are no obvious similarities in these cDNA sequences.

Using the synthetic dodecamer primer, we had some trouble identifying the first few nucleotides following the common 12-nucleotide sequence represented by

the primers. Double-labelling (^{32}P-dATP and ^{32}P-dGTP) with relatively high
levels of dideoxytriphosphate gave sequences from nucleotide 14 (1-12 being the
primer), and some results with different subtypes are shown in Fig. 4.
Nucleotide number 13 will not be seen unless ^{32}P-labelled dideoxynucleoside
triphosphates are used. However, when cDNA synthesis was carried out in a

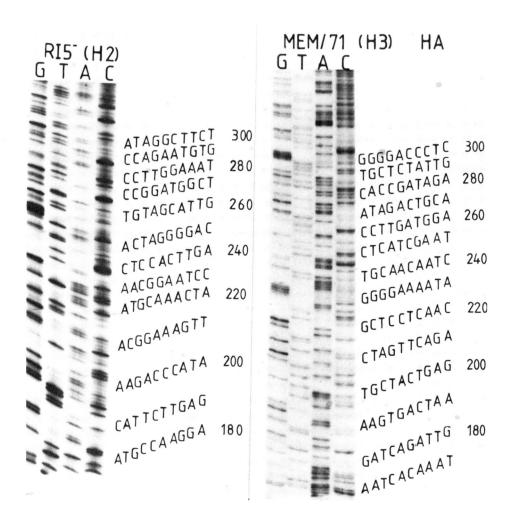

Fig. 3. Autoradiographs of long runs on 8% polyacrylamide gels showing
nucleotide sequences of cDNA transcribed from RNA segment 4 (hemagglutinin gene)
of influenza A strains RI/5⁻/57(H2N2) and Mem/1/71(H3N2). As before,
nucleotides are numbered from the A which is complementary to the 3' U of the
viral RNA strand.

reaction mix which contains dGTP and ddGTP, but no other nucleoside triphosphates, the "G" band at position 14 still appears, inferring that position 13 is also G, in subtypes H0 (PR8), H1 (Mem/10/78) and H3 (Mem/71) as it is in an H2 strain (RI5⁻)[6].

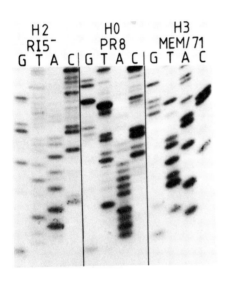

Fig. 4. Radioautograph of a 12% polyacrylamide gel from a double-label experiment to determine the sequence following the end of the 12-nucleotide primer. The sequences, which can be read from nucleotide 14, are:

                14
PR8   G-A-A-A-A-T-A-A-A-A-A

            ‾ 14
RI5   G-T-T-A-T-A-C-C-A-T

              14
Mem/71 G-A-T-G-A-T-T-C-T-A-T-T-A

The hemagglutinin is known to be synthesised as a single polypeptide which is processed to the mature surface antigen by removal of a "signal" peptide, glycosylation, and cleavage into HA1 and HA2, although the order in which these events occur is unknown. Skehel and Waterfield[19] determined the N-terminal amino acid sequence of HA1 from several strains of influenza A viruses of subtypes H0, H1 and H2. The N-terminus of H3 hemagglutinin is blocked, and has recently been shown to be a cyclized glutamine residue[16]. Therefore for these subtypes of hemagglutinin it is possible to identify the N-terminal sequence coded in the cDNA, and hence, by reading back to an A-T-G triplet in the same reading frame, to delineate the "signal peptide" which is cleaved off during processing[17]. By reading on from the approximately 9 amino acids of the known sequences, we can predict the further amino acid sequences of HA1 of the various subtypes, and nucleotide and amino acid sequences of hemagglutinin of influenza A virus of subtypes H0, H2 and H3 are shown in Fig. 5. In the H0 strain (PR8) and the H2 (RI5⁻) sequence[6] there is only one possible initiating A-T-G sequence in the cDNA. In the H3 sequence (Mem/71) there are two A-T-G sequences in the same reading frame as the known amino acid sequence of the HA1 peptides (Fig. 4). In Fig. 5 we have implied that the second A-T-G (nucleotides 30-32) is the initiating codon, but maybe the first, at nucleotides 15-17 (Fig. 4), is used[12] in this strain. The cDNA sequence of another H3 strain (Victoria/75, as represented by A/CSL Vic/77) has only one A-T-G in this region, at nucleotides 30-32.

The sequences shown in Fig. 5 have been aligned to maximise homology at the

```
                    10              20                          40
PR8    A G C A A A A G C A G G G G A A A A T A A A A A C A A C C A A A A T G A A G G C A A A C C T A C T G
                                                                   Met   Lys  Ala  Asn  Leu  Leu
             10              20                          40
RI5⁻   A A G C A G G G G T T A T A C C A T C G A C A A C C A A A A G C A A A A C A A T G G C C A T C A T T
                                                                           Met  Ala  Ile  Ile
          30              40              50              60              70
Mem/71 T A A C C A T G A A G A C C A T T A T T G C T T T G A G C C A C A T T T T C T G T C T G G T T C T C
             Met  Lys  Thr  Ile  Ile  Ala  Leu  Ser  His  Ile  Phe  Cys  Leu  Val  Leu


                                                          80                          100
PR8    G T C C T G T T A T G T G C A C T T G T A G C T G C A G A T G C A G A C A C A A T A T G T A T A G G
       Val  Leu  Leu  Cys  Ala  Leu  Val  Ala  Ala  Asp  Ala ▲ Asp  Thr  Ile  Cys  Ile  Gly
                   60                          80                          100
RI5⁻   T A T C T C A T T C T C C T G T T C A C A G C A G T G A G A G G G G A C C A G A T A T G C A T T G G
       Tyr  Leu  Ile  Leu  Leu  Phe  Thr  Ala  Val  Arg  Gly ▲ Asp  Gln  Ile  Cys  Ile  Gly
                          80                          100                         120
Mem/71 G G C C A A T A C C T T C C A G G A A A T G A C A A C A G C A C A G C A A C G C T G T G T C T G G G
       Gly ▲ Gln  Tyr  Leu  Pro  Gly  Asn  Asp  Asn  Ser  Thr  Ala  Thr  Leu  Cys  Leu  Gly


                        120                         140
PR8    C T A C C A T G C G A A C A A T T C A A C C G A C A C T G T T G A C A C A G T A C T C G A G A A G A
       Tyr  His  Ala  Asn  Asn  Ser  Thr  Asp  Thr  Val  Asp  Thr  Val  Leu  Glu  Lys
                        120                         140
RI5⁻   A T A C C A T G C C A A T A A T T C C A C A G A G A A G G T C G A C A C A A T T C T A G A G C G G A
       Tyr  His  Ala  Asn  Asn  Ser  Thr  Glu  Lys  Val  Asp  Thr  Ile  Leu  Glu  Arg
                                140                         160
Mem/71 A C A T C A T G C A G T G C C A A A C G G A A C A C T A G T G A A A A C A A T C A C A A A T G A T C
       His  His  Ala  Val  Pro  Asn  Gly  Thr  Leu  Val  Lys  Thr  Ile  Thr  Asn  Asp


                        160                         180                         200
PR8    A T G T G A C A G T A A C A C A C T C T G T T A A C C T G C T C G A A G A C A G C C A C A A C G G A
       Asn  Val  Thr  Val  Thr  His  Ser  Val  Asn  Leu  Leu  Glu  Asp  Ser  His  Asn  Gly
              160                         180                         200
RI5⁻   A C G T C A C T G T G A C T C A T G C C A A G G A C A T T C T T G A G A A G A C C C A T A A C G G A
       Asn  Val  Thr  Val  Thr  His  Ala  Lys  Asp  Ile  Leu  Glu  Lys  Thr  His  Asn  Gly
                     180                         200                         220
Mem/71 A G A T T G A A G T G A C T A A T G C T A C T G A G C T A G T T C A G A G C T C C T C A A C G G G G
       Gln  Ile  Glu  Val  Thr  Asn  Ala  Thr  Glu  Leu  Val  Gln  Ser  Ser  Ser  Thr  Gly


                        220                         240
PR8    A A A C T A T G T A G A T T A A A A G G A A T A G C C C C A C T A C A A T T G G G G A A A T G T A A
       Lys  Leu  Cys  Arg  Leu  Lys  Gly  Ile  Ala  Pro  Leu  Gln  Leu  Gly  Lys  Cys  Asn
                        220                         240
RI5⁻   A A G T T A T G C A A A C T A A A C G G A A T C C C T C C A C T T G A A C T A G G G G A C T G T A G
       Lys  Leu  Cys  Lys  Leu  Asn  Gly  Ile  Pro  Pro  Leu  Glu  Leu  Gly  Asp  Cys
                            240                         260
Mem/71 A A A A T A T G C A A C A A T C C T C A T C G A A T C C T T G A T G G A A T A G A C T G C A C A C C
       Lys  Ile  Cys  Asn  Asn  Pro  His  Arg  Ile  Leu  Asp  Gly  Ile  Asp  Cys  Thr  Pro
```

Fig. 5. Nucleotide sequences of cDNA transcribed from the 3' end of the hema-gglutinin gene (RNA segment 4) and predicted amino acid sequences of hemagglutinin of influenza A viruses of subtypes H0 (PR/8/32), H2 (RI/5⁻/57) and H3 (Mem/1/71). The presumed initiating ATG codons are underlined, and arrows indicate the final cleavage which generates the amino terminus of the mature HA1 polypeptide [16,19]. The nucleotide sequence of H1 strains (FW/1/50 and Mem/10/78) are almost identical to the H0(PR8) sequence shown here.

$^{Leu}_{Ile}$-Cys-$^{Leu}_{Ile}$-X-X-His-Ala sequence[19] close to the N-terminus of H0 and H2 subtypes, although 10 residues further from the N-terminus of the H3 hemagglutinin[16]. As noted for the nucleotide sequences shown in Fig. 3, there are very few similarities in nucleotide or amino acid sequences when the H2 and H3 subtype hemagglutinins are aligned.

Sequences have also been obtained from Hl hemagglutinins (A/Mem/10/78,HlNl and A/FW/1/50,HlNl). In 250 nucleotides of cDNA only two differences can be seen between the 1978 Mem/10 strain and the 1950 FW strain, and these differences do not alter the amino acid sequence.

More surprisingly, there is also remarkable conservation when the Hl sequence

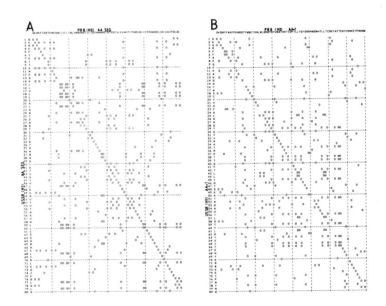

Fig. 6. Computer matching[20] of amino terminal sequences. A. Comparison of amino acid sequences read in the correct reading frame from the hemagglutinin genes of PR8 (H0) and Mem/10/78("USSR",Hl). These sequences are almost identical. B. Comparison of "amino acid sequences" read in a reading frame displaced one nucleotide from the correct one. The high degree of homology retained shows that there are only 18 nucleotide differences between H0 and Hl hemagglutinins in this region (approximately 14% of the gene).

is compared with H0. Since comparisons of nucleotide sequences are difficult to interpret (because the random background "match rate" is 1 in 4), we have compared amino acid sequences. Where there is high homology, "amino acid sequences" read from a reading frame displaced one nucleotide from the real one can be used to test whether there are significant numbers of third position changes in codons. Some results are shown in Fig. 6. The amino acid sequences of the H0 and H1 strains are nearly identical, and when "wrong" reading frame sequences are compared, this near identity remains. Therefore both protein and nucleic acid sequences are very highly conserved through the H0 and H1 subtype hemagglutinins.

Fig. 7 shows the comparison of PR8 (H0) and RI5⁻ (H2) hemagglutinin sequences. There is high homology in the mature HA1 sequence, but this homology is almost invisible when the "wrong" reading frame is used. The conclusion is

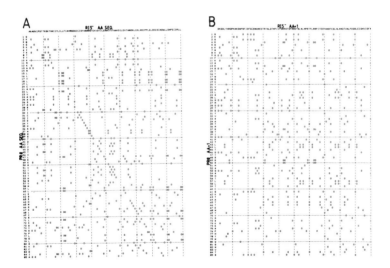

Fig. 7. A. Comparison of amino acid sequences read from the nucleotide sequence of the hemagglutinin genes from RI5⁻ (H2) and PR8(H0). There is good homology from the N-terminus of the mature HA1, but none in the signal peptide. B. Comparison of the wrong "amino acid sequences" as in Fig. 6B. The lack of significant homology indicates that although the amino acid sequences are very similar (A), there are many changes in the third nucleotide of the codons used.

that there is strong pressure to conserve the amino acid sequence, but the nucleotide sequence is more variable. The regions coding for the signal peptide are thus entirely different, and in the HA1 coding sequence there are many differences in the codons used.

The percent homologies in amino acid sequences between subtypes of influenza A hemagglutinin are shown in Table 1.

TABLE 1

PERCENTAGE AMINO ACID SEQUENCE HOMOLOGIES IN THE N-TERMINAL 70-80 AMINO ACIDS (INCLUDING THE SIGNAL PEPTIDE) BETWEEN HEMAGGLUTININS OF DIFFERENT SUBTYPES OF INFLUENZA A VIRUSES

	PR8(H0)	Mem/78(H1)	RI5(H2)	Mem/71(H3)
PR/8/34	100	95.6	56.9	19.8
Mem/10/78		100	56.3	19.3
RI/5⁻/57			100	21.0
Mem/1/71				100

ACKNOWLEDGEMENTS

This work was supported in part by Grant AI 15343 from the National Institutes of Health, U.S.A. and the Australian Government Poultry Industry Trust Fund. Anne Mackenzie and Sally Campbell provided expert technical assistance.

REFERENCES

1. Sanger, F., Nicklen, S. and Coulson, A.R. (1977) Proc. Nat. Acad. Sci. 74, 5463-5467.
2. Sippel, A.E. (1973) Europ. J. Biochem. 37, 31-40.
3. Lewandowski, L.J., Content, J. and Leppla, S.H. (1971) J. Virol. 8, 701-707.
4. Skehel, J.J. and Hay, A.J. (1978) Nucl. Acids Res. 5, 1207-1219.
5. Both, G.W. and Air, G.M. (1979) Europ. J. Biochem. 96, 363-372.
6. Air, G.M. (1979) Virology 97, 468-472.
7. Simoncsits, A., Brownlee, G.G., Brown, R.S., Rubin, J.R. and Guilley, H. (1977) Nature 269, 833-836.
8. Donis-Keller, H., Maxam, A.M. and Gilbert, W. (1977) Nucl. Acids Res. 4, 2527-2538.
9. Stanley, J. and Vassilenko, S. (1978) Nature 274, 87-89.
10. Laver, W.G. (1969a) In Fundamental Techniques in Virology (Eds. K. Habel and N.P. Salzman), pp. 82-86.
11. Sanger, F. and Coulson, A.R. (1978) FEBS Letters 87, 107-110.
12. Kozak, M. (1978) Cell 15, 1109-1123.
13. Porter, A.G., Barber, C., Carey, N.H., Hallewell, R.A., Threlfall, G. and Emtage, J.S. (1979) Nature, 282, 471-477.

14. Rancaniello, V.R. and Palese, P. (1979) J. Virol. 29, 361-373.
15. Lamb, R.A. and Choppin, P.W. (1979) Proc. Natl. Acad. Sci. 76, 4908-4912.
16. Ward, C.W. and Dopheide, T.A. this volume.
17. Waterfield, M.D., Espelie, K., Elder, K., and Skehel, J.J. (1979) Brit. Med. Bull. 35, 57-64.
18. Laver, W.G., Gerhard, W., Webster. R.G., Frankel, M.E., and Air, G.M. (1979) Proc. Natl. Acad. Sci. 76, 1425-1429.
19. Skehel, J.J. and Waterfield, M.D. (1975) Proc. Natl. Acad. Sci. 72, 93-97.
20. Gibbs, A.J. and McIntyre, G.A. (1970) Europ. J. Biochem. 16, 1-11.

DISCUSSION

Salser: Are the changes in the M gene silent and those in the genes for HA and NA the result of positive selection?

Air: That is not what we see.

Brownlee: The third position of codons are frequently non-random so a change in these could still represent selection.

Air: The questions we are asking are whether the surface antigen genes have some mutator function and change faster, or whether all flu genes mutate fast and most changes get selected out, or whether there is less pressure for conservation in the flu systems.

Scholtissek: Using hybridization technique we find about 30% RNAse protection when A and B segment 7's are compared, so perhaps your sample size is too small.

Air: That may be right - since the B genes are longer, we may just be looking at the extra sequence.

Sambrook: I am surprised there are so few deletions in these sequences. Why are there?

Air: I am surprised there are so many, since nucleotides have to be inserted or deleted in multiples of 3. We don't see a region where the reading frame is different, and then comes back, we see simple amino acid insertions or deletions.

Sambrook: There is less deletion than in "ordinary" viruses like adenovirus.
Gibbs: How do you know they are deletions not insertions?
Sambrook: We don't. There is no way of telling.

THE SYNTHESIS AND CLONING OF LARGE INFLUENZA A cDNAS USING SYNTHETIC DNA PRIMERS

IAN CUMMINGS[+] AND WINSTON SALSER[+,++]
[+]Institute of Molecular Biology, University of California, 405 Hilgard Avenue, Los Angeles, California 90024; [++]Department of Biology, University of California, 405 Hilgard Avenue, Los Angeles, California 90024

INTRODUCTION

Detailed analysis of the structure and organization of the influenza A virus genome will be crucial to the understanding of its unique place in nature. Such investigations can most easily be carried out upon recombinant DNAs derived from the viral RNAs. We describe in this paper the generation of large double stranded cDNAs from A/USSR/90/77 (H1N1) and their propagation as recombinant DNAs in the E. coli strain X1776. Our approach is unique in that the first strand reverse transcriptase product was primed by a twelve nucleotide synthetic DNA primer which is complementary to the conserved 3' termini of all eight genome RNA segments.[1] Because these twelve nucleotides are found at the 3' termini of the genome fragments of all influenza A strains studied to date, this approach should provide a simple means of cloning any isolate encountered.

MATERIALS AND METHODS

Virus and virus purification. A/USSR/90/77 (H1N1) was a gift from R. Webster. The virus was grown at 37°C in twelve day chicken embryos for two days. Harvested virus was then purified after pelleting from allantoic fluid on 20-60% (w/v) linear sucrose gradients in a Beckman SW27 rotor. Viral RNAs were isolated by a standard phenol-chloroform-SDS extraction after proteinase K treatment.

Bacterial strain and cloning vehicle. E. coli X1776 was obtained from R. Curtiss III.[2] The cloning vehicle, pBR322, has been described previously.[3]

Enzymes. Restriction endonuclease Pst I was purified by the method of Greene et al.[4] Avian myeloblastosis virus reverse transcriptase was obtained from the Office of Program Resources and Logistics of the Viral Cancer Program, National Cancer Institute, Bethesda, Maryland 20014. DNA polymerase I (Klenow fragment) was purchased from Boehringer-Mannheim. Nuclease S_1 was obtained from Miles Research Laboratories. Adenyl transferase was purified by the method of Sippel.[5] Proteinase K was purchased from Merck.

Radioactive nucleoside triphosphates. alpha ^{32}p deoxycytidine triphosphate was purchased from New England Nuclear.

Plasmid DNA purification. Plasmid DNAs were isolated from one liter growths by the method of Humphreys et al.[6]

Synthetic DNA primer. A dodecamer reverse transcriptase primer of the nucleotide sequence 5'- AGCAAAAGCAGG-3' was kindly provided by T. Hozumi, R. Arentzen and K. Itakura at the City of Hope Medical Center, Duarte, California.

cDNA synthesis. The dodecamer primer (above) was used to specifically prime influenza cDNA in reverse transcription of the cloned cDNAs. Other viral RNA was in vitro tailed by adenyl transferase by the method of Sippel[5] as modified by Alan Davis for synthesis of cDNA using oligo dT primers. Viral RNA templates were pretreated with methyl mercury hydroxide by the method of Payvar and Schimke prior to use as template.[7] Double stranded cDNA was synthesized from viral minus strands by the method of Buell et al[8], except that the Klenow fragment of E. coli DNA polymerase I was substituted for polymerase I and each nucleoside triphosphate was present at 2 mM concentration.

Size fractionation of cDNAs. Double stranded cDNAs were fractionated by size on a 10-40% (w/v) sucrose gradient in 100mM NaCl 10mM Tris HCl 2mM EDTA pH 7.4 at 36K for 24 hours at 25° C in a Beckman SW 41 rotor. This fractionation removed low molecular weight material prior to cloning. Transcripts larger than one kilobase in size were pooled after collecting drop fractions by bottom puncture and ethanol precipitated after adding magnesium chloride to 10mM concentration.

Insertion of cDNAs into pBR322. Influenza A cDNAs were dC

tailed and inserted into dG tailed Pst I linearized pBR322 DNA by the method of Goeddel et al.[9]

Transformation into X1776 host. Transformation of X1776 with the dG-dC hybrid DNA was carried out by a modification of the method of L. Villa-Komaroff[10] as developed by J. Browne in this laboratory.

Colony hybridization. Colonies obtained from the transformation were tested for ampicillin or tetracycline resistances on minimal agar plates with the respective drug at 20 micrograms per milliliter. All clones were then picked onto nitrocellulose grids and prepared for hybridization by the method of Grunstein and Hogness.[11] Radioactive first strand cDNA probe was prepared as described above except that the 2mM unlabelled deoxycytidine triphosphate was replaced with ^{32}P deoxycytidine triphosphate at 2 millicuries per milliliter (approximate specific activity 700 Ci/mM). After removal of unincorporated triphosphates this cDNA was hybridized to the colony hybridization filters in 5X SSC, 1% polyvinylpyrollidone, 1% ficoll, 1% bovine serum albumin at 65° C for 24 hours. Positive colonies were detected after washing the filters in 1XSSC 0.1%SDS at 62° C for 3 hours by autoradiography on Cronex-4 X-ray film (Dupont).

Gel electrophoresis. Plasmid DNAs were run on 0.8% agarose gels in 80mM Tris·HCl 10 mM sodium acetate 2mM EDTA pH 7.8 with 0.5 micrograms per milliliter of ethidium bromide present in the running buffer. Other DNAs were electrophoresed on 2.2% polyacrylamide 0.6% agarose 6M urea gels as described by Floyd et al.[12]

RESULTS

cDNA synthesis. High molecular weight double stranded cDNA was synthesized from methyl mercury hydroxide pretreated viral minus strand RNAs. The average yield during first strand cDNA synthesis was 40-50% by mass (40-50 nanograms first strand per 100 nanograms template) as estimated by trichloroacetic acid-precipitable radioactivity. Little or no cDNA synthesis was observed when the dodecamer primer DNA was omitted. Second

150

strand synthesis by the Klenow fragment of DNA polymerase I yielded 60-80% by mass. The radioactive nucleotides incorporated into the double stranded cDNA product were 90% resistant to S_1 nuclease during cleavage of the hairpin loop left by reverse transcriptase.[13,14,15] The S_1 nuclease product was found to be less than 5% resistant to further S_1 nuclease treatment after denaturation at 100° C followed by quick cooling to 4° C. Similarly treated DNA polymerase I product was 95% S_1 resistant prior to hairpin cleavage. Electrophoresis of the reverse transcriptase, DNA polymerase and S_1 nuclease products upon 2.2% polyacrylamide 0.6% agarose 2M urea gels revealed major cDNA bands of 2.10, 1.75, 1.55, 1.45, 1.05 and 0.87 kilobases size in each reaction (see figure 1). These lengths are consistent with those estimated for these viral RNA segments by Sleigh, Both and Brownlee[16].

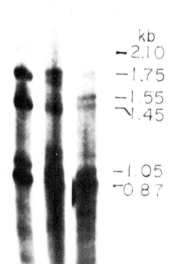

kb
— 2.10
— 1.75
— 1.55
⬎ 1.45

— 1.05
— 0.87

Fig. 1. Autoradiograph of 2.2% polyacylamide 0.6% agarose 6M urea gel electrophoresis of specific dodecamer primed ^{32}P-labelled cDNAs: A) reverse transcriptase product B) DNA polymerase I Klenow fragment product C) S_1 nuclease product. Sizes of discrete bands (as determined from coelectrophoresed ethidium bromide stained marker DNAs) are indicated in the gel margin.

The effect of pretreatment with methyl mercury hydroxide on

cDNA product size was evaluated by generating S₁-cleaved double stranded cDNA as above, except for the omission of this pretreatment. In these reactions double stranded cDNA was synthesized from oligo dT-primed *in vitro* polydenylated and dodecamer primed viral RNAs. These products were compared to those obtained with the dodecamer primer on methyl mercury hydroxide treated template by sedimentation through 10-40% (w/v) sucrose gradients. The pretreatment with methyl mercury hydroxide causes a dramatic increase in the size of the product: the peak mass-average product size (peak of radioactivity unadjusted for chain length) increases from 300 to 900 base pairs upon pretreatment (see figure 2).

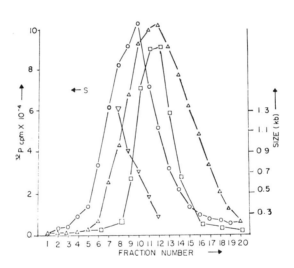

Fig. 2. 10-40% (w/v) sucrose gradient profiles of ³²P labelled double stranded S₁ treated cDNAs generated from: □ , *In vitro* polyadenylated-oligo dT primed viral RNA without methyl mercury hydroxide treatment; Δ , specific dodecamer primed viral RNA without methyl mercury hydroxide treatment; and ◯ , specific dodecamer primed methymercury hydroxide treated viral RNA. Size marker mobilities were estimated from parallel gradients and are indicated from the scale on the right ordinate by the symbol ▽ .

Molecular cloning of influenza cDNA. After dC-tailing, the sucrose gradient size selected cDNA product was annealed to dG-tailed Pst 1-linearized pBR322 DNA. The annealed DNAs were transformed into calcium shocked X1776 with an efficiency of 8 x 10^5 transformants per microgram of intact pBR322. Several thousand tetracycline resistant transformants were obtained from 20 nanograms of cDNA; more than 80% of these colonies were found to be ampicillin sensitive, indicating the possible interruption of the penicillinase locus by an insert molecule. All clones were screened by colony hybridization using radioactive first strand cDNAs as probe. Approximately 50 positive colonies were obtained from among 150 total clones screened. The presence of non-hybridizing clones may be the result of contaminating embryo cellular DNAs in the viral RNA preparation. An autoradiograph of the colony hybridization is shown in figure 3.

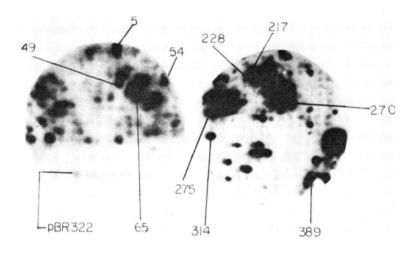

Fig. 3. Autoradiograph from colony hybridization filter of A/USSR/90/77 (H1N1) cDNA clones derived from cDNA shown in Figure 1. 8 x 10^6 cpm ^{32}P-labelled first strand cDNA was used as probe. The clone designations of the five representative positive clones chosen for further analysis are indicated with arrows. 7 negative controls (colonies carrying uninserted pBR322) appear in a line near the filter bottom.

One liter growths of many positive clones were obtained. Pst 1 digestions of the recombinant DNAs were electrophoresed on 0.8% agarose gels to determine the length of excisible inserts. Inserts were detected corresponding to all of those gene copy sizes shown in figure 1 except for the 0.87 kilobase fragment (cDNA transcripts of this size and smaller were discarded in the sucrose gradient fraction step). In thirty six out of forty clones examined the insert sizes agreed precisely with the sizes of cDNA bands in figure 1, suggesting that this cloning procedure may efficiently and reproduceably give full size clones. Figure 4 illustrates the sizes of ten representative Pst 1 cleaved plasmids obtained from the ten colonies indicated in figure 3.

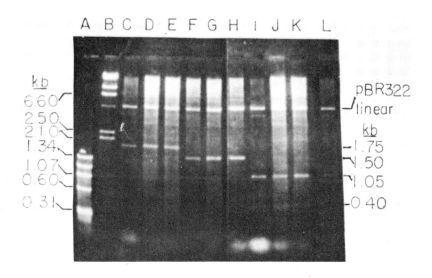

Fig. 4. 0.8% agarose gel electrophoresis of Pst 1 cleaved clone DNAs. Sizes of standard DNAs are shown in the left margin. Insert bands are indicated by dark triangles. Tracks: A) Hind III cleaved wild type lambda bacteriophage DNA; B) Hae III cleaved ØX 174 am3 bacteriophage DNA; C) pD49; D) pD270; E) pD228; F) pD5; G) pD217; H) pD389; I) pD65; J) pD275; K) pD314 and L) pD54.

Plasmids pD49, pD228 and pD270 have inserts of 1.75 kb with

154

internal Eco R_1 sites in identical map positions (data not shown). Plasmids pD5, pD217 and pD389 have inserts of 1.55 kb. Plasmids pD65, pD275 and pD314 have inserts which contain a single Pst 1 site such that the excised inserts migrate as two fragments of 1.05 and 0.40 kb. These three plasmids have Bam H1 sites in identical map positions with respect to the internal Pst 1 site (data not shown). Plasmid pD54 has an insert of 1.05 kb. Further analysis of these clones is now in progress, including absolute gene segment assignments by hybridization, restriction endonuclease mapping and DNA sequence analysis.

ACKNOWLEDGMENTS

The authors wish to thank Dennis Kleid, Keiichi Itakura, Toyohara Hozumi and Rene Arentzen for helpful discussions and for synthesizing and providing the primer used in this work. Alan Davis and Debi Nayak are thanked for helpful discussions. We also wish to thank Dean Gilbert and Jocyndra Wright for their skilled technical assistance. This work was funded in part by Genentech Inc., South San Francisco, California.

REFERENCES

1. Skehel, J.J. and Hay, A.J. (1978) Nucleic Acids Res., 5, 1207-1219.
2. Curtiss, R. III et al. (1977) in Molecular Cloning of Recombinant DNAs (Scott, W.A. and Werner, R. ed.), Academic Press, New York, pp. 99-111.
3. Bolivar, F., Rodriguez, R.C., Greene, P.J., Betlach, M.C., Heyneker, H.C., Boyer, H.W., Crosa, J.H. and Falkow, S. (1977) Gene, 2, 95-113.
4. Greene, P., Heyneker, H.L., Bolivar, F., Rodriguez, R.L., Betlach, M.C., Covarrubias, A.A., Backman, K., Kussel, D.J., Tait,R. and Boyer,H.W. (1978) Nucleic Acids Res. 5, 2373-2380.
5. Sippel, A.E. (1973) Eur. J. Biochem., 37, 31-40.
6. Humphreys, G.O., Willshaw, G.A. and Anderson, E.S. (1975) Biochim. Biophys. Acta. 383, 457-463.
7. Payvar, F. and Schimke, R.T. (1979) J. Biol. Chem., 254, 7636-7642.
8. Buell, G.N., Wickens, M.P., Payvar, F. and Schimke, R.T. (1978) J. Biol. Chem., 253, 2471-2482.
9. Goeddel, D.V., Heyneker, H.L., Hozumi, T., Arentzen, R., Itakura, K., Yansura, D.G., Ross, M.J., Miozzari, G., Crea, R. and Seeburg, P. (1979) Nature, 281, 544-548.
10. Villa-Komaroff, L., Efstratiadis, A., Broome, S., Lomedico,

P., Tizard, R., Nabers, S.P., Chick, W.L. and Gilbert, W. (1978) Proc. Natl. Acad. Sci. USA, 75, 3727-3731.

11. Grunstein, M. and Hogness, D. (1975) Proc. Natl. Acad. Sci. USA, 72, 3961-3972.

12. Floyd, R.W., Stone, M.P. and Joklik, W.K. (1974) Anal. Biochem. 59, 599-609.

13. Salser, W.A. (1974) Ann. Rev. Biochem.,, 43, 923-965.

14. Efstratiadis, A., Kafatos, F.C., Maxam, A.M. and Maniatis, T. (1976) Cell, 7, 279-288.

15. Monahan, J.J., McReynolds, L.A. and O'Malley, B.W. (1976) J. Biol. Chem., 251, 7355-7362.

16. Sleigh, M.J., Both, G.W. and Brownlee, G.G. (1979) Nucleic Acids Res., 6, 1309-1321.

(See DISCUSSION on following page)

DISCUSSION

Palese: Do you think the methyl mercury hydroxide treatment
   might introduce errors in the reverse transcription?

Salser: We reverse it with sulphydryl reagents, otherwise it
   would not function as a template and the equilibrium
   constant favors the dissociation.

Brownlee: There could be a minor side reaction which would
   interfere with transcription.

Salser: The transcriptase tends to stop at modified bases, rather
   than to insert or mismatch.

Both: In our case with ds synthesis with reverse transcriptase,
   the first strand is made very rapidly, but the second takes
   5 hours. This does not fit with your model.

Brownlee: The loopback model seems not to be general, since
   second strand synthesis varies a lot between molecules and the
   self-priming reaction can occur.

Sleigh: And there is no problem in copying right to the ends
   because this has been often used to sequence the ends.

Bean: Why is methyl mercury hydroxide treatment better than heat-
   quickchill?

Cummings: Schimke has also shown this is better - heating gives
   more counts incorporated, but shorter products.

Gething: With the Jap HA gene it made no difference at all.

THE CLONING AND EXPRESSION IN ESCHERICHIA COLI OF AN INFLUENZA
HAEMAGGLUTININ GENE

SPENCER EMTAGE, WILLIAM TACON AND NORMAN CAREY
Searle Research and Development, Division of G. D. Searle & Co. Ltd.,
P. O. Box 53, Lane End Road, High Wycombe, Bucks HP12 4HL, England

INTRODUCTION

Influenza is still a major disease of man although severe illness and death
are confined mostly to the elderly.   The disease is usually mild in healthy
individuals and, at worst, results in days off work.   However, in England the
Hong Kong outbreak of 1968-1970 produced some 25 million lost working days in a
four month period,[1] while in the U.S. the effect of the Hong Kong variant of
1968-1969 was costed at 3.8 billion dollars.[2]   Thus, prevention of influenza
epidemics and pandemics would be of value both economically and socially.

The main structure involved in immunity against influenza is the
haemagglutinin (HA) surface glycoprotein.[3,4]   The functional HA subunit, one of
the spikes on the virus surface, is a triangular rod-shaped glycoprotein with a
MW of ∿250,000 and is comprised of 3 HA monomers.[5]   The HA monomers are
synthesised as single polypeptide chains containing an 18-amino acid precursor
peptide at the N-terminus.[6]   During maturation and virus assembly the pre-HA is
further processed to HA1 and HA2 which remain linked by disulphide bridges.[7,8]

Recent advances in genetic engineering and our knowledge of the structure and
sequence of bacterial operons and control elements now allow the construction of
new bacterial strains with the potential of synthesising large quantities of
viral proteins (antigens) which may ultimately be useful as vaccines.   In this
paper we describe the construction of expression plasmids based on the
tryptophan operon and demonstrate their use by producing haemagglutinin antigen
from an HA gene cloned in E. coli;   this is the first step towards testing the
feasibility of large scale antigen production by these means.

MATERIALS AND METHODS

A complete description of this work, giving full experimental detail and
methodology, will be published elsewhere.   The preparation of synthetic
influenza genes has already been described[9] while manuscripts describing the

cloning and sequencing of the Fowl Plague Virus Haemagglutinin gene,[6] the construction of the trp expression plasmids,[10] and the expression experiments[11] are in press.

RESULTS

Construction and Properties of expression vectors

Our approach to expressing eucaryotic genes in bacteria is based on the following rationale: a) ensure that transcription of the eucaryotic gene is efficient and controllable by providing a powerful bacterial promoter upstream of the gene to be expressed and b) ensure effective translation by using a bacterial ribosome binding site and initiator AUG to produce, in the first instance, a fused protein consisting of an N-terminal bacterial protein sequence followed by the eucaryotic sequences. The tryptophan regulatory region fulfils these requirements. Cells containing trp plasmids should synthesise low levels of gene products when grown in medium supplemented with tryptophan and should be derepressed for trp transcription by the addition of 3β-indoleacrylic acid.[12]

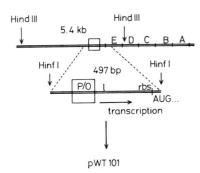

Fig. 1. The trp operon showing the promoter/operator region (P/O) and the five structural genes. The 5.4 Kb Hind III fragment contained in ptrp ED5-1 was the source of the 497 bp Hinfl fragment.

The trp operon is shown schematically in Fig. 1. It contains the E, D, C, B and A genes linked in tandem to the promoter/operator region. We have previously cloned the Hind III fragment containing the trp regulatory region, the trp E gene and part of the trp D gene.[13] This plasmid, ptrp ED5-1 was the progenitor of the new expression vectors. From ptrp ED5-1 we isolated a DNA fragment bounded by Hinfl restriction sites (Fig. 1.) and containing the trp promoter/operator region as well as the nucleotides specifying the leader sequence and first seven amino acids of trp E. The Hinfl ends of this fragment were repaired with DNA polymerase I, Hind III linkers attached to the resulting blunt ends and the fragment cloned into the Hind III site of pBR322.

Cloning into the Hind III site of pBR322 inactivates the tetracycline promoter[14] thereby rendering any transformants tetracycline sensitive unless the DNA inserted has its own promoter transcribing into the tetracycline genes. It was expected that transformants receiving a plasmid in which the Hinfl fragment was cloned in the orientation allowing transcription through the tetracycline gene region would exhibit a tet-r phenotype. This proved to be the case and from these transformants we isolated one plasmid, pWT101, for further characterisation.   Restriction enzyme analysis confirmed the orientation of the trp promoter with respect to the tetracycline genes. Further we showed that the degree of tetracycline resistance could be altered by the level of transcription from the trp promoter.   In the presence of excess tryptophan (100 µg/ml) HB101 cells containing pWT101 had an efficiency of plating on tetracycline supplemented minimal agar of 8.0 µg/ml tetracycline (this is the tetracycline concentration at which 50% of the cells survive). This value was raised to 15.5 µg/ml in the absence of tryptophan and to 46.5 µg/ml when induced with 3β-indoleacrylic acid or in the tryptophan repressor minus strain ED8689.

To convert pWT101 into a plasmid vector suitable for fusing foreign genes to the trp E fragment at its Hind III site it was necessary to remove the other Hind III site.   To accomplish this, pWT101 was digested with EcoRI, incubated with exonuclease III, digested with SI-nuclease to remove the 5'-protruding tails produced by the exonuclease and finally incubated with DNA polymerase I to produce perfect blunt ended molecules.   This DNA was recircularised with T4 DNA ligase and used to transform HB101 cells employing a double antibiotic selection (ampicillin and tetracycline) to ensure the continued expression of both the β-lactamase and tetracycline genes (the latter from the trp promoter). Eight transformants were selected at random for restriction analysis.   All eight plasmids had lost both the Hind III and EcoRI sites and the total DNA deleted varied from 51-361 base pairs.   The plasmid with the smallest deletion, pWT111 (Fig. 2.) was chosen as the Hind III expression vector with a cleavage position designated "0".[15]

pWT111 is designed to permit translation of DNA inserted at the Hind III site as a fused polypeptide in one reading frame only.   To produce the second reading frame the Hind III site of pWT111 was opened, repaired with DNA polymerase I and a second Hind III linker cloned into this position.   This adds 14 base pairs of DNA and gives a new Hind III site with a reading frame altered by plus one nucleotide ("+1" in the O'Farrell designation).[15]   This plasmid was called pWT121 and is shown in Fig. 2.

The third reading frame was obtained by repeating the same series of reactions on pWT121. The resulting plasmid, pWT131, provides the final reading frame ("-1").

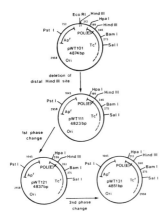

Fig. 2. Restriction maps of pWT101, pWT111, pWT121 and pWT131 illustrating the order of plasmid construction (Reproduced from Tacon et al.[10])

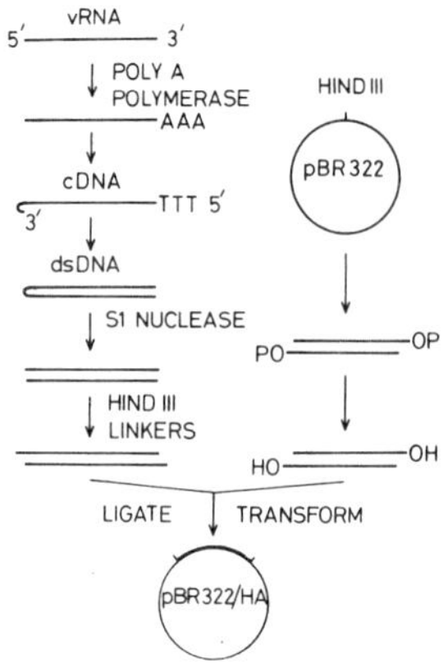

Fig. 3. Schematic diagram for the polyadenylation and reverse transcription of FPV RNA and insertion of ds DNA into bacterial plasmids using chemically synthesised restriction site linkers.

Cloning the HA gene of Fowl Plague Virus (FPV)

The segmented nature of the influenza viral genome[16] greatly facilitated the cloning of this gene. The enzymatic steps involved in the production and cloning of synthetic HA genes are shown in Fig. 3. Briefly, the eight viral RNA segments of unfractionated FPV RNA were polyadenylated in vitro and the complementary DNA strand made with reverse transcriptase and oligo(dT) as primer. Following the removal of the RNA template with alkali the second DNA strand was produced. As with other synthetic genes the two strands are covalently joined at this stage and must be converted to true double-stranded DNA with S1 nuclease.

Part of our strategy was to clone the HA gene in such a way that it could be transferred easily from one plasmid vector to another; for example, by using linker molecules containing restriction enzyme sites.[17] A prerequisite for this technique to be successful is that the gene of interest lacks sites for the enzyme in question. Since the synthetic FPV genes contained substantial numbers of full length or almost full length copies of all eight RNA segments it was possible to demonstrate that the HA gene contained no sites for the enzyme Hind III. Thus the SI-nuclease treated double-stranded FPV DNA was incubated with DNA polymerase I to produce "blunt ends", ligated to Hind III linkers and restricted with Hind III. This procedure produces molecules with Hind III "sticky ends" suitable for cloning into a Hind III vector such as pBR322. By these means we isolated a plasmid, named $pBR322/FPV_{4-10}$, containing an insert of ∿1700 nucleotides which hybridised specifically to a ^{32}P-labelled gene 4 probe (this is the haemagglutinin gene).

The complete nucleotide sequence of the cloned DNA has now been determined and will be presented in detail elsewhere at this meeting. However, to follow the experimental design it is necessary to describe the sequence of the cloned DNA containing the N-terminus of the HA gene. Fig. 4. shows this nucleotide sequence and the predicted amino acid sequence of the start of the pre-HA protein. The cloned DNA consists of Hind III linker, a stretch of 19 A:T base pairs originating from the poly (A) tail added to the vRNA and the oligo(dT) primer used during reverse transcription, 21 base pairs corresponding to the non-translated 5' region of the mRNA and finally the initiator AUG and coding region.

Thus the experimental design for expression was clear. We would transfer the HA gene to the Hind III site of the pWT plasmid series and assay for expression. As there are no stop codons in phase with the AUG of the HA gene one of the plasmids should produce a hybrid polypeptide containing the HA sequence.

```
                            ↓
pWT111:-ATG,CAA,ACA,CAA,AAA,CCG,ACT,CCA,AGC,TT...
       .MET GLN THR GLN LYS PRO THR, PRO SER
                    TRP E SPECIFIED          ↓
pWT121:-ATG,CAA,ACA,CAA,AAA,CCG,ACT,CCA,AGC,TCC,AAG,CTT,..
       .MET GLN THR GLN LYS PRO THR, PRO SER SER LYS LEU
                    TRP E SPECIFIED
       ↓                            10        20
FPV-HA:-AAGCTTGGTTTTTTTTTTTTTTTTTTTAGCAAAAGCAGGGGTTACAAA
        ATG,AAC,A....
        MET ASN

FPV-HA GENE CLONED INTO pWT121 IN THE R-ORIENTATION:-
        -50       -40       -30       -20
    ATG,CAA,ACA,CAA,AAA,CCG,ACT,CCA,AGC,TCC,AAG,CTT,GGT,
   .MET GLN THR GLN LYS PRO THR, PRO SER SER LYS LEU GLY
        -10               10        20
    TTT,TTT,TTT,TTT,TTT,TTT,AGC,AAA,AGC,AGG,GCT,TAC,AAA,
    PHE PHE PHE PHE PHE PHE SER LYS SER ARG GLY TYR LYS
    ATG,AAC,A....
    .MET ASN
    FPV PRE-HA
```

Fig. 4. Predicted nucleotide sequences around the Hind III sites of pWT111, pWT121 and the FPV-HA gene. Arrows (↓) indicate the position of the Hind III sites and only the sequence of the coding strand is shown. (Reproduced from Emtage et al.[11]).

Expression of the haemagglutinin gene

From the nucleotide sequences of the HA gene and the Hind III sites of the pWT series it was clear that, if inserted at the Hind III site of pWT121 in the correct orientation, the HA gene would be translated by readthrough from the trp E fragment (Fig. 4). The protein resulting from initiation at the trp E AUG would be a hybrid consisting of the following fragments in order: i) an N-terminus of 7 amino acids from anthranilate synthetase; ii) 6 amino acids specified by linker DNA; iii) 6 phenylalanine residues from the $(T)_{19}$ region of the cloned FPV DNA; iv) 7 amino acids from the normally non-translated 5'-portion of the HA gene; v) 558 amino acids comprising the haemagglutinin gene and its prepeptide and, finally vi) 5 amino acids specified by Hind III linker at the C-terminus. This is a total of 589 amino acids with a molecular weight of 69,000 daltons.

It was also clear that the HA gene should not be expressed from the initiator AUG of the trp E fragment in pWT111 or pWT131. Recognition of the ribosome binding site and initiator AUG of the HA gene was not anticipated. Similarly we did not expect expression of the HA gene inserted at the Hind III site of pBR322 in either orientation.

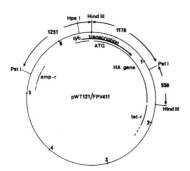

Fig. 5. The structure of pWT121/FPV411(R). The plasmid shown contains the FPV-HA gene cloned at the Hind III site of pWT121 in the R orientation. (Reproduced from Emtage et al.[11])

The HA gene was cloned into the Hind III sites of pWT111, pWT121 and recloned into pBR322 and new plasmids, containing the gene in the two orientations, identified by restriction enzyme analysis. One of these, pWT121/FPV411(R), is shown in Fig. 5. The correct phasing of the HA gene in pWT121/FPV411(R) with the trp E AUG was confirmed by nucleotide sequencing.[18] The determined nucleotide sequence showed one difference from the predicted one; nucleotide -36 was an A instead of a G (Fig. 4). This was also the case for the corresponding position in pWT111. This position corresponds to the

3'-terminal nucleotide of the Hind III linker and the difference might be due
either to micro-heterogeneity or incomplete deblocking after chemical synthesis
at the 3'-ends of these molecules.

E. coli colonies containing representatives of the plasmids described above
were screened for FPV-HA antigen using a solid-phase immunological method.   As
indicated in Table 1, immune activity was detected from all colonies containing
an FPV-HA gene inserted into the pWT plasmids and from pBR322 containing the HA
gene in the L orientation.   Neither of the parent plasmids nor pBR322
containing the HA gene in the R orientation produced any immune reacting
material.

TABLE 1

RADIOIMMUNOASSAY OF FPV-HA IN LYSATES OF E. COLI CONTAINING INFLUENZA GENES

Plasmid	Orientation of Gene[a]	Phenotype	HA content[b]
pWT121/FPV411	R	Tc^r	20.3
pWT121/FPV412	L	Tc^s	5.0
pWT111/FPV502	R	Tc^r	4.1
pWT111/FPV503	L	Tc^s	2.1
pBR322/FPV604	L	Tc^s	3.6
pBR322/FPV605	R	Tc^s	0
pWT121	–	Tc^r	0
pBR322	–	Tc^r	0

[a]We define the R and L orientations in terms of the direction of transcription
required for HA production.   That is, a gene in the R orientation required
rightward transcription for expression;   in the pWT series this is the
orientation for expression from the trp promoter.   (Reproduced from Emtage
et al.[11]).

[b]HA content, in ng/50 μl, was measured on lysates of bacteria grown in M9
medium.

It was interesting to find expression of HA antigen from one orientation of
pBR322/FPV.   The Hind III site of pBR322 lies in the promoter region of the
tetracycline gene and it is known that cloning at the Hind III site destroys
this rightward transcribing promoter.[14]   We therefore propose that a
previously unknown promoter which transcribes in the leftward direction exists
on the tetracycline gene site of the Hind III site of pBR322.   It is
necessary to postulate the existence of this promoter to explain the

expression of the HA gene in pBR322/FPV604(L), pWT121/FPV412(L) and pWT111/FPV503(L). The possibility that there is a pseudo-promoter sequence in the HA gene itself, for example the $(T_{19}):(A_{19})$ sequence, is ruled out as the plasmid pBR322/FPV605(R) does not express its HA gene. (Table 1).

The above postulated promoter explains the transcription of the HA gene in the L-oriented plasmids. How is translation explained? Inspection of the nucleotide sequence around the tetracycline - HA gene junction of pBR322/FPV604(L) reveals nonsense triplets in all three translation phases. This leads to the conclusion that the bacterial translational system is recognising a nucleotide sequence on the HA mRNA itself and initiating protein synthesis at the AUG of the pre-peptide. Indeed, we have compared the sequence of the untranslated region of the HA gene with that of the 3' end of prokaryotic 16S ribosomal RNA[19] and found surprising complementarity (Fig. 6). Consistent with this interpretation is the expression of HA antigen in pWT111/FPV502(R). In this case the HA gene is in the wrong phase to be translated from the trp E AUG; protein synthesis initiating at the trp E AUG is terminated by the now in phase UGA triplet at position 23-25 in the HA gene. Thus we conclude that initiation is from the natural HA AUG at position 22-24 (Fig. 4).

FPV-HA   A G C <u>A G G G G T</u> T A C A A A A T G - 3'

β-LACTAMASE   T G A A A <u>A A G G A</u> A G A G T A T G - 3'

TRP E   A A T T A <u>G A G</u> A A T A A C A A T G - 3'

COMPLEMENT OF
16S RNA 3' END   5' - T A A G G A G G T G A T C - 3'

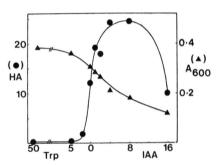

Fig. 6. The HA gene contains a region similar to prokaryotic ribosome binding sites. The nucleotide sequences of the 5'-untranslated regions of HA, β-lactamase[20] and trp E[21] and the complement of the 3'-end of 16S RNA are shown. Regions of homology with 16S RNA are underlined.

Fig. 7. The control of HA production from the trp promoter. Cultures of pWT121/FPV411(R) were grown in M9 medium containing either tryptophan or β-indoleacrylic acid (concentration given in μg/ml). After 2 hr, cells were harvested, lysed and assayed for HA content (μg/ml). (Reproduced from Emtage et al.[11]).

As discussed above the transcription of any gene inserted into the Hind III site of the pWT series should be under <u>trp</u> control; that is the production of gene product should be low in the presence of tryptophan and maximal after induction with β-indoleacrylic acid. That this is so for the HA gene is shown in Fig. 7. 5 μg/ml tryptophan was sufficient for complete repression while 4-8 μg/ml β-indoleacrylic acid produced maximal HA synthesis.

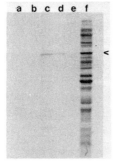

Fig. 8. Immunoprecipitation of the haemagglutinin-like protein. The figure shows immunoprecipitable proteins from cells containing the following plasmids a) pWT121+IAA, b) pWT121/FPV411(R) + trp, c) pWT121/FPV411(R) + IAA, d) pWT111/FPV502(R) + IAA, e) pWT121/FPV412(L) + trp, f) contains an extract from induced cells containing pWT121/FPV411(R). (Reproduced from Emtage et al.[11]).

Finally we have used SDS-polyacrylamide gel electrophoresis to examine the size of immunoprecipitable products in cells containing various plasmids after induction or repression of <u>trp</u> transcription. No immunoprecipitable proteins were present in induced cells containing pWT121 or in repressed cells containing pWT121/FPV411(R) (Figure 8; a & b, respectively). However, induced cells containing pWT121/FPV411(R) or pWT111/FPV502(R) and repressed cells containing pWT121/FPV412(L) all produced a band with molecular weight 61,000 daltons. (Figure 8, c, d & e, respectively). Our experimental design predicted that the HA-like protein synthesised from pWT121/FPV411(R) would have a molecular weight of 69,168 daltons and that the products from pWT121/FPV502(R) would be 26 amino acids smaller at the N-terminus. As the three products are in fact the same size, it seems probable that the primary gene product has been processed and a portion of the polypeptide removed. Evidence for processing was also obtained when the products of these plasmids were examined in minicells.

CONCLUSIONS

We have demonstrated the feasibility of producing controlled amounts of influenza antigenic determinants by genetic engineering. It now remains to determine whether proteins made in this manner are antigenically active and produce a virus neutralising antibody.

ACKNOWLEDGMENT

We thank Alan Porter for confirming the nucleotide sequence of specific
regions of our plasmids, Graham Catlin and Brian Jenkins for support in the
gene synthesis and cloning, John Oxford for providing antiserum to the
haemagglutinin and Dr. A. J. Hale for providing the research facilities.

REFERENCES

1. Schild, G.C. (1977) in Chemoprophylaxis and Virus Infections of the
   Respiratory Tract, Oxford, J.S. ed., CRC Press, Cleveland, Ohio,
   Vol. 1, pp 63-101.
2. Kavet, J. (1972) Ph.D. Thesis, Harvard University, Cambridge, USA.
3. Drzeniek, R., Seto, J.T. and Rott, R. (1966) Biochim, Biophys. Acta, 128,
   547-558.
4. Laver, W.G., and Kilbourne, E.D. (1966) Virology, 30, 493-501.
5. Wiley, D.C., Skehel, J.J. and Waterfield, M.D. (1977) Virology, 79,
   446-448.
6. Porter, A.G., Barber, C., Carey, N.H., Hallewell, R.A., Threlfall, G.
   and Emtage, J.S. Nature, in press.
7. Skehel, J.J. and Schild, G.C. (1971) Virology, 44, 396-408.
8. Laver, W.G. (1971) Virology, 45, 275-288.
9. Emtage, J.S., Catlin, G.H. and Carey, N.H. (1979) Nucleic Acids Res. 6,
   1221-1240.
10. Tacon, W.C.A., Carey, N.H. and Emtage, J.S. Molec. & Gen. Genet., in press.
11. Emtage, J.S., Tacon, W.C.A., Catlin, G.H., Jenkins, B., Porter, A.G. and
    Carey, N.H. Nature, in press.
12. Morse, D.E., Mosteller, R.D. and Yanofsky, C. (1969) Cold Spring Harbor
    Symp. Quant. Biol., 34, 725-740.
13. Hallewell, R.A., and Emtage, J.S. Gene, in press.
14. Rodriguez, R.L., West, R.W., Heyneker, H.L., Bolivar, F. and Boyer, H.W.
    (1979) Nucleic Acids Res., 6, 3267-3287.
15. O'Farrell, P.H., Polisky, B. and Gelfand, D.H. (1978) J. Bacteriol., 134,
    645-654.
16. McGeogh, D., Fellner, P. and Newton, C. (1976) Proc. Natl. Acad. Sci.
    USA, 73, 3045-3049.
17. Scheller, R.D., Dickerson, R.E., Boyer, H.W., Riggs, A.D. and Itakura, K.
    (1977) Science, 197, 177-180.
18. Maxam, A. and Gilbert, W. (1977) Proc. Natl. Acad. Sci. USA, 74, 560-564.
19. Steitz, J.A. and Jakes, K. (1975) Proc. Natl. Acad. Sci. USA, 72,
    4734-4738.
20. Sutcliffe, J.G. (1978) Cold Spring Harbor Symp. Quant. Biol. 42, 77-90.
21. Lee, F., Bertrand, K., Bennett, G. and Yanofsky, C. (1978) J. Molec. Biol.,
    121, 193-217.

DISCUSSION

Sambrook: Do you know why expression is inefficient - is the messenger degraded, or is the promoter not working?

Emtage: We don't know.

Air: Do you expect the product to be soluble?

Emtage: With triton lysis it is. If you just sonicate, most of the HA is in the membrane.

Laver: Mightn't you be getting good expression but fail to detect the product because it is not fully antigenic?

Emtage: We don't know, but when whole cell extracts from induced cells are electrophoresed, 2-2½ of protein is in new bands.

Brownlee: Could the long T-rich region before the start of the HA coding sequence act as an attenuator for transcription?

Emtage: We have two AUG's flanking the T-rich region and we can cut with HindIII, then exoIII, S1 and re-ligate, hoping that the two AUG's become coincident. So far we don't have this, but we do have colonies which express more efficiently.

Sambrook: In other cases eukaryotic genes in E.coli have not been expressed very efficiently.

Emtage: Goodman's group with growth hormone have in their clone the whole of the trp E gene. Therefore you can look at the amount of trp E produced with respect to growth hormone. The growth hormone produced is only about 10% of trp E.

Rott: Has the product cell-absorbing activity and is it cleaved by trypsin?

Emtage: There is no cell-absorbing activity; we don't know about trypsin.

Krug: Is it possible that the antigenic activity detected is not due to intact HA?

Emtage: That's stretching it a bit.

Lai: Is the low expression due to codon utilisation?

Sambrook: Can you put it upstream of some essential E.coli gene to force
  expression?

Emtage: Maybe, but we should be able to find out quite easily if the problem is,
  for instance, codon usage of mRNA and once we know the problem, it is probably
  easily overcome.

3'-TERMINAL SEQUENCES OF HEMAGGLUTININ AND NEURAMINIDASE GENES OF DIFFERENT INFLUENZA A VIRUSES

ULRICH DESSELBERGER, PAUL ZAMECNIK* and PETER PALESE
Mount Sinai School of Medicine, Fifth Avenue and 100th Street,
New York, N.Y. 10029; *Worcester Foundation for Experimental
Biology, Inc., 222 Maple Avenue, Shrewsbury, MA 01545

INTRODUCTION

Influenza A viruses possess a genome of eight single-stranded RNA segments of negative polarity. It was previously reported that the 3' terminal sequences of the RNA segments of several strains were conserved and that they were partially complementary to the 5' terminal sequences[1,2,3]. In addition, it was found that the 5' as well as the 3' terminal sequences of both influenza B and C virus RNAs were similar to those of influenza A virus RNAs.[3]

In the present paper we report 3' terminal nucleotide sequences which extend beyond the region common to all RNA segments. The hemagglutinin and neuraminidase genes of influenza A/PR/8/34 (HON1), A/WSN/33 (HON1) and X-31 (H3N2) viruses were used in this study. The sequence data for the hemagglutinin genes of these three strains are compared with those obtained by Air[4] and Porter et al.[5] for the hemagglutinin genes of A/RI/5⁻/57 and FPV viruses.

The dideoxy DNA sequencing method[6] was used to determine the sequence of the first 100-200 nucleotides of each RNA segment. Reverse transcriptase and a synthetic deoxy-oligonucleotide primer which is complementary to the twelve 3' terminal nucleotides of the hemagglutinin and neuraminidase genes were employed for transcription of the vRNA segment into cDNA. Since the cDNA is of the same polarity as virus-coded mRNA, amino acid sequences can be predicted from the cDNA sequences.

MATERIALS AND METHODS

Viruses and Cells. The following influenza A viruses were used in the study: A/PR/8/34 (HON1; England variant), A/WSN/33 (HON1) and the recombinant X-31 [A/Aichi/2/68(H) - A/Aichi/2/68 (N)] which was prepared by E.D. Kilbourne.[7] Viruses were grown in 10-11 day old embryonated chicken eggs. Purification of viruses followed established procedures.[8,9,10]

RNA Isolation. The RNA of purified virus (vRNA) was extracted according to published procedures,[8,9] and subsequently electro-phoresed on 2.6% polyacrylamide gels at $26°C$. Wet gels were stained with ethidium bromide (5-10 μg/ml) and RNA segments were electrophoresed out of the gel slices into 0.5 M Tris acetate buffer pH 6.[11] The RNAs were purified by ethanol and by per-chloric acid[12] precipitation. This was followed by a second ethanol precipitation. We estimate that less than 0.5 μg of each RNA segment was recovered from each 10 μg sample of total viral RNA.

Synthesis and sequencing of complementary DNA (cDNA). Origi-nally developed for sequencing of DNA, the "dideoxy" sequencing method has been used extensively for sequencing RNA.[13,14,15,4] To prime the synthesis of cDNA an approach similar to that of Hamlyn et al.[13] and of Stephenson and Zamecnik[16] was employed. A dodecamer, [d(AGCAAAAGCAG)rG], was custom-synthesized by Colla-borative Research, Inc., (Waltham, Mass. 02154). This oligonu-cleotide, which is complementary to the conserved 3' end of in-fluenza A virus RNA segments,[1,2,3] was found to efficiently prime influenza virus RNA in a reverse transcriptase reaction. With whole RNA it was found that amounts as small as 1 to 10 ng could be efficiently primed. Our conditions for cDNA synthesis were as

follows: 50 mM Tris-HCl pH 8.3, 60 mM NaCl, 20 mM DTT, 12 mM
MgCl$_2$, 0.05 mM of dCTP, dGTP and dTTP, 0.001 mM (α-^{32}P)-dATP
(300-2000 Ci/mMol), a sufficient amount of vRNA segment (estimated 10-50 ng) and 1 mM of dodecamer (50 ng/10 µl) in a total
volume of 10 µl. The dideoxy compounds were added in ratios of
ddNTP:dNTP of 1:1 to 1:5. These ratios were empirically determined. 0.5 µl of reverse transcriptase (final concentration:
500 units/ml) were added and the reaction mix was incubated at
37°C for 30 min., followed by a 'chase' with 0.05 mM dATP for 10
min. at room temperature. 8 µl of formamide dye mix (90% formamide, deionized with mixed bed resin AG501-X8(D) purchased from
Bio-Rad Labs., Richmond, CA; 0.15% xylene cyanol FF and bromo-
phenol blue, 10 mM EDTA pH 7) were added and the mixture was
boiled for 3 min. prior to application to gels. Avian myeloblastosis virus reverse transcriptase was generously supplied by
Dr. J.W. Beard (Division of Cancer Cause and Prevention, National
Cancer Institute).

Polyacrylamide electrophoresis for DNA sequencing. 8% Polyacrylamide slab gels (40 x 20 x .04 cm) were prepared as described[17] and 3 µl of reaction mixture were applied per slot.
Electrophoresis was at 1200 V and approximately 25-30 mA for 2-6
hours in a Tris-borate EDTA buffer system.[18]

Chemicals. [α-^{32}P]-dATP (2000-3000 Ci/mMol) was obtained from
Amersham Radiochemical Center (Arlington Heights, Ill. 60005).
Other nucleoside triphosphates and 2',3'-dideoxynucleoside tri-
phosphates were from P.-L. Biochemicals (Milwaukee, Wisc. 53205).
RESULTS AND DISCUSSION

Sequences of the hemagglutinin (HA) genes. RNA from purified
A/PR/8/34 (HON1) virus was extracted and the genes were separated

by electrophoresis on a 2.6% polyacrylamide gel. The gene coding
for the HA was eluted from the gel and purified (see Materials and
Methods). The isolated RNA segment was then mixed with the dodecamer [d(AGCAAAAGCAG)rG] and the nucleotide sequence was determined
using the dideoxy chain termination technique. Fig. 1 shows an
example of an autoradiogram of a gel on which the reaction mixture
was separated. The sequence of nucleotides 20-198 was obtained by
electrophoresing the mixtures on polyacrylamide gels for various
time periods. The results of these experiments, including the sequence of the first 20 nucleotides which was obtained previously,[3]
are shown in Table 1. At position 33-35 is a possible initiation
codon and, based on the available nucleotide data, a sequence of
65 amino acids for the A/PR/8/34 HA is predicted (Table 1). Previously Waterfield et al.[19,20] reported the N-terminal sequences
of the HA's of two HON1 strains, A/Bel/42 and A/Weiss/43 viruses.
The first 10 amino acids of these proteins exactly correspond to
amino acids 18-27 of the A/PR/8/34 HA sequence shown in Table 1.
The 17 amino acids preceding this sequence are mostly hydrophobic
(Table 1) and very likely represent a presequence, as postulated
by the signal peptide hypothesis.[21]

In order to compare the A/PR/8/34 HA sequence with that of another HON1 strain, we purified the RNA of A/WSN/33 virus and sequenced its HA gene. Analysis shows that there is an identical
stretch of 18 amino acids (amino acid positions 18-35) coded for
by these two hemagglutinin genes with only one difference in the
nucleotide sequence (nucleotide position 116). This region most
likely represents the N-terminal of both HA molecules. In contrast, 5 out of the 17 amino acids in the two presequences are different (amino acid positions 4, 10, 12, 13 and 15). Even more

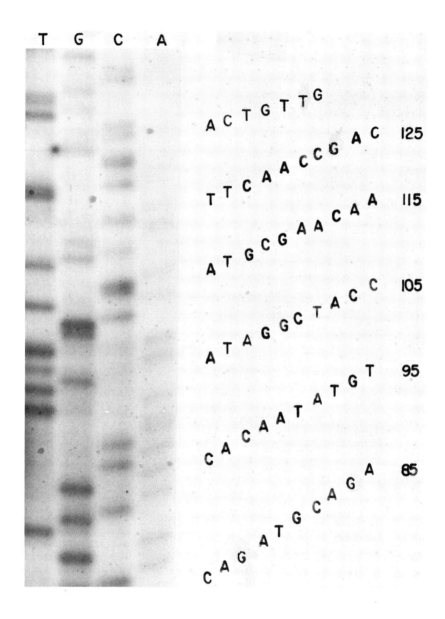

Fig. 1. The sequence from nucleotide 76 to 132 of cDNA complementary to the 3' end of the hemagglutinin gene of A/PR/8/34
(HON1) influenza virus. Conditions for synthesis and termination
of cDNA are described in Materials and Methods. Letters T, G, C,
A at the top of the lanes designate the respective dideoxy nucleoside triphosphates used for termination of the reaction.

changes are observed among the signal sequences of the HA genes of A/RI/5⁻/57, FPV and A/PR/8/34 viruses. Of the 17-18 amino acids of the presequences only residues 6 and 7 are identical in the HA genes of A/PR/8/34 and FPV viruses (Table 1 and ref. 5). Only three amino acids are common to the predicted presequences of A/RI/5⁻/57 and A/PR/8/34 HA genes. Similarly, there is very little homology between the predicted presequences of the A/PR/8/34 and X-31 HA genes (Table 1). Since the N-terminal sequence of the X-31 HA is not known at this time, we can only speculate as to the precise cleavage site of the presequence. However, since the presequences of the influenza virus hemagglutinins examined are 15, 17 and 18 amino acids long (Table 1 and refs. 4 and 5) and since cleavage of the presequence usually involves a small amino acid, position 16 is a likely candidate for the C-terminal of the presequence of the X-31 HA.

The N-terminal amino acids of the HAs of A/PR/8/34 (HON1) and A/WSN/33 (HON1) viruses are very similar, as pointed out above, but there is only limited homology among the N-terminal amino acids of the HO, H2 and Hav1 hemagglutinins derived from A/PR/8/34, A/RI/5-/57[4] and FPV viruses, respectively (Table 1). Comparison of the predicted terminal amino acid sequences of the HO (A/PR/8/34 virus) and the H3 hemagglutinin (X-31 virus) suggests no homology at all (Table 1).

Sequences of the neuraminidase (NA) genes. Table 2 shows the nucleotide sequences of cDNAs complementary to the 3' ends of one N2 and two N1 neuraminidase genes derived from X-31, A/WSN/33 and A/PR/8/34 viruses respectively. Sequences were obtained by following the procedures described for the analysis of the HA genes. The 20 terminal nucleotides of the A/PR/8/34 NA segment were

Table 1. Comparison of the 3' Ends of Hemagglutinin Genes from Different Influenza A Viruses

Strain	Sequences of									

First segment (positions 1–50)

position markers: 10 20 30 40 50

A/PR/8/34 (HON1)
cDNA: AGCAAAAGCAGGGGAATATAAAAACAACCAAA ATG AAG GCA AAC CTA CTG GTC CTG TTA
amino acids: met lys ala asn leu leu val leu leu

A/WSN/33 (HON1)
cDNA: ·······AXAAAAACXACCAAA ATG AAG GCA AAA CTA CTG GTC CTG TTA
amino acids: met lys ala lys leu leu val leu leu

X-31 (H3N2)
cDNA: ·······TTAATC ATG AAG ACG ATG ATT GCT TTG AGC TAC
amino acids: met lys thr met ile ala leu ser tyr

A/RI/5⁻/57* (H2N2) amino acids: met ala ile ile tyr leu ile leu leu

FPV* (HavlN1) amino acids: met asn thr gln ile leu val phe ala

Second segment (positions 60–110)

position markers: 60 70 80 90 100 110

A/PR/8/34
AGT GCA CTT GCA GCT GCA GAT GCA ▶GAC ACA ATA TGT ATA GGC TAC CAT GCG AAC AAT TCA
ser ala leu ala ala ala asp ala asp thr ile cys ile gly tyr his ala asn asn ser
(10 … 20 … 100 … 110)

A/WSN/33
TAT GCA TTT GTA GCT ACA GAT GCA ▶GAC ACA ATA TGT ATA GGC TAC CAT GCG AAC AAC TCA
tyr ala phe val ala thr asp ala asp thr ile cys ile gly tyr his ala asn asn ser
(60 … 70 … 80 … 90 … 100 … 110)

X-31
ATT GTC TGT GCT CTG GCT CTC GGC ▶CAA GAC CTT CCA ▶GGA AAT GAC AAC AGC ACA GCA ACG
ile val cys ala leu ala leu gly gln asp leu pro gly asn asp asn ser thr ala thr
(60 … 70 … 80 … 90 … 100 … 110)

A/RI/5⁻/57*
phe ile ala val arg gly ▶asp gln ile cys ile gly tyr his ala asn asn
(10 … 20)

FPV*
leu val ala val ile pro thr asn ala ▶asp lys ile cys leu gly his his ala val ser
(10 … 20)

(continued on next page)

Table 1. (continued)

Strain	120		130		140		150		160		170	
A/PR/8/34	ACC GAC ACT GTT	GAC ACA	CTC GAG AAG AAT	GTG ACA GTG ACA CAC TCT GTT AAC CTG								
	thr asp thr val	asp thr	val leu glu lys	asn val thr val thr his ser val asn leu								
	30			40								

	120		130		140							
A/WSN/33	ACC GAC ACT GTT	GAC ACA	ATA TTC									
	thr asp thr val	asp thr	ile phe									
	30											

FPV* asn gly thr lys val asn thr leu thr glu arg gly val glu val val asn ala thr glu
      30   40

	180		190	
A/PR/8/34	CTC GAA GAC AGC CAC AAC G			
	leu glu asp ser his asn			
	50			

FPV* thr val glu arg thr asn
      50

*The amino acid sequences of the hemagglutinins of A/BI/5⁻/57 virus and of FPV were those
of Air⁴ and Porter et al.⁵

The nucleotide sequences of cDNAs transcribed from the 3' ends of isolated HA segments
were determined using the "dideoxy" sequencing technique. Nucleotides and amino acids
different from those of the A/PR/8/34 virus HA gene are underlined. Sequences of the
different genes are aligned with respect to the initiation codon ATG (AUG). Arrows indicate
the predicted C-termini of the signal presequences.

Table 2. Comparison of the 3' Ends of Neuraminidase Genes from Different Influenza A Viruses

Strain	Sequences of

```
                                                20                  30              40            50
A/PR/8/34   cDNA        AGCGAAAGCAGGGGTTTAAA ATG AAT CCA AAT CAG AAA ATA ATA ACA ACC ATT GGA TCA
(HON1)      amino acids                      met asn pro asn gln lys ile thr thr ile gly ser
                                                                                      10

                                               20                 30                 40            50
A/WSN/33    cDNA        .............AT ATG AAT CCA AAC CAX AAA ATA ATA ACT ATT GGG TCA
(HON1)      amino acids                 met asn pro asn     lys ile thr ile gly ser
                                                   his                          10

                                           20                 30            40              50
X-31        cDNA        ..........AA ATG AAT CCA AAT CAA CTA ATA ACA ATT CGC TCT
(H3N2)      amino acids               met asn pro asn gln lys ile thr ile gly ser
                                                       thr leu               10  arg


             60                        70                 80                   90              100            110
A/PR/8/34   ATC TGT CTG GTA GTC GGA CTA ATT AGC ATA TTG CAA ATA GGG AAT ATA ATC TCA ATA ATA
            ile cys leu val val gly leu ile ser ile leu gln ile gly asn ile ser ile
                                               20                             100                     30

             60                        70                 80                   90              100            110
A/WSN/33    ATC TGT TTG GTA GTC GGC TTC ATT AGC CTA TTG CTG ATT GGG ATC ATC TCA CCA
            ile cys leu val val gly phe ile ser leu leu leu ile gly ile pro ser pro
                                       phe               20  leu              thr          30  leu

             60                        70                 80                   90              100
X-31        GTC TCT CTG ACC ATT GCX ACA GTA TGC TTC CGC CTG CTG GCC XTC CTG
            val ser leu thr ile ala thr val cys phe leu leu ala leu
            leu              thr  ile 20      arg


             120                       130                140          150
A/PR/8/34   TGG ATX AGC CAT TCA ATT CAA ACT GGA AGT CAA AAC
            trp ile ser his ser ile gln thr gly ser gln asn
            met                                       40

             120           130
A/WSN/33    CGG AXX AGC CAT TCX
            arg         ser his ser
```

The nucleotide sequences of cDNAs transcribed from the 3' ends of isolated NA genes were determined using the dideoxy sequencing technique. Nucleotides and amino acids different from those found for the A/PR/8/34 NA gene are underlined. Sequences of the different genes are aligned with respect to their first initiation codon ATG (AUG).

determined by direct RNA sequencing and have been reported previously.[3] Starting from the first ATG (AUG) triplet in position 20-22 or 21-23 the sequence data reveal the coding information for 44, 36, and 27 amino acids in the NA genes of A/PR/8/34 virus, A/WSN/33 virus and X-31 virus, respectively. The two N1 genes are highly conserved for the first 130 nucleotides, whereas the N1 and N2 genes have few sequences in common beyond position 65.

ACKNOWLEDGEMENTS

We are very thankful to G.N. Godson for teaching us the "dideoxy" sequencing technique and we acknowledge the excellent technical assistance of Ronald Taussig. U.D. is a recipient of a Fulbright Fellowship and P.P. is a recipient of an I.T. Hirschl Career Research Award. This work was supported by Grant AI-11823 from the NIH, grant PCM 78-07844 from the NSF and grant MV-23A from the American Cancer Society.

REFERENCES

1. Skehel, J.J. and Hay, A.J. (1978) Nucl. Acids Res. 5, 1207-1219.
2. Robertson, J.S. (1979) Nucl. Acids Res. 6, 3745-3756.
3. Desselberger, U., Racaniello, V.R., Zazra, J.J. and Palese, P. (1979) Gene, vol. 8, in press.
4. Air, G.M. (1979) Virology 97, 468-472.
5. Porter, A.G., Barber, C., Carey, N.H., Hallewell, R.A., Threlfall, G. and Emtage, J.S., (1979) Nature, in press.
6. Sanger, F., Nicklen, S. and Coulson, A.R. (1977) Proc. Natl. Acad. Sci. USA 74, 5463-5467.
7. Kilbourne, E.D., Schulman, J.L., Schild, G.C., Schloer, G., Swanson, J. and Bucher, D. (1971) J. Infect. Dis. 124, 449-462.
8. Palese, P. and Schulman, J.L. (1976) Proc. Natl. Acad. Sci. USA 73, 2142-2146.
9. Ritchey, M.B., Palese, P. and Schulman, J.L. (1976) J. Virol. 20, 307-313.
10. Desselberger, U., Nakajima, K., Alfino, P., Pedersen, F.S., Haseltine, W.A., Hannoun, C. and Palese, P. (1978) Proc. Natl. Acad. Sci. USA 75, 3341-3345.
11. Young, J.F., Desselberger, U. and Palese, P. (1979) Cell 18, 73-83.
12. Jeppesen, P.G.N., Barrell, B.G., Sanger, F. and Coulson, A.R. (1972) Biochem. J. 128, 993-1006.

13. Hamlyn, P.H., Brownlee, G.G., Cheng, Ch.-Ch., Gait, M.J. and Milstein, C. (1978) Cell 15, 1067-1075.
14. McGeoch, D.J. and Turnbull, N.T. (1978) Nucl. Acids Res. 5, 4007-4024.
15. Both, G.W. and Air, G.M. (1979) Eur. J. Biochem. 96, 363-372.
16. Stephenson, M.L. and Zamecnik, P.C. (1978) Proc. Natl. Acad. Sci. USA 75, 285-288.
17. Sanger, F. and Coulson, A.R. (1978) FEBS lett. 87, 107-110.
18. Peacock, A.C. and Dingman, C.W. (1968) Biochemistry 7, 668-674.
19. Waterfield, M.D., Espelie, K., Elder, K., and Skehel, J.J. (1979) Brit. Med. Bull. 35, 57-63.
20. Skehel, J.J. and Waterfield, M.D. (1975) Proc. Natl. Acad. Sci. USA 72, 93-97.
21. Blobel, G. and Dobberstein, B. (1975) J. Cell Biol. 67, 835-851.

DISCUSSION

Klenk: How do you explain this heterogeneity in the signal sequence? The signal sequence interacts with receptors in the membrane so one would expect it to be highly conserved.

Brownlee: It has been found that signal peptides from a number of different proteins differ in sequence and that only their hydrophobicity is common.

THE 5' ENDS OF INFLUENZA VIRAL MESSENGER RNAs ARE DONATED BY CAPPED CELLULAR
MESSENGER RNAs

ROBERT M. KRUG, MICHELE BOULOY AND STEPHEN J. PLOTCH
Memorial Sloan-Kettering Cancer Center, New York, New York 10021 USA

INTRODUCTION

One feature distinguishing influenza virus from other nononcogenic RNA viruses is that the functioning of the host nuclear RNA polymerase II is required
for virus replication, specifically for viral RNA transcription.[1-3] Our recent
studies of viral RNA transcription have provided an explanation for this requirement for RNA polymerase II. We have shown that capped eukaryotic mRNAs
strongly stimulate viral RNA transcription in vitro and donate their 5' terminal methylated cap and a short stretch of internal nucleotides to the 5' end of
the viral RNA transcripts.[4-6] A similar mechanism appears to operate in vivo,
because we have found that the viral messenger RNAs (mRNAs) synthesized in the
infected cell contain a short stretch of nucleotides at their 5' end, including
the cap, that are not viral-coded.[7] The need for newly synthesized host mRNA
primers to stimulate viral RNA transcription would explain the requirement for
the proper functioning of host RNA polymerase II in the infected cell. Here
we will summarize some of the results of these recent studies.

MATERIALS AND METHODS

These have been detailed elsewhere[4-10], as will be indicated in the legends
to the figures and tables.

RESULTS AND DISCUSSION

We had proposed a few years ago[8-10] that viral RNA transcription in vivo
requires initiation by primer RNAs synthesized by RNA polymerase II and that
the 5' terminal cap found on in vivo viral mRNA[11] is derived from these primer
RNAs. These proposals were based on two sets of data: (i) the strong stimulation by a primer dinucleotide, ApG or GpG, of viral RNA transcription in vitro
catalyzed by the virion-associated transcriptase[8,9,12]; and (ii) the absence of
detectable capping and methylating enzymes in virions.[10]

Our later experiments essentially proved these proposals. We first identified primer RNAs in rabbit reticulocyte extracts, where they were shown to be
globin mRNAs.[4] We showed that beta-globin mRNA, purified by polyacrylamide gel

electrophoresis, stimulated viral RNA transcription about 80-fold and, on a molar basis, was about 2000 times more effective as a primer than ApG.[4] Other capped eukaryotic mRNAs were also found to be extremely effective primers.[4-6] The viral RNA transcripts primed by these eukaryotic mRNAs functioned as viral mRNAs in cell-free systems.[4]

To determine whether the cap of the primer mRNA was physically transferred to the viral mRNA during *in vitro* transcription, we used as primer a mRNA containing radiolabel only in its cap. Globin mRNA containing ^{32}P only in its cap was prepared by enzymatically recapping β-eliminated globin mRNA in the presence of $(\alpha-^{32}P)$ GTP and S-adenosylmethionine (AdoMet).[4] With this globin mRNA as primer in the presence of unlabeled nucleoside triphosphates, the resulting viral mRNA segments were shown to contain ^{32}P derived from the primer (Fig. 1A, lane 1). All of the ^{32}P in the viral mRNA segments was in cap struc-

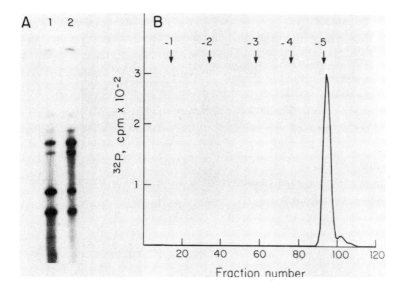

Fig. 1. Transfer of the ^{32}P-labeled cap of globin mRNA to influenza viral mRNA during transcription *in vitro*. (A) Gel electrophoresis of deadenylated *in vitro* viral mRNA. Experimental procedures were as previously described.[5,8,9] The viral mRNA was synthesized in transcriptase reaction mixtures containing: lane 1, unlabeled nucleoside triphosphates and globin mRNA containing 32P only in the cap; lane 2, (α-32P) GTP as labeled precursor and unlabeled globin mRNA. (B) DEAE-Sephadex chromatography of the RNAase T2 digest of the RNA eluted from the bands in lane 1. From reference 5.

tures, and none was in internal residues: DEAE-Sephadex chromatography of the RNase T2 digest of the viral mRNA segments showed that all of the ^{32}P eluted at a charge of -5 or -6 (Fig. 1B), where cap structures elute. A similar experiment was done with reovirus mRNAs containing ^{3}H label only in their caps; these mRNAs were synthesized in vitro with reovirus cores in the presence of (methyl-^{3}H) AdoMet.[6] Again, the influenza viral mRNAs contained label (^{3}H) derived from the primer mRNAs, and this ^{3}H-label was shown to be in the cap structure m^{7}GpppG^{m}, identical to that found in the reovirus mRNA primers.[6] Thus, the cap was indeed physically transferred to influenza viral mRNA from globin mRNA or reovirus mRNA primers.

To determine whether sequences in addition to the cap were transferred from a primer mRNA to influenza viral mRNA, we compared the size of the eukaryotic mRNA-primed viral mRNA segments to that of the ApG-primed viral mRNA segments. If the mRNA-primed segments contain additional sequences at their 5' ends, we would expect that these segments would be larger than those primed by ApG, as the latter segments initiate exactly at the 3' end of the virion RNA (vRNA) templates.[13-16] First we compared the electrophoretic mobility of the globin mRNA-primed and ApG-primed viral mRNA segments after enzymatic deadenylylation of the segments (Fig. 2A). The globin mRNA-primed segments (lane 3) migrated slightly slower than the ApG-primed segments (lane 1). This difference in mobility was confirmed by electrophoresing a mixture of these two RNAs (lane 2): doublets can be observed which are most evident at the position of the two smallest segments. These relative mobilities were unaffected by prior treatment with glyoxal to eliminate secondary structure in the RNAs[5,17] (Fig. 2B), or by prior decaping of the globin mRNA-primed segments.[6] From the difference in mobility, we estimated that the globin mRNA-primed segments were 10-15 nucleotides larger than the ApG-primed segments. Other experiments established that these extra nucleotides were at the 5' end of the viral mRNA segments.[5] A similar mobility difference was observed when a mixture of ApG-primed and reovirus mRNA-primed segments were analyzed by gel electrophoresis (Fig. 3, lane 6).[6] In fact, when the influenza viral mRNA segments primed by globin mRNA and by reovirus mRNA were mixed (lane 4), no doublets were evident. Thus, gel electrophoretic analyses indicated that approximately the same number of nucleotides, about 10-15, were transferred to influenza viral mRNA from either globin or reovirus mRNA primers.

To obtain further evidence for the transfer of some internal nucleotides from the primer mRNA to influenza viral mRNA, we used uniformly ^{32}P-labeled

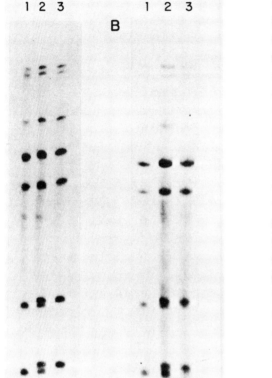

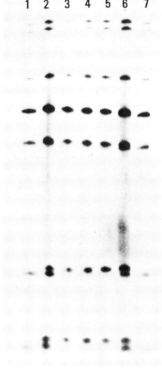

Fig. 2. Gel electrophoresis of viral mRNA, after deadenylation, synthesized in reaction mixtures containing (α-^{32}P) GTP as labeled precursor and either ApG (lane 1) or globin mRNA (lane 3) as primers. Lane 2 contains a mixture of the viral mRNA of lanes 1 and 3. The deadenylylated viral mRNAs were electrophoresed directly (A) or after treatment with glyoxal (B). From reference 5.

Fig. 3. Comparison of the electrophoretic mobility of the influenza viral mRNAs primed by reovirus mRNA, globin mRNA, and ApG. The viral mRNAs, synthesized with (α-^{32}P) GTP as labeled precursor, were deadenylated prior to electrophoresis. Lanes 1 and 7: ApG-primed viral mRNA. Lane 3: reovirus mRNA-primed influenza viral mRNA. Lane 5: globin mRNA-primed viral mRNA. Lane 2: mixture of ApG-and reovirus mRNA-primed influenza viral mRNAs. Lane 4: mixture of reovirus mRNA-and globin mRNA-primed influenza viral mRNAs. Lane 6: mixture of ApG-and globin mRNA-primed viral mRNAs. From reference 6.

reovirus mRNA as a primer in a transcriptase reaction mixture containing unlabeled CTP, ATP and UTP, and ^{3}H-labeled GTP. As shown in Fig. 4A, lane 2,
the three m and s influenza viral mRNA segments contained ^{32}P derived from
the reovirus mRNA primer. When the s segments were eluted from the gel,
digested with RNase T2, and the hydrolyzate analyzed by DEAE-Sephadex chromatography (Fig. 4B), ^{32}P-radiolabel was found in both internal residues at a

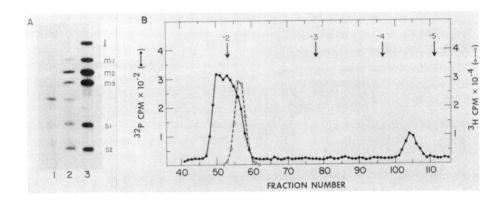

Fig. 4 Transfer of the cap and internal nucleotides from uniformly ^{32}P-labeled
reovirus mRNA to influenza viral mRNA during transcription in vitro. Experimental procedures were described in the text and in a previous publication.[6]
(A) Gel electrophoresis of the influenza viral mRNA after deadenylation (lane
2). Lane 1: the ^{32}P-reovirus mRNA primer. Lane 3: deadenylylated influenza
viral mRNA synthesized in a transcriptase reaction containing unlabeled globin
mRNA and (α-^{32}P) GTP as labeled precursor. (B) DEAE-Sephadex chromatography
of the RNase T2 digest of the s size influenza viral mRNAs of lane 2. From
reference 6.

charge of -2 and in the cap at -4.6. The number of chains of influenza viral
mRNA synthesized can be estimated from the ^{3}H-radiolabel at -2. The results
indicated that approximately one cap and 25 internal residues of reovirus
mRNA were transferred to each chain of influenza viral mRNA. This estimation
is in close agreement with that obtained from gel electrophoresis, especially
considering the possible inaccuracies in the two types of analyses.

These studies did not allow us to identify which bases of the primer mRNA
were transferred. To accomplish this, we (in collaboration with H. Robertson
and E. Dickson of Rockefeller University) used ^{125}I-globin mRNA as primer and
sequenced the ^{125}I-labeled region transferred to the viral mRNA. These results

will be published elsewhere, and we will only present the conclusions here. A set of identical ^{125}I-labeled sequences were found at the 5' end of all eight viral mRNA segments. The predominant sequence, representing 75% of the transferred oligonucleotides, indicated that the first 12, 13 or 14 nucleotides at the 5' end of beta-globin mRNA were transferred to the 5' end of the viral mRNAs. The minor ^{125}I-labeled RNase Tl-resistant oligonucleotides found in the viral mRNA molecules indicated that shorter 5' terminal pieces of beta-globin mRNA were at times transferred and also suggested that the transferred sequences were linked to G as the first base inserted by transcription.

The sequence transferred from beta-globin mRNA is not complementary to the vRNA template (whose sequence is 3'UCGUU...[13-16]), indicating that this beta-globin mRNA sequence does not hydrogen-bond to the template. In addition, other recent data strongly favor a mechanism of priming that does not involve hydrogen-bonding between the primer mRNA and the template vRNA: (i) capped fragments of globin mRNA too short to contain an AG sequence (or any other sequence complementary to the 3' end of the vRNA) effectively stimulate viral RNA transcription (unpublished results); and (ii) capped, synthetic ribopolymers lacking AG also stimulate transcription (unpublished results in collaboration with A. Shatkin's laboratory of Roche Institute). Therefore, in the absence of hydrogen-bonding, a likely mechanism for priming is that a capped 12-14 nucleotide fragment is cleaved from the 5' end of the primer mRNA and that this fragment then undergoes a specific interaction with the transcriptase which causes stimulation of transcription concomitant with the linking of the primer to the first base transcribed.

This specific interaction most probably involves the 5' terminal methylated cap of the primer mRNA, as priming activity requires the presence of the terminal m^7G of the cap.[5] Chemical (β-elimination) or enzymatic removal of the cap of globin or other mRNAs eliminates essentially all their priming activity, and most of this activity can be restored by enzymatically recapping the β-eliminated mRNAs. The cap apparently must contain methyl groups, since reovirus mRNAs with 5' terminal GpppG ends are not active as primers.[6] Indeed, in other experiments, we have recently shown that each of the two methyl groups in the cap, the 7-methyl in the terminal G and the 2'-0-methyl in the penultimate base, strongly influences the priming activity of a mRNA (unpublished experiments).

If a similar priming by host RNAs operates in vivo, then the viral mRNA synthesized in the infected cell should contain 10-15 nucleotides at its 5' end, including the cap, which are not viral-coded. This is exactly what we found. First, when compared by gel electrophoresis (Fig. 5), the in vivo viral mRNA segments were larger (migrated slower) than the ApG-primed in vitro mRNA segments[7], identical to the mobility difference between the segments of eukaryotic mRNA-and ApG-primed in vitro mRNA (see Figs. 2 and 3). In addition, when ^{3}H-methyl-labeled in vivo viral mRNA was hybridized to vRNA, the 5' terminal cap structure of the mRNA was not protected against pancreatic or T1 RNase digestion (Fig. 6).[7] All of the cap (the -4.4 to 5.2 charge species) was released from the double-strands by the nuclease digestion. Only internal m^6A residues (charge -2) remained in the double-strands, although approximately one-third of these residues were released. As each molecule of in vivo viral mRNA contains an average of three m^6A residues[11], these results indicate that one of these m^6A's is in the 5' terminal sequence that is not viral coded.[17] Thus, our results strongly suggest that host cell mRNAs and/or their precursors serve as primers for viral RNA transcription in the infected cell, and that they donate their cap and 10-15 internal nucleotides, one of which is m^6A, to the resulting viral mRNA molecules.

The synthesis of these host cell mRNA primers can be presumed to constitute the α-amanitin-sensitive step (RNA polymerase II function) required for viral RNA transcription. A critical, unanswered question is why new and continuous synthesis of these host mRNA primers is required. It may be that this requirement is due at least in part to the site of viral RNA transcription in the infected cell. Some data suggests that the nucleus is the site of primary transcription.[3,18] If this is the case, then the need for continued host cell mRNA synthesis may reflect the fact that the amount of available cellular mRNA and/or its precursors in the nucleus is limited and rapidly depleted. Clearly, it will be of great interest to establish definitively where both primary and amplified transcription occurs in the cell.

ACKNOWLEDGEMENTS

We thank Barbara Broni and Paul Simonelli for expert technical assistance. This research was supported by U.S. Publich Health Service Grants AI 11772 and CA 08748, and by U.S. Public Health Service International Fellowship TW02590-01 to M.B.

188

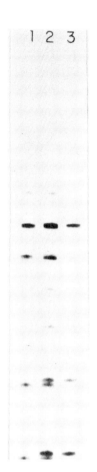

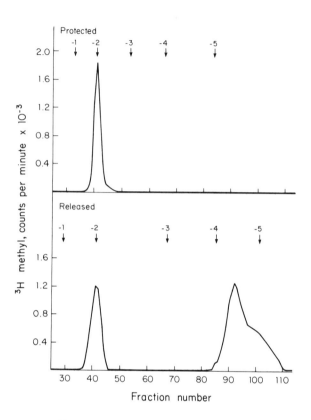

Fig. 6. ³H-methyl-labeled species retained in (protected) or released from vRNA: in vivo viral mRNA hybrids by pancreatic RNase digestion. The in vivo viral mRNA contained the ³H-methyl label. The hybrids were digested with pancreatic RNase, and the RNase-resistant double-strands and RNase-released material were collected as described previously.[7] The double-strands (after heating and fast-cooling) and the released material were digested with RNase T2, and the hydrolyzates were analyzed by DEAE-Sephadex chromatography. From reference 7.

Fig. 5. Comparison of the electrophoretic mobility of in vivo and ApG-primed in vitro viral mRNA. The two viral mRNAs, isolated as previously described[7-9], were deadenylylated prior to electrophoresis. Lane 1: ApG-primed in vitro viral mRNA. Lane 3: in vivo viral mRNA. Lane 2: a mixture of the viral mRNAs of lanes 1 and 2. From reference 7.

REFERENCES

1. Lamb, R.A. and Choppin, P.W. (1977) J. Virol. 23, 816-819.
2. Spooner, L.L.R. and Barry, R.D. (1977) Nature 268, 650-652.
3. Mark, G.E., Taylor, J.M., Broni, B. and Krug, R.M. (1979) J. Virol. 29, 744-752.
4. Bouloy, M., Plotch, S.J. and Krug, R.M. (1978) Proc. Nat. Acad. Sci. USA 75, 4886-4890.
5. Plotch, S.J., Bouloy, M. and Krug, R.M. (1979) Proc. Nat. Acad. Sci. USA 76, 1618-1622.
6. Bouloy, M., Morgan, M.A., Shatkin, A.J. and Krug, R.M. (1979) J. Virol., in press.
7. Krug, R.M., Broni, B.A. and Bouloy, M. (1979) Cell 18, 329-334.
8. Plotch, S.J. and Krug, R.M. (1977) J. Virol. 21, 24-34.
9. Plotch, S.J. and Krug, R.M. (1978) J. Virol. 25, 579-586.
10. Plotch, S.J., Tomasz, J. and Krug, R.M. (1978) J. Virol. 28, 75-83.
11. Krug, R.M., Morgan, M.M. and Shatkin, A.J. (1976) J. Virol. 20, 45-53.
12. McGeoch, D. and Kitron, N. (1975) J. Virol. 15, 686-695.
13. Skehel, J.J. and Hay, A.J. (1978) Nucleic Acids Res. 4, 1207-1219.
14. Both, G.W. and Air, G.M. (1979) Eur. J. Biochem. 96, 363-372.
15. Air, G.M. (1979) Virology 97, 468-472.
16. Robertson, J.S. (1979) Nucleic Acids Res. 6, 3745-3757.
17. McMaster, G.K. and Carmichael, G.G. (1977) Proc. Nat. Acad. Sci. USA 74, 4835-4838.
18. Barrett, T., Wolstenholme, A.J. and Mahy, B.W.J. (1979) Virology 98, 211-225.

(See DISCUSSION on following page)

DISCUSSION

Salser: As the transferred sequences are linked to the G, would you predict
that a clone made from this would differ by one nucleotide at the end?

Krug: I wouldn't predict that - we don't know that every messenger cuts at
exactly the same position. In β globin we get 12, 13 and 14 as major species,
and others may be different.

Salser: But the first G put in opposed to a U in the vRNA may lead to a reverse
transcript with a difference.

Krug: But another possibility is that most cuts are at A and so regenerate the
AGC sequence.

Lai: Both clones we obtained had A.

Krug: But your primer already has the A and even if the other strand has G, it
may not lead to errors.

Sambrook: Have you tried flu in one of the systems for active transcription in
a semi-purified system to find out if new caps are being made?

Krug: No.

Barry: Is it just the cap that is recognised or are some of the succeeding
nucleotides important?

Krug: There is enormous heterogeneity in the sequences.

THE STRUCTURE OF THE HEMAGGLUTININ AND NEURAMINIDASE GENES AS
REVEALED BY MOLECULAR HYBRIDIZATION

CHRISTOPH SCHOLTISSEK
Institut für Virologie, Justus-Liebig-Universität Giessen,
6300 Giessen, Germany

INTRODUCTION

The antigenic variability of influenza viruses can be explained
by the peculiar structure of the genes coding for the surface
glycoproteins, hemagglutinin (HA) and neuraminidase (NA). It will
be shown that these genes consist of a relatively small highly
conserved region or regions presumably involved in the functional
integrity of the gene products, and a large variable region or
regions presumably involved in the antigenic properties. These
conclusions were obtained by applying the technique of molecular
hybridization, which has been calibrated by introducing random
mismatching by treatment of the ^{32}P-labelled virion RNA (vRNA)
with HNO_2 prior to hybridization with the homologous complementary
RNA (cRNA).

METHODS AND RESULTS

By molecular hybridization it is possible to measure the relative base sequence homology between related genes. The technique
applied to influenza virus RNA genes is as follows[1]: A ^{32}P-
labelled RNA segment of vRNA is hybridized with a surplus of non-
labelled cRNA isolated from microsomes of chick embryo cells 5 hrs
after infection. After digestion with RNase A the acid precipitable radioactivity is measured. In the homologous system under
standard conditions (2 x SSC, 20°, 20 min) this is identical with
the input radioactivity. In the heterologous system the amount of
RNase-resistant radioactivity depends on the base sequence homology between the allelic genes as well as on the distribution of
mismatching along the molecule, and on the salt- and temperature
conditions used for digestion. The latter conditions measure the
stability of the heteroduplex molecule after hybridization. Thus,
if there is a 50% base sequence homology between two allelic
genes we can construct the two extreme situations shown in

Figure 1: In the upper part the homologous base pairs are evenly distributed over the total length of the molecule. Such a molecule should be extremely unstable and should be completely digested by RNase under relatively mild conditions (low temperature, low salt concentration). In the lower part the homologous base pairs are clustered in a few blocks making them extremely stable, while the residual regions do not show any base pairing and should be digested under mild conditions. Thus, under standard conditions the molecule depicted in Figure 1A would not be protected at all against RNase digestion, while the molecule in Figure 1B would be protected by 50% in spite of the fact that in both cases the base sequence homology is 50%.

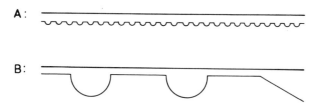

Fig. 1. Scheme for the distribution of 50% mismatching at random (A) or in 3 clusters (B).

In Figure 2 the relative stability of heteroduplex molecules obtained after hybridization of segment 4, which is the HA gene of fowl plague virus (A/FPV/Rostock/34; Hav1N1), with homologous and heterologous cRNA is shown. On the left graph data are presented obtained after digestion of the double-stranded RNA molecules by RNase A in 2 x SSC at different temperatures. After hybridization with cRNA of A/turkey/England/63 (Hav1Nav3) there is complete protection at 10°, while at 20° (standard conditions) the protection is only 90%. At higher temperatures the molecule is almost completely digestable. Under these conditions, however, also the homologous hybrid is not completely stable. If the cRNA of the serologically unrelated strain virus N (A/chick/Germany/N/49; Hav2Neq1) is used for hybridization, the protection never exceeds

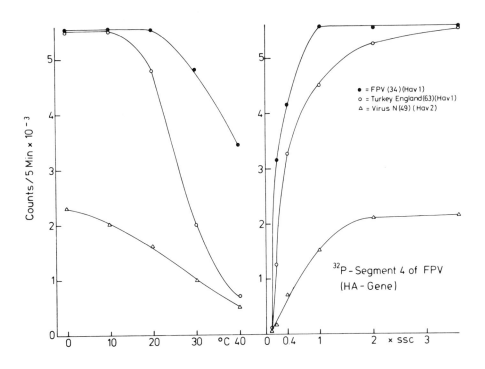

Fig. 2. RNase protection of hybrid molecules of ^{32}P-segment 4 of
FPV under various conditions of digestion. Left: Aliquots were
digested for 20 min in 2 x SSC at different temperatures (abscissa).
Right: Aliquots were digested at 10° for 20 min at different concentrations of SSC (abscissa).

40% and the residual homologous part is somewhat more stable when
compared with the turkey England-FPV hybrid. (Single-stranded RNA
is digested at 0° by at least 96%, at 20° by at least 98%). On the
right graph data are shown obtained after digestion of double-
stranded RNA at 10° and at different salt concentrations (SSC =
0.15 M NaCl; 0.015 M Na-citrate). At 0.1 x SSC also the homologous
hybrid RNA is completely digested. At high salt the turkey England-
FPV hybrid is completely protected, while protection after hybridi-

zation with cRNA of virus N does not exceed 40%. Corresponding observations have been made, when melting profiles of heteroduplex molecules of the HA and NA genes were determined[1,2]. All these results are compatible with the idea that the genes coding for the surface glycoproteins consist of a relatively small (30% for HA; 20% for NA) highly conserved region(s), and a relatively large variable region(s).

In order to substantiate this idea we have calibrated the hybridization technqiue by introducing random mismatching by treatment of the ^{32}P-labelled vRNA with nitrous acid at pH 4.1 according to Schuster and Schramm[3]. By this treatment cytidine (C) is converted to uridine (U); adenosine (A) to inosine (I), which behaves like guanosine (G) during base pairing; G is converted to xanthosine (X), which behaves like G; and U is not affected. By determination of the base composition after treatment with HNO_2 we can evaluate the percentage of mismatching introduced in this way. (The conversion of a GC-pair to a GU-pair has been regarded as mismatching). In Figure 3 the correlation between mismatching, RNase protection and melting profiles is demonstrated for two RNA segments with different contents of C+G (segments 8 and 5 of FPV). The percentage of mismatching increases linearly with time of treatment with HNO_2. According to the C+G-content the melting point of the hybrid RNA of segment 5 is $2°$ higher. The melting point of segment 8 is $87°$, which agrees with that of the HA and NA gene[2]. Thus we can compare these data with our results obtained with RNA segment 4 and 6 of FPV.

In Figure 4 melting profiles are presented of hybrid molecules of segment 6 of FPV. Except for the A/duck/Ukraine/63 strain (Hav7Neq2) the other strains have a N1 neuraminidase like FPV. Accordingly, these latter strains exhibit after hybridization a relatively high RNase protection at $20°$. The melting points obtained from these curves (between $73°$ and $76°$) are $2°$ to $3°$ higher than expected from the RNase protection indicating that the mismatching in the hybrid molecules is nearly, but not completely, distributed at random over the total length of the molecule. The theoretical RNase protection calculated from the melting point of the hybrid with the duck Ukraine strain should be about 94%. Since it is only 20% it is clear that about one fifth of the molecule

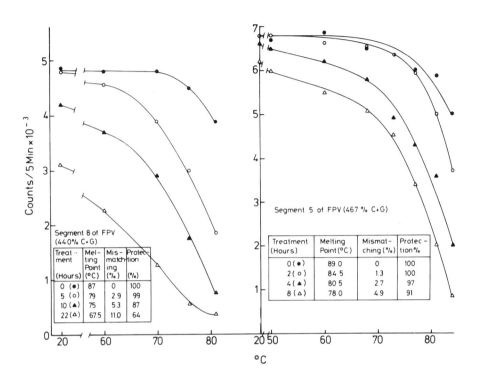

Fig. 3. Calibration of the hybridization technique by introducing random mismatching with HNO₂. ^{32}P-labelled vRNA segments 8 (left) or 5 (right) were treated for different length of time with HNO₂. The reisolated RNA was hybridized with saturating concentrations of the homologous cRNA. Aliquots were heated for 8 min in 1 x SSC containing 1% formaldehyde at the desired temperature (abscissa) and were digested in 2 x SSC at 20° with RNase.

exhibits a base sequence homology of more than 95%, while the base sequence homology of the residual 80% is not much higher than that found with an unrelated RNA. Corresponding results have been obtained with the hemagglutinin gene[2] indicating that within the HA gene there is a region, or regions, of altogether 30% of the total length, which are highly conserved. We can calculate from these data, that the highly conserved block(s) of the HA gene consists of about 600 nucleotides, and that of the NA gene of about 300

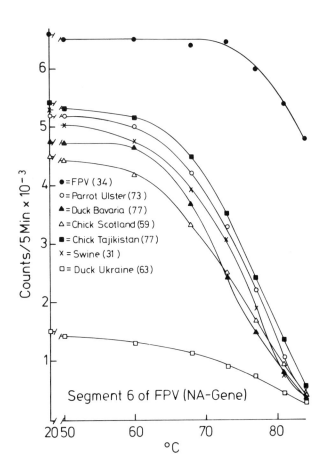

Counts/5 Min × 10⁻³

● = FPV (34)
○ = Parrot Ulster (73)
▲ = Duck Bavaria (77)
△ = Chick Scotland (59)
■ = Chick Tajikistan (77)
× = Swine (31)
□ = Duck Ukraine (63)

Segment 6 of FPV (NA-Gene)

°C

Fig. 4. Melting profiles of hybrid molecules obtained after hybridization of ³²P-segment 6 (NA-gene) of FPV with saturating concentrations of cRNA of various influenza strains. For experimental
conditions see legend of Figure 3.

nucleotides. Since mismatching is supposed to be about 5% within

these regions we can calculate, that for the HA gene about 30 bases and for the NA gene only about 15 bases vary within the conserved part of these genes.

The sensitivity of the method to differentiate between highly related genes can be estimated as follows: The melting point of a homologous hybrid can be determined with an accuracy of $\pm$ 1°. Since 1.3% mismatching causes already a difference in the melting point of 4.5° (Fig. 3, right) mismatching of 0.5% should be detectable. This means that 10 point mutations within a gene of the size of the HA should be discovered.

In Figure 5 the melting profiles of hybrid molecules obtained with ^{32}P-labelled segment 6 (NA gene) of the human strain A/PR/8/34 (HON1) are shown. It can be seen that the human A/FM/1/47 (H1N1) strain is closer related to PR8 than the human A/FW/1/50 isolate. The human H1N1 virus which was isolated 7 years later (A/Loy/4/57; H1N1) is again less related to PR8 when compared to the FW-strain. This clearly indicates that there is a drift within the N1 gene. The swine virus (A/swine/1976/31; Hsw1N1) which is supposed to be a survivor of the Spanish influenza of 1918/19 is even less related to the NA gene of PR8 than that of the Loy strain. The NA gene of A/FPV/Rostock/34 (Hav1N1) exhibits the lowest relatedness to the NA gene of PR8. Our serological data are in agreement with the genetic data.

DISCUSSION

The structural feature of having a small highly conserved portion and a large variable portion has been found only with the genes coding for the surface glycoproteins of influenza viruses. In contrast, the genes coding for the proteins surrounded by the lipid bilayer (the three P-proteins, NP and M) are highly conserved[2]. According to the calibration curves of Figure 3, in these genes the relatively little mismatching is scattered over the total length of the molecule. For the HA- and NA-genes it has been found, that the conserved regions are located always at the same sites within the molecules when different strains were compared[4]. These observations are interpreted to mean that the conserved parts of the HA- and NA-genes are involved in the functional integrity of the gene products. Most mutations in these regions would be lethal. The variable part might be involved in the im-

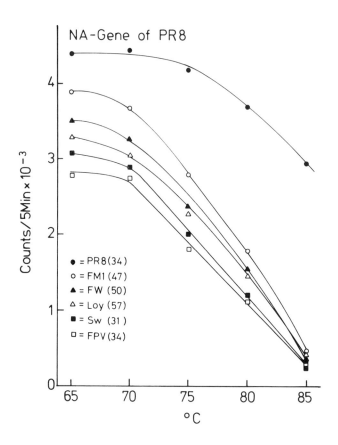

Fig. 5. Melting profiles of hybrid molecules obtained after hybridization of ^{32}P-segment 6 (NA) gene of PR8 with saturating concentrations of cRNA of various influenza strains. For experimental
conditions see legend of Figure 3.

munological properties. Mutations there sould be tolerated, and

the immune response would select always for such mutants which

have   changed their immunological properties to a certain extent.

In this way we can explain the unusual antigenic drift quite easily. Given enough time, a serologically completely different strain
will finally emerge. However, since only a limited number of
antigenically different strains have evolved we have to assume
that certain restrictions, perhaps concerning the shape of the
molecule, are involved in the evolution of influenza A virus
strains.

ACKNOWLEDGMENTS

I thank V. von Hoyningen-Huene for providing me with the ^{32}P-
labelled vRNA segments. The work was supported by the Sonderforschungsbereich 47, Virology, of the Deutsche Forschungsgemeinschaft.

REFERENCES

1. Scholtissek, C., Harms, E., Rohde, W., Orlich, M. and Rott, R. (1976) Virology 74, 332-344.
2. Scholtissek, C. (1979) Virology 93, 594-597.
3. Schuster, H. and Schramm, G. (1958) Z. Naturforsch. 13b, 697-704.
4. Scholtissek, C., Rohde, W. and Harms, E. (1977) J. Gen. Virol. 37, 243-247.

(See DISCUSSION on following page)

DISCUSSION

White: I would like to comment on 70-80% of the HA gene being variable. It is
inconceivable that 70-80% of the molecule could be antigenically active,
therefore either most changes are silent or are inducing conformational
changes in the antigenic site.

Porter: Do you have data comparing segment 8 of FPV to H0 and H3?

Scholtissek: In FPV segment 8 of human strains RNAse protection is about 85%.
Between human influenza strains the homology is extremely high and they form
one group. In avian strains there are two groups.

Porter: The homology in segment 8 between our fowl plague sequence and Gillian
Air's H2 sequence is about 90%, over the first 150 nucleotides.

Choppin: How about between A and B viruses?

Scholtissek: Between A and B the RNAse protection is quite low - about 20%, but
there are sequence homologies.

STUDIES ON STRUCTURE - FUNCTION RELATIONSHIPS OF INFLUENZA VIRUS
GLYCOPROTEINS

RUDOLF ROTT
Institut für Virologie, Justus-Liebig-Universität Giessen,
6300 Giessen, Germany

INTRODUCTION

Formation of hemagglutinin (HA) of orthomyxoviruses is ac-
companied by cotranslational and posttranslational modifications
such as proteolytic cleavage and glycosylation. There is evidence
that initial translation products contain a N-terminal presequence,
which after insertion into the membrane of the endoplasmatic reticulum is subsequently removed to form native HA polypeptide[1].
Glycosylation starts on the nascent polypeptide by transfer of a
carbohydrate core from a preformed oligosaccharide pyrophosphoryl-
dolichol. It is completed during transport of the HA molecule
from rough to smooth membranes[2,5]. The final stage in the formation of active hemagglutinin involves cleavage by a host specific
protease to produce a molecule containing the polypeptide components HA1 and HA2 (for review see[6])

In this paper I would like to give a contribution to the biological consequences resulting from these modifications of the HA
molecule.

ROLE OF POSTTRANSLATIONAL PROTEOLYTIC CLEAVAGE OF HEMAGGLUTININ
FOR INFECTIVITY

Recent studies[7-9] clearly showed that the structure of the HA as
coded for by the viral genome determines whether a host proteolytic enzyme will be capable of performing the cleavage necessary
for infectivity of the virus particle. Only virions with a cleaved
HA are infectious, while virus particles containing uncleaved HA
are non-infectious. Viruses formed as non-infectious particles
in a given host cell system can be converted into infectious
particles by treatment in vitro with trypsin or trypsin-like
enzymes which characteristically cleave the hemagglutinin. Since
viruses formed with uncleaved HA are capable to adsorb to receptors of the host cell, hemagglutinin, in addition to its role
in adsorption, must have a decisive function for virus penetration.

It has been suggested that penetration takes place by fusion of the viral envelope with the cell membrane. This concept is supported by the following observations:

1. Comparative studies using nuclear magnetic resonance spectra of chicken fibroblasts exposed to influenza virus carrying either cleaved or uncleaved HA indicates that the virus containing the cleaved HA induces an alteration in the fluidity of the lipid bilayer of the plasma membrane early after infection which is not seen when cells are infected with virus particles containing an uncleaved HA[10].

2. Primed T lymphocytes exert a cytotoxic effect when the target cells are incubated with infectious or UV-inactivated influenza virus containing cleaved HA. Cytotoxicity cannot be observed, however, if virus particles containing uncleaved HA are merely adsorbed to the surface of a potential target cell. Trypsin-mediated cleavage of the latter cell-adsorbed virions is followed by strong cytolysis[11].

3. More direct evidence for fusion between the viral envelope and plasma membrane of the host cell being dependent on a cleaved HA comes from studies with liposomes carrying the viral glyco-proteins on their surface. Such liposomes can be prepared by mixing viral glycoproteins with lipids in the presence of octyl-glucoside, which is easily removed by dialysis[12]. Electron microscopic studies showed (Fig. 1) that liposomes containing cleaved HA fuse with cell membranes. Liposomes with uncleaved HA are merely adsorbed to the cell surface and fusion occurs only after _in vitro_ treatment with trypsin. This membrane inter-action is followed by transfer of the liposomal contents into the cytoplasm, as was proved by staining of the cytoplasm with fluorescein labelled dextran which was trapped in liposomes (Fig. 2). Interestingly, native virus particles could be shown to fuse with liposomes which were prepared containing a crude extract of host membrane components. Virus was able not only to adsorb to these liposomes, but electron microscopic observations showed that viral spikes had become incorporated and exposed on

the liposomal membrane. Hence it could be inferred that an event equivalent to virus penetration had occurred. Such liposomes again fuse with the host cell membrane[13].

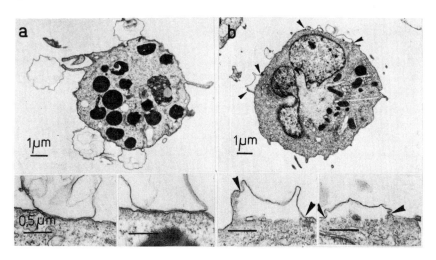

Fig. 1. Interaction of chick embryo cells with liposomes containing uncleaved (a) or cleaved (b) hemagglutinin of virus N. Liposomes were reacted with cells for 30 min at room temperature.

Surprisingly, preliminary studies gave evidence that HA alone even in the cleaved form is not able to induce fusion. Liposomes coaded with cleaved HA without neuraminidase are strongly adsorbed to cell membranes (Fig. 3). However, fusion occurs only when soluble neuraminidase - viral or even V. cholerae enzyme - is introduced into the liposome-host cell mixture. This might indicate that both viral glycoproteins, the HA and the neuraminidase, are required for penetration and infectivity of influenza virus. This conclusion is in contrast to previous findings where infection of influenza virus was not prevented by anti-neuraminidase antibodies[14,15]. It might be that a residual enzyme activity after the antigen-antibody reaction is sufficient to aid fusion.

The nature of the receptor responsible for virus penetration, i.e. membrane fusion, is not biochemically defined. These results suggesting a cooperative role of neuraminidase for penetration should help us to shed light on the mechanism underlying virus penetration.

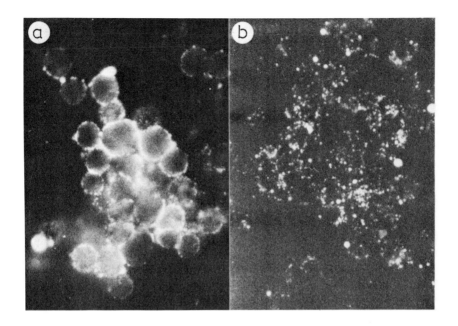

Fig. 2. Interaction of chick embryo cells with fluorescein-dextran loaded liposomes containing cleaved (a) or uncleaved (b) HA of virus N.

STRUCTURE OF THE HA AND PATHOGENICITY

A comparative analysis performed on a large number of naturally occurring avian influenza strains has demonstrated that the susceptibility of the HA to proteolytic cleavage correlates with host range and with pathogenicity of these viruses for the chicken[16]. Only those viruses which are produced in an infectious form in a broad range of host cells are pathogenic. It should be emphasized that there are not only differences in cleavability of the HA glycoprotein and pathogenicity between the different HA-subtypes but even within a single subtype. Although all strains in the subtype Hav1 have a serologically closely related hemagglutinin, they differ in cleavability and pathogenicity. Analyses of the genetic relatedness of the HA gene of these viruses show significant differences in their base sequence homology (v. Hoyningen and Scholtissek, personal communication). Differences in the structure of the HA glycoprotein of the Hav1 strains can also be shown by

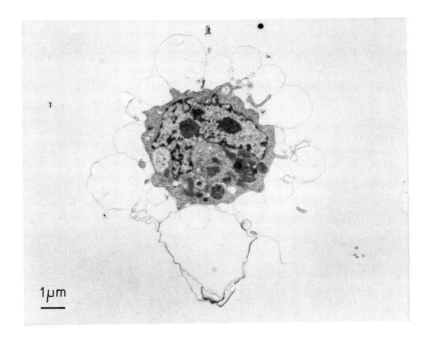

Fig. 3. Adsorption to cell membrane of liposomes containing
cleaved HA of virus N in the absence of neuraminidase.

tryptic peptide analysis and cyanogen bromide fragmentation. Besides the number of common peptides they also contain peptides of
different mobilities. The most significant differences are revealed by isoelectric focusing. In general, the HA of the pathogenic strains have a significantly more basic isoelectric point
than the HA of the non-pathogenic strains. These different isoelectric points are due to differences in the structure of the HA1
subunit rather than HA2. This became evident in the isoelectric
focusing patterns of the 2 HA subunits derived from HA of the
pathogenic strains cleaved in vivo and the HA of non-pathogenic
strains which had been treated with trypsin (Table 1) (Bosch,
unpublished results).

TABLE 1

DETERMINATION OF ISOELECTRIC POINTS OF THE HA OF PATHOGENIC AND
NON-PATHOGENIC AVIAN INFLUENZA VIRUSES OF SUBTYPE Hav1

Virus strain	Pathogenicity for chicken	Isoelectric points[*]		
		HA	HA1	HA2
A/FPV/Rostock	+	7.35	>8.5	5.3
A/FPV/Dutch/27	+	7.3	>8.5	5.3
A/FPV/turkey/Engl./63	+	7.4	>8.5	5.3
A/parrot/Ulster/73	−	6.35	6.6	5.35
A/turkey/Oregon/71	−	6.6	7.0	5.3

[*] Because of the heterogenicity of HA and its subunits mean values
are given.

The findings pointing to the prime significance of the HA for
pathogenicity do not contradict the results obtained with recombinants of influenza A viruses obtained in vitro. In an analysis
of a large number of such recombinants, it became evident that
pathogenicity of influenza viruses depends not only on the HA but
also on an opitmal gene composition which varies and is determined
by the parental viruses used for reassortment. It was observed
that a concomitant transfer of the genes coding for viral polymerase activity is critical for pathogenicity (for review see[17]).
One has to keep in mind that the recombinants obtained in vitro
can be looked as artificially constructed viruses. It appears that
in the avian host, only viruses with an optimal gene composition
survive. If in addition to carrying such an optimal gene composition, the viruses possess HA which is cleaved in different types
of host cells, they are pathogenic.

INFLUENCE OF CO- AND POSTTRANSLATIONAL MODIFICATIONS ON THE ANTI-
GENICITY OF HEMAGGLUTININ

The question whether co- and posttranslational processing influences the antigenicity of HA was examined using radioimmune
precipitations (Kaluza, Klenk and Rott, in preparation). It could

be shown that uncleaved HA is precipitated with antisera against uncleaved as well as cleaved HA. Similarly, cleaved HA is also precipitated with both kinds of antisera. Furthermore, antibodies for both forms of HA could be removed by absorption with excess of uncleaved HA. Experiments were undertaken to prove whether glycosylation influences the antigenic reactivity of the HA. Non-glycosylated HA was obtained by treatment of infected cells with 2-deoxy-D-glucose, which is known to inhibit glycosylation[18,19]. Antisera against glycosylated HA precipitate the non-glycosylated equally well as the glycosylated HA (Fig. 4). Virus preparations with glycosylated HA absorbed antibodies against both glycosylated and non-glycosylated HA. Furthermore, a mutant of fowl plague virus (FPV) with a temperature-sensitive defect in the HA has been ana-lyzed. This mutant has a block in the transport from rough to smooth membranes, proteolytic cleavage does not occur and glyco-sylation is incomplete[5]. Antiserum against the wild type FPV pre-cipitated the mutant HA synthesized at the non-permissive tempera-ture as well as that formed at the permissive temperature.

CONCLUSION

The antigenic structure of HA is expressed on the HA polypeptide chain and neither glycosylation nor cleavage change its reactivi-ty. This structural stability should allow the isolation of HA antigen(s) as fragments of relatively low molecular weight. The biological significance of glycosylation is still unknown. It seems quite clear that glycosylation is not required for membrane insertion of HA. The unglycosylated HA migrates in the cytoplasm in the same manner as the glycosylated molecule[20]. It might be that carbohydrates are necessary for metabolic stability and that they are responsible for the hydrophilic properties of the HA molecule. Proteolytic cleavage is a fundamental step in the formation of in-fectious influenza virus. By cleavage a hydrophobic region, which seems to promote penetration, becomes accessible on the N-terminus of HA. All data available are in agreement with the concept that penetration occurs by fusion of the viral envelope with the cell membrane. There is some evidence that the fusion process represents a cooperative function between cleaved HA and neuraminidase. The mechanism by which neuraminidase acts in penetration is still

unknown. Cleavage of HA in different types of cells in the organism
enables the virus to spread rapidly and determines the outcome of
an infection.

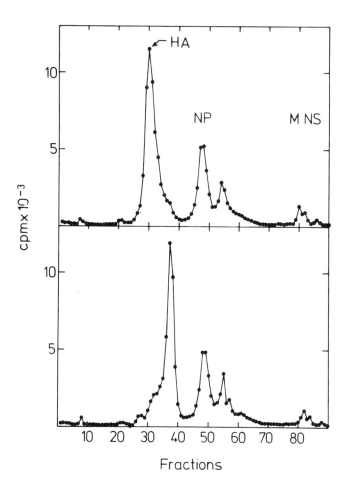

Fig. 4. Indirect radioimmune precipitation of virus N proteins
extracted from infected cells with antiserum against virus N.
Cell extracts were prepared from infected cells treated with 1 mM
2-deoxy-D-glucose (lower panel) or not treated (upper panel) and
labelled 5 hrs after infection for 30 min with [3H]-amino acids.
The extracts were precipitated by antibodies against virus-specific proteins present in infected cells.

ACKNOWLEDGMENTS

Original work was done in cooperation with Miss M. Orlich, and Drs. F. X. Bosch, R. T. C. Huang, G. Kaluza, H.-D. Klenk, C. Scholtissek, and K. Wahn. It was supported by the Deutsche Forschungsgemeinschaft (Sonderforschungsbereich 47).

REFERENCES

1. Waterfield, M. D., Espelie, K., Ebler, K. and Skehel, J. J. (1979) Brit. Med. Bull. 35, 57-63.
2. Schwarz, R. T., Schmidt, M. F. G., Anwer, U. and Klenk, H.-D. (1977) J. Virol. 23, 217-226.
3. Klenk, H.-D., Schwarz, R. T., Schmidt, M. F. G. and Wöllert, W. (1978) Top. Infect. Dis. 3, 83-99.
4. Nakamura, K. and Compans, R. W. (1979) Virology 93, 31-47.
5. Lohmeyer, J. and Klenk, H.-D. (1979) Virology 93, 134-145.
6. Klenk, H.-D. and Rott, R. (1980) Curr. Top. Microbiol. Immunol., in press.
7. Klenk, H.-D., Rott, R., Orlich, M. and Blödorn, J. (1975) Virology 68, 426-439.
8. Lazarowitz, S. G. and Choppin, P. W. (1975) Virology 68, 440-454.
9. Klenk, H.-D., Rott, R. and Orlich, M. (1977) J. gen. Virol. 36, 151-161.
10. Nicolau, C., Klenk, H.-D., Reimann, A., Hildenbrand, K. and Bauer, H. (1978) Biochim. Biophys. Acta 511, 83-92.
11. Kurrle, R., Wagner, H., Röllinghoff, M. and Rott, R. (1979) Eur. J. Immunol. 9, 107-111.
12. Huang, R. T. C., Wahn, K., Klenk, H.-D. and Rott, R. (1979) Virology 97, 212-217.
13. Huang, R. T. C., Wahn, K., Klenk, H.-D. and Rott, R. (1980), submitted.
14. Seto, J. T. and Rott, R. (1966) Virology 30, 731-737.
15. Webster, R. G. and Laver, W. G. (1967) J. Immunol. 99, 49-55.
16. Bosch, F. X., Orlich, M., Klenk, H.-D. and Rott, R. (1979) Virology 95, 197-207.
17. Rott, R. (1979) Arch. Virol. 59, 285-298.
18. Kaluza, G., Scholtissek, C. and Rott, R. (1972) J. gen. Virol. 14, 251-259.
19. Klenk, H.-D., Scholtissek, C. and Rott, R. (1972) Virology 49, 723-734.
20. Klenk, H.-D., Wöllert, W., Rott, R. and Scholtissek, C. (1974) Virology 57, 28-41.

(See DISCUSSION on following page)

DISCUSSION

Salser: Do your experiments rule out the possibility that some antigenic determinants are dependent on glycosylation?

Rott: I think so.

Ward: Have you looked at immunogenicity of uncleaved HA?

Rott: No. It is very difficult to isolate non-glycosylated HA, and we could not be sure HA was not cleaved before antibody production starts.

Laver: What does antibody do to the fusion of the liposomes?

Rott: We haven't looked.

Rott: When we treat virus with monospecific antisera against neuraminidase, we only inhibit 95-98% of neuraminidase activity and maybe there is still enough left to aid fusion. Palese and Compans have shown that virus particles are not liberated if neuraminidase is completely inhibited. When we do the experiments there is always a little neuraminidase activity left. Even with protease treatment you cannot be sure you have eliminated all neuraminidase.

Gandhi: Why is it difficult to isolate non-glycosylated HA?

Rott: Because the non-glycosylated HA is destroyed by cellular enzymes.

Choppin: Do you think your liposomes are behaving like virus particles?

Rott: The liposomes have HA activity, and intact virus particles can fuse with liposomes which are coated with cell receptors.

Palese: When you add neuraminidase inhibitor to the virus, you do not inhibit virus penetration.

Compans: But you could have, for example, charge repulsion between the liposome membrane and cell membrane if sialic acid is present, but this may not have anything to do with viruses.

Rott: All I can say is that liposomes coated with HA alone will not fuse to cell membrane, but if you add soluble neuraminidase you get fusion.

Wiley: It seems sensible that the HA has to unbind from a sialic acid containing receptor if it is to end up on the surface of the cell, therefore it must be a 2-step process.

Rott: That's why I asked Purnell if there were two receptors, and we are also thinking in terms of two receptors, one for HA1 and one for HA2. We know we can unmask the structures of the cell surface with neuraminidase, we can unmask antigens which are not normally exposed, and it is possible that the neuraminidase acts by unmasking the receptor responsible for attachment of HA2.

PROCESSING OF THE HEMAGGLUTININ: GLYCOSYLATION AND PROTEOLYTIC CLEAVAGE

HANS-DIETER KLENK
Institut für Virologie, Justus-Liebig-Universität Giessen,
6300 Giessen, Germany

INTRODUCTION

The biosynthesis of the hemagglutinin involves translation at membrane-bound ribosomes, insertion into the membrane of the rough endoplasmic reticulum, and transport to the plasma membrane[1]. Insertion into the rough endoplasmic reticulum appears to be mediated by a signal sequence at the amino-terminus (Skehel this meeting). Little is known about the mechanism responsible for transport to the plasma membrane. Virus mutants with a temperature-sensitive defect in hemagglutinin transport should be valuable tools for throwing light on this problem[2].

Processing of the hemagglutinin involves proteolytic cleavage and glycosylation. Proteolytic cleavage removes at the cotranslational level the signal sequence and converts at the posttranslational level the precursor HA into the fragments HA_1 and HA_2. Cleavage of HA which is essential for the infectivity of the virus appears to be exerted by cellular proteases. Depending on the presence of an appropriate enzyme in a given cell, virus particles with cleaved or with uncleaved hemagglutinin may be formed[3,4]. Glycosylation occurs also in a stepwise manner, with different saccharide residues added in distinct cellular compartments. It is initiated at the rough endoplasmic reticulum by the en bloc transfer of oligosaccharides containing mannose and glucosamine from a polyisoprenol derivative to the nascent polypeptide chain. After a trimming process, fucose and galactose are attached presumably in the Golgi apparatus[2,5,6].

This contribution is concerned primarily with the arrangement of the oligosaccharide side chains on the hemagglutinin and with some molecular details of the cleavage of HA into HA_1 and HA_2.

MATERIALS AND METHODS

Viruses. 18 Influenza A strains containing most of the hemagglutinin serotypes known to date have been analyzed. Viruses were grown in the chick embryo, in chick embryo fibroblasts, and in MDBK cells. Virus growth, labeling with radioactive isotopes, virus purification, and isolation of the hemagglutinin by preparative polyacrylamide gel electrophoresis were done as described elsewhere[5].

Carbohydrate analyses. Glycopeptides were prepared by Pronase digestion and isolated by chromatography on Biogel P6 columns[5,7]. Constituent sugars were determined by gas liquid chromatography[8] and by labeling with radioactive precursor sugars[5]. The nature of the carbohydrate-protein linkage was determined by procedures described elsewhere[7].

Analysis of amino acid sequences. Amino-terminal sequences were determined either by a microscale modification of the dansyl-Edman degradation of unlabeled polypeptides[9] or by Edman degradation of polypeptides that were specifically labeled with radioactive amino acids. Carboxy-termini were determined by digestion with carboxypeptidases A and B followed by amino acid analysis of the released residues.

RESULTS AND DISCUSSION

The carbohydrate side chains of the hemagglutinin are exclusively asparagine-linked oligosaccharides similar to those found in other viral glycoproteins and in serum glycoproteins. The side chains can be isolated in the form of glycopeptides that are obtained after Pronase digestion. Table 1 shows the gross composition of the glycopeptides that are obtained from the hemagglutinin of most influenza A strains when grown in chick embryo cells. Two major types are found: the complex type I and the mannose-rich type II. With each type at least 2 subtypes (A,B) can be distinguished. Whereas both types appear to be distinct structural entities, the subtypes may be modifications of the same basic structure that differ from each other only by microheterogeneity. This is suggested by the observation that all 4 subtypes are obtained from HA$_2$ of Hav1, even though this glycoprotein contains only one complex and one mannose-rich side chain (see below). Detailed structural analyses of the various types of side chains are presently under way.

TABLE 1
STRUCTURAL PROPERTIES OF THE GLYCOPEPTIDES OBTAINED FROM INFLUENZA VIRUS HEMAGGLUTININ[5,7,8]

	Type I A	Type I B	Type IIA	Type II B
Constituent sugars	GlcNAc, Man, Gal, Fuc		Man	GlcNAc
Molecular weight	3,000	2,400	1,800	1,100
Number of amino acids	ca. 3	ca. 3	ca. 2	?
Number of sugars	ca. 15	ca. 12	ca. 9	?
Protein - CH linkage	Asparagine-N-Acetylglucosamine			
Binding to Concanavalin A	weak		strong	

Number of side chains. Based on the total carbohydrate content of the hemagglutinin and on the size of the glycopeptides, estimates have been made of 5 - 6 side chains on Hav1[5] and 4 - 5 side chains on HO[10]. A more accurate procedure for the determination of the number of side chains is based on the following principle. Inhibitors of glycosylation, such as 2-deoxyglucose or glucosamine, interfere with the formation of lipid-linked oligosaccharides. Glycoproteins synthesized under conditions of partial inhibition have a reduced sugar content. This reduction is due to the lack of whole carbohydrate chains[5]. Depending on the number of eliminated side chains, different subspecies of a given glycoprotein can be resolved on polyacrylamide gels. Using this procedure it was found that HA_2 of serotypes Hav1 and Hav2 contains 2 oligosaccharides, whereas HA_2 of serotypes HO and H3 contains only 1 oligosaccharide[11].

Localization of the side chains on the polypeptide. The determination of the nucleotide sequence of the Hav1 gene (Porter, this meeting) allows the localizing of possible carbohydrate attachment sites (Asn-x-Thr or Asn-x-Ser) on the hemagglutinin polypeptide. HA_2 contains 2 such sites which are located on different tryptic peptides. Since one side chain is complex and the other one mannose-rich (see below), the respective tryptic peptides can be separated from each other by differential affinity to agarose-bound Concanavalin A. By specifically labeling each polypeptide with a radioactive amino acid not present in the other glycopeptide it could be demonstrated that Hav1 has a side chain of type II in position 424 and a side chain of type I in position 496.

TABLE 2

THE GLYCOPEPTIDES DERIVED FROM HEMAGGLUTININ SUBUNITS HA_1 and HA_2 OF DIFFERENT INFLUENZA A STRAINS

Strain	Serotype of hemagglutinin and neuraminidase	HA_1		HA_2	
		type I	II	type I	II
A/PR/8/34	HON1	+	−	+	−
A/FM/1/47	H1N1	+	−	+	−
A/Asia/M/1468	H2N2	+	+	+	−
A/MRC/11	H3N1	+	+	+	−
A/Swine/Shope/31	Hsw1N1	+	−	+	−
A/equine/Miami/1/63	Heq2Neq2	+	+	+	−
A/FPV/Rostock	Hav1N1	+		+	+
A/FPV/Dutch/27	Hav1Neq1	+	−	+	+
A/fowl/Victoria/75	Hav1Neq1	+		+	+
A/turkey/Ore/71	Hav1Nav2	+	−	+	+
A/chick/Ger/49	Hav2Neq1	+	+	+	+
A/duck/Eng/56	Hav3Nav1	+	+	+	−
A/duck/CSSR/56	Hav4Nav1	+	−	+	−
A/turkey/Ont/7732/66	Hav5Nav6	+	+	+*	−
A/chick/Scot/59	Hav5N1	+		+*	
A/duck/Ukr/1/63	Hav7Neq2	+	+ (?)	+	−
A/turkey/Ont/6116/68	Hav8Nav4	+		−	−
A/turkey/Wis/66	Hav9Neq1	+	+	+	−

* Type I without fucose

Host specific variations. The size of the oligosaccharide side chains depends on the host cell. This can be demonstrated by a comparison of virus grown in MDBK cells with virus grown in chick embryo fibroblasts. Type I glycopeptides derived from virus grown in

MDBK cells are significantly larger than those from virus grown in chick embryo fibroblasts. No such differences are observed with type II glycopeptides. Thus, host-specific variations appear to be restricted to type I side chains[11].

Strain specific variations. A comparative analysis of the hemagglutinin glycopeptides of 18 influenza A strains of mammalian and avian origin including most of the hemagglutinin subtypes known to date has been carried out. All strains were grown in chick embryo fibroblasts. Table 2 demonstrates that there are distinct variations in the distribution of type I and type II side chains on HA_1 and HA_2.

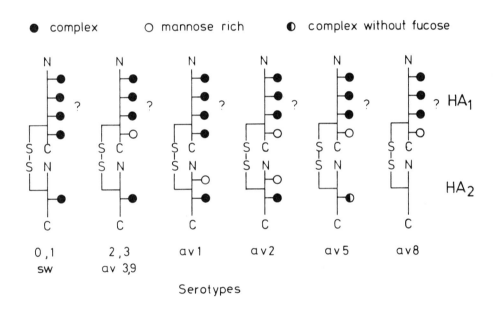

Fig. 1. Oligosaccharide patterns of different serotypes of the influenza A hemagglutinin. Viruses were grown in chick embryo fibroblasts. Number and arrangement of side chains on HA_1 have not been fully elucidated yet.

The data described so far are summarized in Fig. 1 showing the arrangement of the oligosaccharides on the hemagglutinin of different influenza A strains. With most serotypes, there is one side chain of type I on HA_2. With other serotypes, HA_2 contains 2 side chains, one of each type, and in at least one instance HA_2 is completely carbohydrate-free. The situation is less clear as far as the number and arrangement of the side chains on HA_1 is concerned. Thus, it has to be expected that with increasing information more than the 6 distribution patterns shown here will emerge. It should be pointed out that in the present study variations in the carbohydrate pattern have not been observed within a given serotype and that closely related serotypes (e.g. HO, H1, Hsw1 or H3, Heq2, Hav7) usually also have similar carbohydrate patterns. However, there are exceptions to this rule. E.g., Hav2 and Hav3, even though serologically related, have different carbohydrate patterns. Our observations together with a similar study by Nakamura and Compans[12] support the notion that the primary structure of the polypeptide is an important determinant for the carbohydrate moiety of the glycoprotein.

Molecular details of the cleavage of HA into HA_1 and HA_2

The cleavage site. The amino acid sequences at the carboxy-terminus of HA_1 and at the amino-terminus of HA_2 have been analyzed on egg-grown FPV hemagglutinin (Hav1) and have been compared with the sequence of the uncleaved FPV hemagglutinin, that has been deduced from the nucleotide sequence of the hemagglutinin gene (Porter, this meeting) (Fig. 2). It is clear that the amino-terminus of HA_2 is formed by Gly 343. Although more work is needed to clearly identify Ser 336 as the carboxy-terminus of HA_1, our data exclude the possibility that this terminus is located at Arg 342. Thus it appears that a basic polypeptide fragment is eliminated

HA (Porter and Emtage, 1979)

```
                    335                  340                    345
NH₂——Val - Pro - Glu - Pro - Ser - Lys - Lys - Arg - Glu - Lys - Arg - Gly - Leu - Phe - Gly - Ala - Ile ———— COOH

NH₂—— x - x - x - x - Ser (?)                          Gly - Leu - Phe - Gly - x - x ———— COOH
                          |                                          |
                         COOH                                       NH₂

              HA₁                                              HA₂
```

Fig. 2. The cleavage site of the FPV hemagglutinin (Hav1).

when HA is cleaved in vivo. If Ser 336 will be verified as the
carboxy-terminus of HA_1, involvement of at least 2 proteases will
have to be postulated, since trypsin-like enzymes (see below) are
able to cleave Arg-Gly, but not Ser-Lys.

TABLE 3

CLEAVAGE AND ACTIVATION OF THE HEMAGGLUTININ OF A/CHICK/GERMANY/49
(Hav2) BY DIFFERENT PROTEASES

Proteases	Cleavage	Activation
Trypsin	+	+
Streptomyces Griseus Protease	+	+
Acrosin*	+	+
Thermolysin	+	0
Chymotrypsin	+	0
Papain	+	0
Elastase	0	0

* Acrosin was a gift of Dr. H. Fritz and Dr. W. Müller-Esterl, Universität München

The amino-terminus of HA_2 after cleavage with different proteases. Proteases of different specificities are able to cleave HA,
but activation is observed only after cleavage with trypsin or
trypsin-like enzymes[4,13]. A number of proteases tested on the hemagglutinin of A/chick/Germany/49 (Hav2) is listed in Table 3.
These observations suggested that cleavage of a specific peptide
bond is required for activation. Therefore comparative sequence
analyses were carried out on Hav2 that has been cleaved either in
vivo or in vitro using proteases of various specificities. Of
prime interest was the amino terminus of HA_2 which is thought to
play a crucial function in penetration because of its structural
similarity to the amino-terminus of F_1 of paramyxoviruses[14]. After
in vitro cleavage with trypsin, the amino-terminus of HA_2 is
identical to that obtained after in vivo cleavage (Fig. 3). It differs, however, by a few amino acids from the amino-terminus of HA_2
obtained after cleavage with non-activating enzymes such as thermolysin or chymotrypsin. These observations suggest that activation

of infectivity requires a highly specific amino acid sequence at the amino-terminus of HA_2.

Cleavage	Activation	Amino-Terminus of HA_2 of Influenza Strain N
In Vivo	+	NH_2 - Gly - Leu - Phe - Gly - Ala - Ile - x - x - x
By Trypsin	+	NH_2 - Gly - Leu - Phe - Gly - Ala - Ile - Ala - Gly - x
Acrosin	+	NH_2 - Gly - Leu - Phe - x - Ala - Ile - x - x - x
By Thermolysin	O	NH_2 - Leu - Phe - Gly - Ala - Ile - x - x - x
By Chymotrypsin	O	NH - Gly - Ala - Ile - Ala - Gly - Phe

Fig. 3. The amino-terminus of HA_2 of virus N [A/chick/Germany/49 Hav2Neq1)] after in vivo cleavage in the egg and after in vitro cleavage by various proteases.

ACKNOWLEDGMENTS

This work was done in collaboration with W. Garten, W. Keil, H. Niemann, R. T. Schwarz and R. Rott. It was supported by the Deutsche Forschungsgemeinschaft (SFB 47).

REFERENCES

1. Compans, R. W. and Klenk, H.-D. (1979) in Comprehensive Virology, H. Fraenkel-Conrat and R. R. Wagner, eds., Plenum, N.Y., Vol. 13, pp. 293-407.
2. Lohmeyer, J. and Klenk, H.-D. (1979) Virology 93, 134-145.
3. Klenk, H.-D., Rott, R., Orlich, M. and Blödorn, J. (1975) Virology 68, 426-439.
4. Lazarowitz, S. G. and Choppin, P. W. (1975) Virology 48, 440-454.
5. Schwarz, R. T., Schmidt, M. F. G., Anwer, U. and Klenk, H.-D. (1977) J. Virol. 23, 217-226.
6. Nakamura, K. and Compans, R. W. (1979) Virology 93, 31-47.
7. Keil, W., Klenk, H.-D. and Schwarz, R. T. (1979) J. Virol. 31, 253-256.
8. Schwarz, R. T., Fournet, J., Montreuil, J., Rott, R. and Klenk, H.-D. (1978) Arch. Virol. 56, 251-255.
9. Weiner, A. M., Platt, T. and Weber, K. J. (1972) J. Biol. Chem. 247, 3242-3251.
10. Nakamura, K. and Compans, R. W. (1978) Virology 86, 432-472.
11. Schwarz, R. T. and Klenk, H.-D. (1979) in Glycoconjugates, R. Schauer et al., eds., Thieme, Stuttgart, pp. 678-679.

12. Nakamura, K. and Compans, R. W. (1979) Virology 95, 8-23.
13. Klenk, H.-D., Rott, R. and Orlich, M. (1977) J. Gen. Virol. 36, 151-161.
14. Gething, M. J., White, I. M. and Waterfield, M. D. (1978) Proc. Natl. Acad. Sci. (USA) 75, 2737-2740.

Summary. The hemagglutinin of influenza A virus contains 2 major types of oligosaccharide side chains, the complex type I and the mannose-rich type II. Analysis of 18 strains revealed wide variations in the distribution of the side chains on the hemagglutinin. So far 6 different distribution patterns can be distinguished. These observations demonstrate that the primary structure of the polypeptide plays a major role in determining the carbohydrate complement of the hemagglutinin. Comparative amino acid sequence analysis of the cleaved and uncleaved FPV hemagglutinin suggest elimination of a small peptide fragment and the involvement of more than one protease in the cleavage reaction. After in vitro cleavage with trypsin, the amino-terminus of HA_2 is identical to that obtained after in vivo cleavage. It differs, however, by a few amino acids from the amino-terminus of HA_2 obtained after cleavage with non-activating enzymes. These data suggest that activation of infectivity requires a highly specific amino acid sequence at the amino-terminus of HA_2.

(See DISCUSSION on following page)

DISCUSSION

Compans: Doesn't the fact that you can get activation with a specific protease suggest that only a single enzyme is used?

Klenk: We can only answer this if we sequence the C-terminus of HA1 after in vitro cleavage. It could of course be Arg anyway, or it might be the same as after in vivo cleavage, where the carboxypeptidase analyses suggest Ser.

Ward: It is surprising that carboxypeptidase A cleaves a Pro-Ser link!

Klenk: Yes, it is surprising.

Wiley: Do you check that no other cuts are introduced by thermolysin or chymotrypsin?

Klenk: The cleavage fragments on polyacrylamide gels are indistinguishable from those obtained after trypsin. The N termini of HA1 are identical.

Bean: Is there any chance that neuraminidase contains protease activity?

Klenk: I don't know.

Wiley: But the HA is activated before it reaches the cell surface.

Ward: If the neuraminidase has a protease you wouldn't be able to activate the HA with trypsin!

STUDIES ON THE STRUCTURE AND FUNCTION OF THE OLIGOSACCHARIDES OF THE INFLUENZA A HEMAGGLUTININ

RICHARD W. COMPANS, KIYOTO NAKAMURA, MICHAEL G. ROTH, WILLIAM L. HOLLOWAY, AND MAURICE C. KEMP

Department of Microbiology, University of Alabama Medical Center, Birmingham, Alabama, 35294 U.S.A.

INTRODUCTION

Several laboratories have characterized the oligosaccharides obtained from the hemagglutinin (HA) glycoprotein of various influenza A viruses following extensive digestion with pronase.[1-5] These observations have indicated that two major types of oligosaccharides are present in HA: complex (type I) oligosaccharides containing glucosamine, mannose, galactose, and fucose, as well as high mannose (type II) oligosaccharides which lack galactose and fucose. The oligosaccharides are synthesized by the en bloc transfer of high mannose type cores to asparagine residues, and subsequently some mannose residues are removed and other sugars are added to the resulting cores to produce the complex oligosaccharides.[6] However, the processing events resulting in formation of complex oligosaccharides occur only at certain glycosylation sites. Analysis of the pronase-derived glycopeptides of HA obtained from various influenza A virus subtypes revealed marked strain dependent differences in the relative amounts of complex and high mannose type oligosaccharides.[3] The high mannose type pronase glycopeptides are often resolved into two size classes by gel filtration,[3] and under certain conditions two size classes of the complex glycopeptides are also resolved.[5] However, it has not been possible to determine the exact number of glycosylation sites on HA by these techniques. We have recently investigated the number of glycosylation sites by analysis of glycopeptides obtained after extensive digestion of HA with trypsin, which produces glycopeptides containing a larger number of amino acid residues.[7] We have also investigated the role of glycosylation of HA in the intracellular migration processes of the glycoprotein and in the selective formation of virions at certain cellular membrane domains in epithelial cell monolayers.

TRYPTIC GLYCOPEPTIDES OF THE A/WSN HEMAGGLUTININ.

The A/WSN (H_0N_1) strain of influenza virus was grown in MDBK cells and purified as described previously.[8,9] The HA_1 and HA_2 glycoproteins were isolated by SDS-polyacrylamide gel electrophoresis of purified virions after mild trypsin treatment to remove neuraminidase (NA) glycoproteins.[2] For preparation of tryptic glycopeptides, the isolated glycoproteins were digested for 24 hr with 1 mg of TPCK trypsin, and the resulting glycopeptides were fractionated by ion exchange chromatography on DE52 cellulose.[7] Three major peaks were obtained from HA_1 (designated I, II, and III) and a single major peak was obtained from HA_2. Further fractionation of the HA_1 glycopeptides on Bio-Gel P-6 revealed that peaks I and III each consisted of two components, designated I-A, I-B, III-A, and III-B, respectively. In contrast, peak II from HA_1 and the single peak from HA_2 yielded a single main peak when analyzed by gel filtration. These results, as well as estimates of the molecular weights of each tryptic glycopeptide before and after digestion with Pronase, are summarized in Table I.

TABLE 1. PROPERTIES OF THE TRYPTIC GLYCOPEPTIDES OF THE A/WSN HEMAGGLUTININ[a]

HA Subunit	Tryptic Glycopeptide Designation	Oligo-saccharide Type	Molecular Weight		Endo-H Sensitivity	Sulfation	Affinity for LCA (% bound)	Affinity for Ricin (% bound)
			Before Pronase	After Pronase				
	I-A	complex	3,500	2,600-2,900	mostly resistant	-	32%	43%
	I-B	high mannose	1,800	1,600-1,800	totally sensitive	-	28%	0%
HA_1	II	complex	3,900	2,800-3,100	resistant	±	18%	56%
	III-A	complex	4,200	3,200	resistant	+	4%	100%
	III-B	intermediate	3,200	2,000-2,500	partially sensitive	+	90%	100%
HA_2	I	complex	3,000	2,900	resistant	-	18%	100%
	II	complex	3,000	2,900	resistant	+	N.D.	N.D.

a. The experimental results from which these data were obtained are presented in detail elsewhere.[7]

Further characterization of these glycosylated tryptic peptides has included determination of their extent of sulfation, sensitivity to digestion with endo-β-N-glucosaminidase H (endo-H), and affinity for lectins.[7] The results of such analyses (Table I) have revealed extensive heterogeneities in these properties, which are thought to be a result of heterogeneity in the oligosaccharide components. These results may be summarized as follows:

Sulfation. Previous studies had indicated that at least a portion of the complex oligosaccharides linked to HA contain covalently bound sulfate.[10, 11] Ion exchange chromatography on DE52 appears to be a feasible method for separation of sulfated and non-sulfated forms of the same glycopeptide type. This was demonstrated clearly with HA_2 tryptic glycopeptides, where the sulfated glycopeptides exhibited much stronger binding to the resin than did the nonsulfated components. The elution profiles of the sulfated and nonsulfated glycopeptides from HA_2 on gel filtration columns were nearly identical, suggesting the presence of a single structural type of glycopeptide that varied only in the content of sulfate. The glycopeptides from HA_1 presented a more complex pattern and the elution profile of sulfate-labeled glycopeptides from the DE52 column was markedly heterogeneous. Nevertheless, the results suggested that most of the sulfation of glycopeptides occurred in the III-A and III-B classes of tryptic glycopeptides, and that populations of these glycopeptides which differed in their extent of sulfation could be separated by ion exchange chromatography.

Endo-H sensitivity. We have previously shown that the high mannose glycopeptides of influenza HA are sensitive to digestion by endo-H, whereas complex glycopeptides are resistant.[3, 6] This enzyme cleaves between the two proximal N-acetylglucosamine residues of asparagine-linked glycopeptides that contain large mannose cores, but complex glycopeptides containing smaller cores are resistant to cleavage.[12, 13] Of the various tryptic glycopeptides, only glycopeptide I-B was completely sensitive to endo-H digestion, indicating the presence of a large oligomannosyl core structure. Glycopeptide III-B was partially sensitive and about 12% of glycopeptide I-A was sensitive to endo-H, whereas the remaining tryptic glycopeptides were resistant to enzymatic cleavage.

Lectin affinity. We examined the affinity of tryptic glycopeptides for two lectins, lens culinaris agglutinin (LCA) and ricinus communis agglutinin (ricin), which bind to α-D-mannopyranosyl and α-D-galactosyl residues, respectively. The results of affinity chromatography with lectins bound to agarose indicate that most of the tryptic glycopeptides were heterogeneous with respect to affinity for these lectins. Glycopeptide III-B bound most effectively to LCA, whereas III-A, III-B and glycopeptide I from HA_2 bound very effectively to ricin. A surprising result was obtained with HA_1 glycopeptide I-B, which did not bind effectively to LCA-agarose despite the apparent presence of terminal mannosyl residues based on radiolabeling data and endo-H sensitivity.

These results indicate that six major glycosylated tryptic peptides can be obtained from the A/WSN hemagglutinin glycoprotein. Five of these glycopeptides are recovered from the HA_1 subunit and one is obtained from the HA_2 subunit. We interpret these results to indicate that the six glycosylated tryptic peptides are obtained from six distinct glycosylation sites on the hemagglutinin glycoprotein molecule. It is likely that the separation of the tryptic glycopeptides by ion exchange chromatography primarily reflects the charge of the peptide portion, since the only negatively charged residue on the oligosaccharides appears to be sulfate which is present only in the glycopeptides eluting in the more retarded fractions from DE52. The tryptic glycopeptides contained in peak II from HA_2 are probably the sulfated form of the glycopeptides in peak I from HA_2, since they have indistinguishable molecular weights. Of the HA_1 glycopeptides, the peptide portions of I-A and I-B appear to be distinct since the extent of their decrease in size after subsequent pronase digestion is markedly different. However, further study is needed to determine if the peptides associated with III-A and III-B are distinct.

The observation that different oligosaccharide types are associated with different tryptic glycopeptide classes suggests that different glycosylation sites may acquire oligosaccharides with distinct structures. This observation supports our previous conclusion that the primary structure of the glycoprotein may determine the type of oligosaccharide which is linked to specific glycosylation sites.[3] However, there appears to be some heterogeneity even among oligosaccharide chains attached to a particular glycosylation site. This was most clearly demonstrated by the use of affinity chromatography on immobilized plant lectins. Each class of tryptic glycopeptide purified by a combination of ion exchange chromatography and gel filtration exhibited heterogeneity when analyzed by such affinity chromatography, indicating that the oligosaccharides attached to any glycosylation site may exhibit some variability in structure.

SEPARATION OF TRYPTIC GLYCOPEPTIDES BY REVERSE PHASE ION PAIR HPLC.

We have also analyzed the tryptic glycopeptides of the A/WSN HA glycoprotein by reverse phase high pressure liquid chromatography (HPLC).[14] The glycopeptides are applied to a column containing a stationary phase consisting of hydrophobic chains bonded to a rigid support, and are eluted by a gradient containing increasing amounts of an organic solvent. Thus the order of elution is primarily determined by hydrophobic interactions between amino acid residues and the stationary phase. Addition of compounds that form ion pairs with the sample is used to increase the recoveries of peptides.

To demonstrate the consistency of the elution profiles of tryptic glycopeptides from HA, we prepared separate samples of glycopeptides labeled with ^{3}H-glucosamine and with ^{14}C-glucosamine. The glycopeptides were mixed, applied to a column of μ Bondapak C_{18}, and eluted with a gradient of acetonitrile . As shown in Fig. 1, a total of about 8 glycopeptide peaks are resolved in the radioactivity profile obtained with either isotope. It is apparent that there is almost exact correspondence between the patterns obtained with ^{3}H and ^{14}C-glycopeptides.

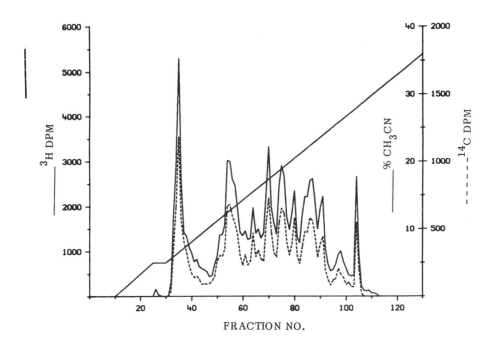

FRACTION NO.

Fig. 1.   Cochromatography of [3]H- and ^{14}C-glucosamine labelled influenza A/WSN tryptic glycopeptides. HA glycoproteins labelled with [3]H- or ^{14}C-glucosamine were isolated by SDS-polyacrylamide gel electrophoresis in the absence of reducing agents and digested with TPCK-trypsin. The labelled tryptic glycopeptides were applied to a C_{18} μ Bondapak column in 0.1% H_3PO_4, pH 2.85, and were eluted from the column by an increasing concentration of 0.1% H_3PO_4:CH_3CN; 40:60,V/V. The flow rate was 2.0 ml/min, 2ml fractions were collected, and radioactivity was determined by liquid scintillation counting. From Kemp et al.[14]

These results demonstrate the feasibility of using HPLC as an analytical or preparative method for characterization of the glycosylation sites of viral glycoproteins, and suggest that up to 8 glycopeptides are obtained from HA of influenza A/WSN. Further studies are needed to determine the correspondence between tryptic glycopeptides separated by ion exchange chromatography and gel filtration (Table 1), and the peaks observed by HPLC. It will also be necessary to obtain data on the peptide portions of these glycopeptides in order to determine if they all represent distinct glycosylation sites, or if some peaks may represent alternative oligosaccharide structures linked to the same glycosylation sites.

GLYCOSYLATION DOES NOT DETERMINE THE VIRAL MATURATION SITE.

Recent studies in several laboratories have utilized glycosylation inhibitors to investigate the role of carbohydrate side chains in determining membrane insertion, intracellular migration and biological activities of viral glycoproteins. In several virus-cell systems, inhibition of glycosylation by tunicamycin did result in inhibition of virion formation.[15-17] However, glycosylation is not necessary for normal transmembrane insertion of glycoproteins,[18] and in other virus-cell systems, normal intracellular migration as well as virion assembly has been observed with unglycosylated viral glycoproteins.[19, 20] The nonglycosylated glycoproteins are more sensitive to proteolytic degradation,[15] and may undergo aggregation at physiological temperatures.[21] Taken together, these results indicate that glycosylation is not a requirement in a positive sense for migration of glycoproteins to the cell surface or for their assembly into virions; however, some polypeptides may require glycosylation in order to assume a conformation which is compatible with remaining in a nonaggregated state, and other proteins may require glycosylation in order to protect them from proteolytic degradation. We have recently investigated[22] whether glycosylation of viral glycoproteins is a determinant of the site of virus maturation in epithelial cell monolayers, in which certain enveloped viruses are observed to form at different domains of the plasma membrane.

Cells of the Madin Darby canine kidney (MDCK) cell line exhibit many of the properties of normal renal tubular epithelial cell. Tight junctions are formed between adjacent cells in monolayer cultures, a spontaneous electrical potential is formed between upper and lower cell surfaces, and a vectorial transport of fluid occurs from apical to basal cell surfaces.[23-27] It has recently been observed that the assembly of certain enveloped viruses occurs selectively at the apical or basolateral plasma membrane domains, which are separated by tight junctions.[28, 29] Vesicular stomatitis virus (VSV) buds at the basolateral cell membrane, whereas influenza and parainfluenza viruses are formed at the free apical surface. Glycoproteins of each virus appeared to be selectively incorporated into the same plasma membrane domain where budding occurred, suggesting that the site of glycoprotein insertion determines the maturation site. Selective budding of virus at the exposed cell surface of chick chorioallantoic membranes had also been observed in early electron microscopic studies of influenza virus maturation.[30]

The viruses that form at apical vs. basolateral surfaces of MDCK cells show a qualitative difference in sialic acid content; VSV possesses a single sialic acid-containing glycoprotein (G), whereas influenza and parainfluenza viruses lack sialic acid presumably due to their neuraminidase activities.[31] Therefore, it seemed plausible that viral oligosaccharides could be involved as determinants of glycoprotein migration processes. To investigate this possibility, we examined the effect of tunicamycin, a potent glycosylation inhibitor, on the maturation site of these viruses. We determined by radiolabeling with ^{3}H-glucosamine that glycosylation of the VSV G protein and influenza HA and NA glycoproteins in MDCK cells was completely inhibited by 0.5 µg/ml of tunicamycin. To analyze the effects of the inhibition of glycosylation on the site of virus maturation, we grew MDCK cell monolayers on plastic films, and cells were fixed and embedded in situ.[32] Cells infected with 10-15 PFU/cell of influenza A/WSN or VSV-Indiana were treated with 1.0 µg/ml of tunicamycin at 2 h.p.i., and fixed and embedded at intervals during the growth cycle. Influenza virions maturing in the presence of tunicamycin budded exclusively from the apical membranes of MDCK monolayers (Fig. 2). The virions were never observed to bud from the basal or from the lateral membranes, but were restricted to the apical surface above the tight junctions for as long as the monolayer remained intact. VSV virions budding in the presence of tunicamycin were observed along the basal membranes or lateral membranes beneath the tight junctions (Fig. 3). Occasionally VSV virions were seen budding inside structures that could be either invaginations of the basal membrane or cytoplasmic vacuoles; this was also true of cells infected in the absence of tunicamycin. VSV virions were not observed budding from the apical surface of intact monolayers in either the presence or absence of tunicamycin. These results indicate that the polarity of virus maturation in MDCK cells is maintained under conditions of complete inhibition of the glycosylation of viral glycoproteins.

Since glycosylation is not essential for determining the site of influenza and vesicular stomatitis virus maturation, it is likely that features of the polypeptide backbones of viral glycoproteins determine their sites of insertion into the plasma

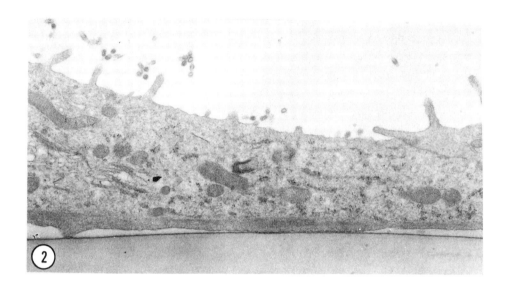

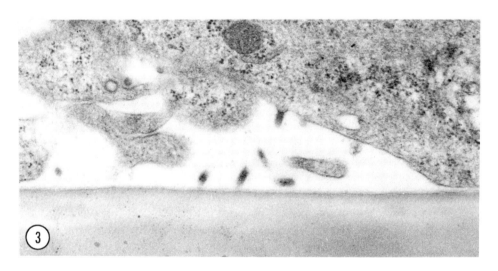

Fig. 2.   Influenza virions associated with the apical cell surface of MDCK cells in the presence of tunicamycin.   Cells were grown on plastic films, and 1.0   g/ml of tunicamycin was added following virus adsorption.   The underlying plastic film and the opposing basal surface of the cell are free of virions.   From Roth et al.[22] Magnification: x 23,000.

Fig. 3.   Vesicular stomatitis virions budding from the basal membrane of an MDCK cell in the presence of 1.0   g/ml of tunicamycin.   The apical cell surface was devoid of virions (not shown).   From Roth et al.[22]   Magnification: x 40,000.

membrane. Several possible mechanisms may be envisioned that could be involved in determining the insertion of glycoproteins into particular membrane domains:

(1) Distinct intracellular membrane systems could exist for all stages of biosynthesis and processing of proteins destined for the apical vs. basolateral membrane, and signal sequences on nascent polypeptides could direct proteins to one set of membranes or the other.

(2) The initial sites of synthesis in rough endoplasmic reticulum may be common, and segration may occur subsequently (e.g. in the Golgi complex) into membrane vesicles destined to be incorporated into distinct plasma membrane domains. Such segregation could be directed entirely by structural features of the proteins molecules themselves, or by secondary effects following their association with cellular components.

(3) The apical and basolateral plasma membranes themselves could have distinct structural properties (e.g. lipid composition) that could result in preferential incorporation of particular glycoproteins. Recognition could occur, for example, by transmembrane segments of glycoproteins in smooth membrane vesicles derived from the Golgi complex.

There is insufficient information at present to distinguish between the possible mechanisms that may be envisioned for determining the membrane localization of glycoproteins; however, further study of the intracellular locations of viral glycoproteins should enable us to determine the cellular level at which these glycoproteins are sorted into distinct compartments. A more difficult problem will be to elucidate the precise molecular features that determine such sorting events; nevertheless studies with viral glycoproteins probably offer the best prospects for obtaining such information, which should contribute new insights not only relevant for understanding virus assembly but also for understanding the biogenesis of cellular membranes.

ACKNOWLEDGMENTS

Research by the authors was supported by Grant No. PCM 78-09207 from the National Science Foundation, AI 12680 from the National Institute of Allergy and Infectious Diseases, and CA 18611 from the National Cancer Institute. M. G. R. is supported by training grant AI 07150 from the National Institute of Allergy and

Infectious Diseases, and M. C. K. is supported by postdoctoral fellowship 1-F32-CA 06086 from the National Cancer Institute.

REFERENCES

1. Schwarz, R. T., Schmidt, M. F. G., Anwer, U., and Klenk, H. -D. (1977) J. Virol. 23, 217-226.
2. Nakamura, K., and Compans, R. W. (1978) Virology 86, 432-442.
3. Nakamura, K., and Compans, R. W. (1979) Virology 95, 8-23.
4. Collins, J. K., and Knight, C. A. (1978). J. Virol. 26, 457-467.
5. Keil, W., Klenk, H. -D., and Schwarz, R. T. (1979) J. Virol. 31, 253-256.
6. Nakamura, K., and Compans, R. W. (1979) Virology 93, 31-47.
7. Nakamura, K., Bhown, A. S., and Compans, R. W. (1980) Submitted for publication.
8. Choppin, P. W. (1969) Virology 39, 130-134.
9. Landsberger, F. R., Lenard, J., Paxton, J., and Compans, R. W. (1971) Proc. Nat. Acad. Sci. U.S.A. 68, 2579-2583.
10. Compans, R. W., and Pinter, A. (1975) Virology 66, 151-160.
11. Nakamura, K., and Compans, R. W. (1977) Virology 79, 381-392.
12. Arakawa, M., and Muramatsu, T. (1974) J. Biochem. (Tokyo) 76, 307-317.
13. Tarentino, A. L., and Maley, F. (1974) J. Biol. Chem. 249, 811-817.
14. Kemp, M. C., Holloway, W. L., Bennett, J. C., and Compans, R. W. (1980) Submitted for publication.
15. Schwarz, R. T., Rohrschneider, J. M., Schmidt, M. F. G. (1976) J. Virol. 19, 782-791.
16. Leavitt, R., Schlesinger, S. and Kornfeld, S. (1977) J. Virol. 21, 375-385.
17. Leavitt, R., Schlesinger, S., and Kornfeld, S. (1977) J. Biol. Chem. 252, 9018-9023.
18. Rothman, J. E., Katz, F. N., and Lodish, H. F. (1978) Cell 15, 1447-1454.
19. Nakamura, K., and Compans, R. W. (1978) Virology 84, 303-319.
20. Gibson, R., Leavitt, R., Kornfeld, S., and Schlesinger, S. (1978). Cell 13, 671-679.
21. Gibson, R., Schlesinger, S., and Kornfeld, S. (1979). J. Biol. Chem. 254, 3600-3607.
22. Roth, M. G., Fitzpatrick, J. P., and Compans, R. W. (1979) Proc. Natl. Acad. Sci. U. S., in press.
23. Leighton, J., Estes, L. W., Mansukhan, S., and Brada, Z. (1970) Cancer 26, 1022-1028.
24. Misfeld, D. S., Hamamoto, S. T. and Pitelka, D. R. (1976) Proc. Natl. Acad. Sci. U. S. A. 73, 1212-1216.
25. Cereijido, M., Robbins, E. S., Dolan, W. J., Rotunno, C. A. and Sabatini, D. D. (1978) J.Cell Biol. 77 , 853-880.
26. Lever, J. E. (1979) Proc. Natl. Acad. Sci. U. S. A. 76, 1323-1327.
27. Rindler, M. J., Chuman, L. M., Shaffer, L., and Saier, M. H., Jr. (1979) J. Cell Biol. 81, 635-648.
28. Rodriguez Boulan, E., and Sabatini, D. D. (1978) Fed. Proc. 37, 1722.
29. Rodriguez Boulan, E., and Sabatini, D. D. (1978) Proc. Natl. Acad. Sci. U. S. A. 75, 5071-5075.
30. Murphy, J. S., and Bang, F. B. (1952) J. Exp. Med. 95, 259-268.
31. Klenk, H. -D., Compans, R. W., and Choppin, P. W. (1970) Virology 42, 1158-1162.
32. Holmes, K. V. and Choppin, P. W. (1968) J. Cell Biol. 39, 526-543.

IDENTIFICATION OF THE SULPHATED OLIGOSACCHARIDE OF A/MEMPHIS/102/72 INFLUENZA VIRUS HEMAGGLUTININ

COLIN W. WARD[*], JEAN C. DOWNIE[+], LORENA E. BROWN[++] AND DAVID C. JACKSON[++]
*CSIRO, Division of Protein Chemistry, 343 Royal Parade, Parkville, 3052, Australia; +National Biological Standards Laboratory, Parkville; ++Department of Microbiology, University of Melbourne, Parkville, Australia.

INTRODUCTION

Influenza virus contains 5-7% carbohydrate[1] in the form of the two glycosylated coat proteins and glycolipid. Since the process of glycosylation is carried out by host cell enzymes, the structure of the resulting viral oligosaccharides should closely resemble those found on host glycoproteins. The presence, in purified preparations of influenza virus, of a host-specific antigen that reacts with antibodies raised against uninfected chick chorioallantoic membranes or allantoic fluid has been recognized for many years.[2-4] The antigen present in uninfected chick embryos has been isolated and shown to be a sulphated mucopolysaccharide.[5-7] A similar sulphated proteoglycan has recently been found loosely associated with whole virions.[8]

Influenza virus also contains carbohydrate that is covalently attached to the hemagglutinin and neuraminidase.[9,10] Depending on the cell type in which the virus is grown, these glycoproteins are capable of interaction with antibodies raised against homologous host tissue[10] and heterologous virus.[11] Compans and Pinter[8] showed that this protein-linked host antigen was also sulphated and estimated that a minimum of 0.5 moles of sulphate was incorporated per mole of HA polypeptide. Recently Downie[12] confirmed this incorporation of inorganic sulphate into influenza HA and showed that there was a direct correlation between the presence of sulphated oligosaccharide, host antigen activity and the stability of HA during isolation in the presence of SDS.

Now that the amino acid sequence and position of the attached oligosaccharide side chains of the Hong Kong hemagglutinin is known (see Ward and Dopheide, this volume) it is of interest to establish the location of the sulphated moiety on A/Mem/72 HA_1 and to see if it has any association with the viral host antigen activity.

METHODS

The production of unlabelled virus, HA, HA_1 and HA_2; and the procedures employed in the purification of peptides resulting from cyanogen bromide and enzymatic cleavages were as described by Ward and Dopheide (this volume). The preparation of ^{35}S-sulphate labelled viral proteins was as described by Downie.[12]

TABLE 1

INCORPORATION OF ^{35}S-SULPHATE INTO INFLUENZA VIRUS A/MEM/71-BEL GROWN IN DIFFERENT HOST CELL TYPES

Host Cell Type	Host Antigen HI Titre[a]	Concentration of $^{35}SO_4$ Inoculated	HA Units Tested	^{35}S-Sulphate Incorporated[b] (CPM)
Embryonated Hen's Egg	1/240	100 μCI/Egg	3000	662
			5000	1089
Embryonated Duck's Egg	<1/10	100 μCI/Egg	3000	36
			5000	70

a. The virus grown in each cell type was titrated against anti-chick CAM serum as described by Laver and Webster, 1966.

b. CPM of ^{35}S-incorporated with acid precipitable material. Based on reference 12.

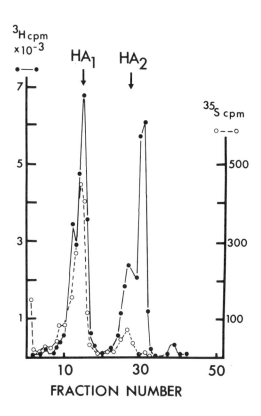

Fig. 1. Polyacrylamide gel electrophoretic profile of A/Mem/102/72 (H3) A/Bel/42 (N1) virus. Virus, grown in eggs in the presence of ^{3}H-amino acids (●—●) and $^{35}SO_4^-$ (O--O), was analysed on a 10% polyacrylamide gel. After electrophoresis, the gel was sliced transversely into 2 mm pieces and the levels of radioactivity determined.

RESULTS AND DISCUSSION

Influenza virus A/Mem/1/71 grown in either whole chick embryos or surviving cells of the chorioallantoic membrane, incorporates inorganic ^{35}S-sulphate into the hemagglutinin sub-units.[12] In contrast virus grown in embryonated duck eggs does not incorporate inorganic sulphate into the hemagglutinin (Table 1) nor does it react with serum raised against chick host antigen.[12] Separation of the ^{35}S-labelled HA into HA_1 and HA_2 by either guanidine hydrochloride density gradient centrifugation[12] or SDS polyacrylamide gel electrophoresis (Fig. 1) showed that most of this sulphate was associated with the HA_1 polypeptide. Furthermore, a quantitative assay using $BaCl_2$ to precipitate inorganic sulphate showed that influenza virus A/Mem/71 grown in chick embryos contained one molecule of sulphate per HA_1 polypeptide chain (Table 2). This report describes the identification of the sulphated oligosaccharide on A/Mem/102/72 HA_1.

TABLE 2

NUMBER OF SULPHATE RESIDUES PER MOLECULE OF INFLUENZA VIRUS A/MEM/71 HEMAGGLUTININ

Glycoprotein	Molecular Wt.	CPM ^{35}S Per µg Protein	No. Molecules x 10^{14}	No. Molecules Sulphate
HA	200,000	25.80	0.774	3.02
HA_1	47,000	15.80	2.02	1.16
HA_2	28,000	36.56	7.82	0.30
Sulphate	35	0.0136	2.34	

Based on reference 12.

A/Mem/72 HA_1 has a molecular weight of 47,000, including approximately 11,500 daltons of carbohydrate.[13] Elucidation of its primary structure has shown that it contains 328 amino acid residues including 4 methionines (residues 168,260,268 and 320). It has also been shown that the carbohydrate occurs in six separate oligosaccharide units attached in N-glycosidic linkage to asparagine residues 8,22,38,81,165 and 285 (see Ward and Dopheide, this volume). The oligosaccharides on residues 8,22,38 and 81 are complex containing N-acetylglucosamine, mannose, galactose and fucose (Table 3) while those on residues 165 and 285 are simple containing only N-acetylglucosamine and mannose (see Ward and Dopheide, this volume). Since the sulphated moiety of influenza virus is believed[12] to resemble a basic corneal keratosulphate unit

TABLE 3

LOCATION AND TYPE OF OLIGOSACCHARIDE UNITS ON A/MEM/102/72 HA_1

Asn Residue Number	Amino Acid Sequence	Carbohydrate Side Chain Type
8	Asn-Ser-Thr	Complex
22	Asn-Gly-Thr	Complex
38	Asn-Ala-Thr	Complex
81	Asn-Glu-Thr	Complex
165	Asn-Val-Thr	Simple
285	Asn-Gly-Ser	Simple

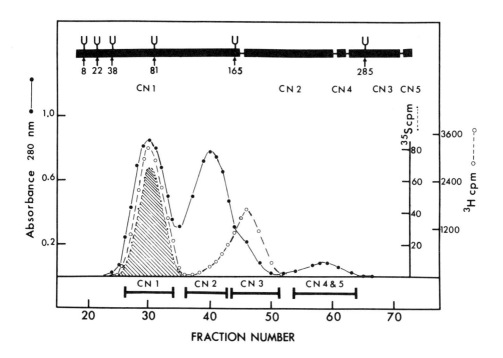

Fig. 2. Separation of cyanogen bromide peptides from ^{35}S-labelled 2-[[3]H-]-S-carboxymethylated HA_1 (600 nmol) on G-100 Sephadex in 50% formic acid. Column size was 140 x 1.0 cm; fraction size was 2.0 ml. 20 µl aliquots were counted for ^{35}S and ^{3}H radioactivity. The elution positions of the five cyanogen bromide fractions are indicated. At the top of the figure is a schematic representation showing size and arrangement of these 5 cyanogen bromide peptides as they occur in the sequence of HA_1 and the location of the size oligosaccharide units.

esterified at position 6 of either N-acetylglucosamine or galactose,[14] the inorganic sulphate would be expected to be incorporated into at least one of the four complex carbohydrate units on A/Mem/72 HA_1.

Cyanogen bromide cleavage of A/Mem/72 HA_1 at the four methionine residues yields five peptides, CN1 to CN5, which can be readily isolated by gel filtration.[1] Polyacrylamide gel electrophoresis (not shown) and gel filtration (Fig. 2) show that the ^{35}S-sulphate is associated exclusively with the N-terminal 168 residue cyanogen bromide peptide CN1. As expected no sulphate was incorporated into the simple carbohydrate unit on CN3.

Tryptic digestion of CN1 yielded 10 major peptides (see Ward and Dopheide, this volume), five of which contain carbohydrate. As shown in Fig. 3 the

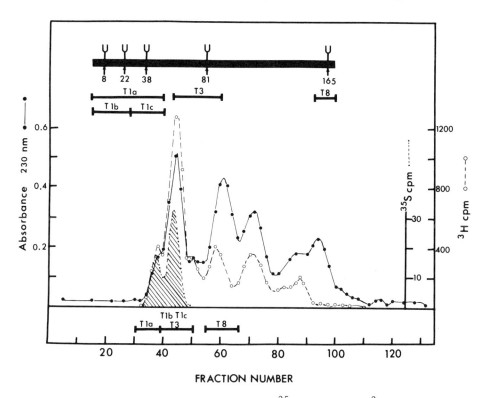

Fig. 3. Chromatography of tryptic digest of ^{35}S-labelled 2-[^{3}H]-S-carboxy-methylated CN1 on two Sephadex G-50 five columns (each 150 x 0.9 cm) connected in series. The columns were eluted with 0.01 M NH_4HCO_3 - 10% isopropanol at a flow rate of 4.4 ml/hr. Fractions (2.2 ml) were monitored by absorbance at 230 nm and radioactively in 50 µl aliquots, and were pooled as shown. The peaks containing the glycopeptides are indicated. The figure also contains a schematic diagram of CN1 showing the location of the five tryptic glycopeptides.

^{35}S-sulphate was associated only with the first two peaks. The large N-terminal 50 residue peptide Tla comprises the first peak and the mixture of Tla, Tlb, Tlc and T3 make up the second. This shows that the sulphate has been incorporated into at least one of the three complex carbohydrate units on peptide Tla, but does not rule out the possibility of additional sulphate incorporation into the complex oligosaccharide on T3.

The tryptic peptides present in fractions 40-50 (see Fig. 3) were digested with chymotrypsin and then subjected to gel filtration as shown in Fig. 4. The major glycoproteins expected from this digest are C1, C2b, C2c and C6 (see Fig. 4). C6 which contains the complex carbohydrate at Asn_{81}, eluted with the tritium label at the trailing edge of the second peak (fractions 62-70) and clearly does not co-migrate with the ^{35}S label. High voltage paper electrophoresis of the material contained in this region confirmed that the sugar

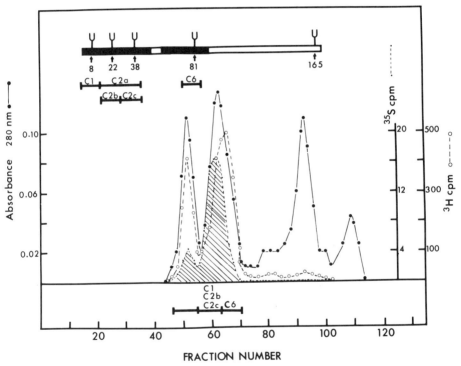

Fig. 4. Chromatography of the chymotryptic digest of the tryptic peptides present in fractions 40-50 of Fig. 3. Column dimensions and elution conditions were as described in Fig. 3. Fractions (2.2 ml) were monitored by absorbance at 230 nm and radioactivity in 100 µl aliquots. The fractions expected to contain the glycopeptides are indicated as are the positions of each chymotryptic glycopeptide in the structure of CN1.

component associated with peptide C6 was not sulphated. Thus the only oligo-saccharides that may be sulphated are those attached to asparagine residues 8, 22 and 38. The three glycopeptides, C1, C2b and C2c which contain these sugar units should[15] all elute at the leading edge of the second peak (fractions 55-65, Fig. 4) where the ^{35}S-sulphate label was located. Experiments are in progress to separate these three chymotryptic glycopeptides to establish which of these are sulphated.

It also remains to be established whether the hemagglutinin-linked host antigen activity is associated with this sulphated oligosaccharide. Preliminary experiments shown in Table 4 demonstrate that only the ^{35}S-sulphate bearing fragments of A/Mem/72 HA are capable of binding to anti-Host Antigen IgG. The smallest of these fragments tested to date is the 168 residue cyanogen bromide peptide CN1 from HA_1 with no activity being associated with the non-sulphated simple carbohydrate containing glycopeptide HA_1-CN3. Experiments are in progress to monitor the enzymic digests of CN1 for anti-host activity.

TABLE 4

BINDING PROPERTIES OF RADIOIODINATED FRAGMENTS OF A/MEM/102/72 HA TO ANTI-(HOST ANTIGEN) IgG

Polypeptide	Sulphated	IgG	
		Anti-Host Antigen	Preimmune
HA	+	27.8	2.4
HABR	+	44	8.8
HA_1	+	49.5	4.3
Pox	+	26.3	1.2
P1	+	43.5	1.9
P2	−	3.3	1.7
CN1	+	17	1.3
CN3	−	2.8	1
A/Bel/42 HA_1	+	18.3	2.1

Equimolar amounts (2 pmoles) of radioiodinated hemagglutinin fragments were incubated with 25 µg IgG for 3 hrs. Antigen-antibody complexes were then detected using protein A-Sepharose and results expressed as the percentage of antigen band.

REFERENCES

1. Frommhagen, L.H., Knight, C.A. and Freeman, N.K. (1959) Virology, 8, 176-197.
2. Knight, C.A. (1944) J. Exptl. Med. 80, 83-99.
3. Schäfer, W., Munk, K. and Armbruster, O. (1952) Z. Naturforsch. 76, 29-33.
4. Harboe, A. (1963) Acta Pathol. Microbiol. Scand. 57, 488-492.
5. Haukenes, G., Harboe, A. and Mortensson-Egnund, K. (1965) Acta Pathol. Microbiol. Scand. 64, 534-542.
6. Howe, C., Lee, L.T., Harboe, A. and Haukenes, G. (1967) J. Immunol. 98, 543-557.
7. Lee, L.T., Howe, C., Meyer, K. and Choi, H.U. (1969) J. Immunol. 102, 1144-1155.
8. Compans, R.W. and Pinter, A. (1975) Virology, 66, 151-160.
9. Smith, W., Belyavin, G. and Sheffield, F.W. (1955) Proc. Roy. Soc. B143, 504-522.
10. Laver, W.G. and Webster, R.G. (1966) Virology, 30, 104-115.
11. Jackson, D.C., Dopheide, T.A., Russell, R.J., White, D.O. and Ward, C.W. (1979) Virology, 93, 458-465.
12. Downie, J.C. (1978) J. Gen. Virol. 41, 283-293.
13. Ward, C.W. and Dopheide, T.A. (1976) FEBS Lett. 65, 365-368.
14. Bhavanandan, V.P. and Meyer, K. (1967) J. Biol. Chem. 212, 4352-4359.
15. Ward, C.W. and Dopheide, T.A. (1980) Virology. In press.

DISCUSSION

Brownlee: Why does that particular ASN get sulphated?

Downie: Maybe there is a signal in the polypeptide sequence.

Ward: It is also the largest carbohydrate group at position 8.

Compans: To some extent, sulphation is host-cell dependent.

Downie: Yes, but it is difficult to isolate HA from tissue-culture grown virus.

Choppin: The paraflu viruses have only 10% of chains sulphated.

MOLECULAR IMMUNE RECOGNITION OF PROTEINS:
THE PRECISE DETERMINATION OF PROTEIN ANTIGENIC SITES HAS LED TO SYNTHESIS OF
ANTIBODY COMBINING SITES AND OTHER TYPES OF PROTEIN BINDING SITES

M. ZOUHAIR ATASSI
Department of Immunology
Mayo Medical School
Rochester, Minnesota 55901

INTRODUCTION

Knowledge of the molecular features responsible for the antigenicity of
certain parts of native protein molecules lies at the basis of understanding
in molecular terms the cellular events of the immune response. The majority
of antigens associated with many immunological disorders are proteins, and
therefore, defining the antigenic sites of these protein antigens will be critical for the manipulation and molecular elucidation of the mechanisms of these
disorders. From a purely chemical perspective, the interaction between protein
antigens and their antibodies and the elegant specificity of this recognition
phenomenon remains one of the most fascinating and challenging frontiers in
biochemistry.

Progress in this field has been very slow, and the elucidation of the entire antigenic structure of a protein had frustrated many attempts. Considerable chemical and technical factors were responsible for the slow progress in
this field, and these have already been discussed in detail (Atassi, 1975;
1977b). In the last few years great advances have been made in the determination and synthesis of the antigenic sites of some proteins. The entire antigenic structures of two proteins, sperm-whale myoglobin (Atassi, 1975) and hen
egg-white lysozyme (Atassi, 1978) have now been determined. Also, most of the
antigenic sites (5 out of 6 sites) of serum albumin have now been localized and
synthesized (Atassi et al., 1979; Sakata and Atassi, 1980a). Our determination
of the antigenic structure of Mb, and then that of lysozyme has answered many
questions relating to the molecular immune recognition of native proteins with
surprising accuracy (Atassi, 1975). Many of the observations and findings
first made from our Mb work (Atassi, 1972, 1975) have since become established
concepts that have been confirmed with a variety of other proteins. However,
it is necessary to stress here the caution that this is a very complex field,
and hence, proper understanding of the immunochemistry of proteins requires
the elucidation of the complete antigenic structures of a few native proteins
(Atassi, 1972, 1975). Already, our precise determination of the entire antigenic structure of lysozyme (Atassi, 1978) has shown fascinating differences
between these two proteins and these will be briefly outlined below.

CHEMICAL STRATEGY FOR THE DELINEATION OF PROTEIN ANTIGENIC (AND OTHER BINDING) SITES

I had considered at the outset that the antigenic structure of a protein cannot be deduced by the exclusive application of a single chemical approach. A strategy was, therefore, developed (Atassi, 1972) which relied on five approaches. This strategy first enabled us to achieve the precise determination of the entire antigenic structure of myoglobin (Atassi, 1975), and we subsequently found it to be equally effective in scoring a similar achievement with lysozyme (Atassi, 1978). These approaches were: (1) to study the effect of conformational changes on the immunochemistry of the protein; (2) to study the immunochemistry and conformation of chemical derivatives of the protein, specifically modified at appropriate amino acid locations; (3) to isolate and characterize immunochemically-reactive fragments that can quantitatively account for the total reaction of the native protein; (4) to study the effect of chemical modification at selected amino acid locations on the immunochemistry and conformation of immunochemically-reactive peptides; (5) after hopefully narrowing down each of the antigenic sites by approaches (1-4) to a conveniently small size, the final delineation would rely on studying the immunochemistry of synthetic peptides corresponding to many overlaps around this region. It is critical to note that each of these chemical approaches has advantages as well as shortcomings. The application, usefulness and shortcomings of these approaches in protein immunochemistry have recently been discussed in considerable detail (Atassi, 1975, 1977a and b). It is also necessary to stress here that none of these approaches by itself is capable of yielding the full antigenic structure. We invariably used the results from one approach to confirm and correct those from the others. The complete structure is a composite, logical coordination of all the information.

It should be noted that the above strategy, although first employed in the delineation of protein antigenic sites, is obviously applicable to the precise delineation and chemical synthesis of other types of protein binding sites. An antigenic site is no different from other protein binding sites, except that its specific binding activity is with antibody. Thus the delineation and synthesis of protein antigenic sites can serve as a prototype for the delineation and synthesis of other types of protein binding sites. Our introduction of the concept of "surface-simulation" synthesis (Atassi et al., 1976b; Lee and Atassi, 1976) has further provided a dimension of versatility by which in principle any type of protein binding sites can now be synthesized after careful chemical characterization. This should open up many investigative fields in protein biological activity.

MAIN FEATURES OF THE ENTIRE ANTIGENIC STRUCTURES OF MYOGLOBIN AND LYSOZYME AND
MOST OF THE ANTIGENIC STRUCTURE OF SERUM ALBUMIN

The derivations of the antigenic structures of myoglobin and lysozyme
spanned numerous publications. A concise review of the antigenic structure of
myoglobin has appeared (Atassi, 1975) and a very comprehensive account of the
derivation has recently been published (Atassi, 1977b). The climax of the
studies on the antigenic structure of lysozyme can be found in the papers
dealing with the synthesis of the three antigenic sites of lysozyme which quantitatively accounted for its entire antigenic reactivity (Atassi et al., 1976b;
Lee and Atassi, 1976, 1977a, b; Atassi and Lee, 1978a, b) and the work has recently been reviewed (Atassi, 1978). Therefore, complete presentation of the
derivation of the antigenic structures will not be given in this article. However, the main features of the antigenic structures of myoglobin (Mb) and of
lysozyme will be outlined below for convenience. Also, the five antigenic
sites of serum albumin that have so far been delineated and synthesized (Atassi
et al., 1979; Sakata and Atassi, 1980a)will be given.

Special Features of the Antigenic Structure of Myoglobin (Mb)

By application of the first four chemical approaches mentioned above, it
was possible to achieve delineation of the antigenic sites in Mb to within 8 to
10 residues. Further delineation by chemical methods could not be pursued due
to the fact that in each case this would have required modification of hydrophobic or nonpolar amino acids which is, of course, not possible. However,
having reached a chemical delineation down to such a conveniently small size,
precise narrowing down of the reactive regions was achieved by the organic
synthesis and immunochemical studies of peptides corresponding to various parts
of the regions. It is necessary here to caution that if synthesis precedes the
orderly chemical narrowing down, it will clearly be wasteful and in fact can
lead to erroneous conclusions.

In our studies, 26 different peptides representing various parts of each
reactive region, as well as control reference peptides corresponding to non-
antigenic locations, have been synthesized, purified, characterized, and their
immunochemistry studied.

This section gives a very brief outline of the first antigenic structure
of a protein to be completed (Atassi, 1975). Readers desiring more detail may
consult a very comprehensive recent review (Atassi, 1977b). On the other hand,
the initial description of our work (Atassi, 1975) offers a convenient and
concise account.

Five antigenic sites are present in the native protein and are situated on:
(a) Sequence 16-21 +1 or 0 residue on one side only of this segment depending
on the antiserum. This antigenic site exhibits a certain degree of 'shift' or
'displacement' and minor variability in size (limited to +1 residue only) from
one antiserum to the next. Its location in the three-dimensional structure is
on the bend between helices A and B; (b) sequence 56-62, on the bend between
helices D and E. This antigenic site has exhibited no variability in size with
the antisera so far studied; (c) sequence 94-99 on the bend between helices F
and G; (d) sequence 113-119, on the end of helix G and only part of the bend
GH; (e) sequence 146-151 (+ lysine 145 with some antisera). This antigenic
site is situated on the end of helix H and part of the randomly-coiled C-terminal pentapeptide. The primary structures of the five antigenic sites are shown
in Figure 1. The locations of the antigenic sites in the three-dimensional
structure of native Mb are shown in a schematic diagram in Figure 2.

Region	Structure and Location	No. of Residues
Region 1	15 16 21 22 (Ala)-Lys-Val-Glu-Ala-Asp-Val-(Ala)	6 (or 7)
Region 2	56 62 Lys-Ala-Ser-Glu-Asp-Leu-Lys	7
Region 3	94 99 Ala-Thr-Lys-His-Lys-Ile	6
Region 4	113 119 His-Val-Leu-His-Ser-Arg-His	7
Region 5	145 146 151 (Lys)-Tyr-Lys-Glu-Leu-Gly-Tyr	6 (or 7)

FIGURE 1. Primary structures of the five antigenic sites of sperm whale Mb.
Residues in parentheses are part of the antigenic site only with some antisera.
Thus for site 1, the reactive region invariably occupies sequence 16 to 21 and
with some antisera Ala-15 is part of the region (which will then correspond
to sequence 15 to 21) while with other antisera Ala-22 is an essential part of
the region (which will then correspond to sequence 16 to 22). This site occupies either six or seven residues depending on antiserum. For sites 2, 3 and
4 no such "displacement" or "shift" to one side or the other has been observed
(at least with the antisera so far studied). In the case of site 5, Lys-145
can be part of the antigenic region only with some antisera and this site will,
therefore, comprise six or seven residues, depending on the antiserum. (From
Atassi, M.Z., Immunochemistry, 12, 423, 1975. With permission).

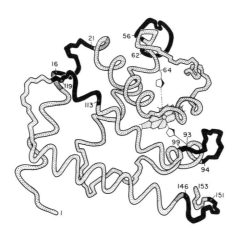

FIGURE 2. A schematic diagram showing the mode of folding of Mb and its anti-genic structure. The solid black portions represent segments which have been shown to comprise accurately entire antigenic sites. The striped parts, each corresponding to one amino acid residue only, can be part of the antigenic site with some antisera. The dotted portions represent parts of the molecule which have been shown exhaustively to residue outside antigenic sites. (From Atassi, M.Z., Immunochemistry, 12, 423, 1975. With permission).

We have previously cautioned (Atassi, 1975; Atassi and Pai, 1975) against the likely formulation of an erroneous conclusion that every bend constitutes an antigenic site. No such statement is made or implied here and indeed exami-nation of Figure 2 immediately reveals that the bends B-C, C-D and E-F do not carry antigenic sites. Also, site 4 (i.e. 113-119) is located mostly on a helical portion.

The antigenic sites are surprisingly small (6-7 residues) and possess sharp boundaries. They may exhibit limited variability in boundaries with various antisera which, when it exists, will be ±1 residue. The size, surface locations and shape of these antigenic sites make them quite accessible for binding with antibody combining sites.

The type of amino acids present in the antigenic sites is to be expected from their surface locations (Atassi, 1972). Lysine is present in four sites (Figure 1) and in the fifth, arginine is present. Three out of five antigenic sites contain asparatic acid or glutamic acid or both. Two sites contain his-tidine. From this and the demonstrated detrimental effect of appropriate modi-fications of these polar residues on the antigenic reactivity, it may be con-cluded (Atassi, 1972 and 1975) that interactions of the Mb antigenic sites with antibody must be predominantly polar in nature. Stabilizing effects are con-tributed by hydroxy and non-polar amino acids through hydrogen bonding and

and hydrophobic interactions (Atassi, 1972). The sequence and three-dimensional structural features that confer immunogenicity on these regions are not too clear.

The sum of the reactivities of these sites accounts quantitatively for the entire (100%) antibody response directed against native Mb (Atassi, 1979a; Twining and Atassi, 1979). The affinity of an antigenic site or its share of the total reactivity of Mb may vary with the antiserum. However, with all the antisera studied so far (at least eight), an antigenic site is invariably an antigenic site, but its potency or efficiency varies with the individual animal immunized (Atassi, 1972).

The findings that purely conformational changes in Mb will influence its reaction with antisera to the native protein (Atassi, 1967b; Andres and Atassi, 1970) and the immunochemical results on numerous peptide fragments have enabled us to conclude (Atassi and Thomas, 1969) that the primary antibody response, at least in early-course antisera, is directed against the native three-dimensional structures of proteins.

An intact antigenic site free of extraneous non-reactive residues would usually react less than when it is isolated as part of a longer peptide (Atassi 1972; Koketsu and Atassi, 1973, 1974a and 1974b). The non-reactive parts may assist the achievement of the correct folding for binding of the antigenic site with antibody combining site (Atassi and Saplin, 1968). On the other hand, recent evidence (Koketsu and Atassi, 1974a and 1974b; Atassi and Pai, 1975) has revealed that non-reactive parts composed of bulky residues linked to an antigenic site may exert unfavorable steric or conformational effects on the ability of the site to bind with antibodies.

Summary of the Features of the Antigenic Structure of Lysozyme

Hen egg-white lysozyme is a "tight" protein (i.e. inaccessible to proteolytic attack and containing disulfide bonds). My interest in the antigenic structure of lysozyme was stimulated by the fact such tight proteins (e.g. lysozyme, ribonuclease) have been difficult to study. Because of the inaccessibility of these tight proteins, it has not been possible to prepare a variety of overlapping peptides without rupturing the disulfide bonds. Investigators, therefore, diverted their effort to study the immunochemistry of preparations with broken disulfide bonds. Unfortunately, these unfolded preparations bear no immunochemical relationship to the native protein. The deadlock was resolved by the finding (Habeeb and Atassi, 1970) that reversible masking of the amino groups by citraconylation rendered the protein completely susceptible to tryptic hydrolysis at the arginyl bonds. This formulated the basis for

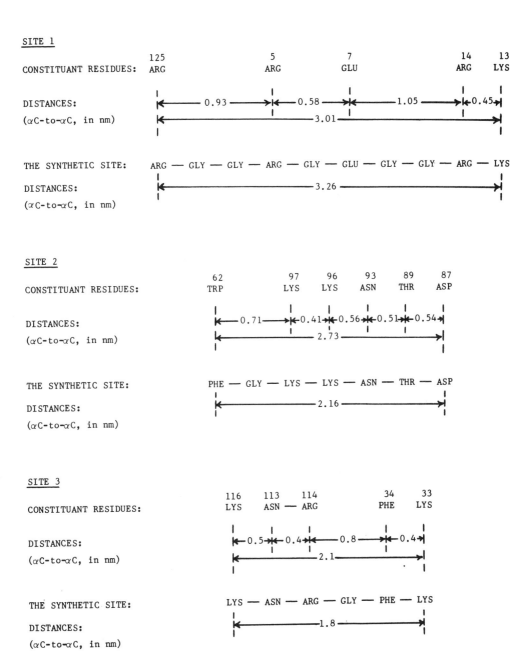

SITE 1

CONSTITUANT RESIDUES:

125 ARG   5 ARG   7 GLU   14 ARG   13 LYS

DISTANCES: (αC-to-αC, in nm)

|←—— 0.93 ——→|←— 0.58 —→|←—— 1.05 ——→|←0.45→|
|←———————————————— 3.01 ————————————————→|

THE SYNTHETIC SITE: ARG — GLY — GLY — ARG — GLY — GLU — GLY — GLY — ARG — LYS

DISTANCES: (αC-to-αC, in nm)

|←———————————————— 3.26 ————————————————→|

SITE 2

CONSTITUANT RESIDUES:

62 TRP   97 LYS   96 LYS   93 ASN   89 THR   87 ASP

DISTANCES: (αC-to-αC, in nm)

|←—0.71——→|←0.41→|←0.56→|←0.51→|←0.54→|
|←———————————— 2.73 ————————————→|

THE SYNTHETIC SITE: PHE — GLY — LYS — LYS — ASN — THR — ASP

DISTANCES: (αC-to-αC, in nm)

|←———————————— 2.16 ————————————→|

SITE 3

CONSTITUANT RESIDUES:

116 LYS   113 ASN — 114 ARG   34 PHE   33 LYS

DISTANCES: (αC-to-αC, in nm)

|←0.5→|←0.4→|←—— 0.8 ——→|←0.4→|
|←———————————— 2.1 ————————————→|

THE SYNTHETIC SITE: LYS — ASN — ARG — GLY — PHE — LYS

DISTANCES: (αC-to-αC, in nm)

|←———————————— 1.8 ————————————→|

(See caption on following page)

248

FIGURE 3. The three antigenic sites representing the entire antigenic structure of lysozyme. The diagram shows the spatially contiguous residues constituting each antigenic site and their numerical positions in the primary
structure. The distances (in nm) separating the consecutive residues and the
overall dimension of each site (in its extended form) are given, together with
the dimension of each surface-simulation synthetic site. The latter assumes
an ideal C^{α}-to-C^{α} distance of 0.362 nm. The precise boundary, conformational
and directional definitions of the sites are described in the text. The
three sites account quantitatively for the entire (96 to 100%) antigenic
reactivity of lysozyme (From Atassi, M.Z. and Lee, C.-L., Biochem. J., 171,
429, 1978. With permission).

obtaining fragments with intact disulfide bonds from tight proteins (Atassi et
al., 1973a). Tryptic hydrolysis may resume at the lysyl peptide bonds after
removal of the citraconyl blocking group. From the tryptic hydrolysate of native lysozyme (i.e. without breaking its disulfide bonds) three fragments were
identified which accounted for 85-90% of the total immunochemical reactivity
of lysozyme (Atassi et al., 1973a).

Through the systematic application of the chemical strategy outlined above,
lysozyme was found to have three antigenic sites, each constituting spatially
adjacent residues (that are otherwise distant in sequence) and describing a
discrete area on the surface topography of the protein (for review, see Atassi,
1978). Although we had proposed the existence of this type of protein antigenic sites quite early (Atassi and Saplin, 1968), we subsequently found that
they did not exist in myoglobin (Atassi and Koketsu, 1975; Atassi, 1975). The
first such site was identified and characterized in lysozyme (Atassi et al.,
1976a). The need for the chemical verification of such sites led us to introduce the concept of "surface-simulation" synthesis, by which the spatially adjacent surface residues constituting a protein binding site are linked directly
via peptide bonds with appropriate spacing where necessary (Atassi et al.,
1976b; Lee and Atassi, 1976). Our introduction of the concept of surface-
simulation synthesis enabled us to precisely delineate and chemically synthesize the three antigenic sites of lysozyme (for review, see Atassi, 1978).
Furthermore, surface-simulation synthesis afforded a powerful new concept in
protein molecular recognition that provided for the first time a chemical strategy for the synthesis of any type of protein binding sites (Atassi et al.,
1976b; Atassi and Lee, 1978b; Atassi, 1978, 1979b; Twining and Atassi, 1978,
Kazim and Atassi, 1980a).

It would perhaps be useful at this stage to present, for the sake of
direct comparison, the highlights of the antigenic structure of lysozyme.
Native lysozyme has three antigenic sites. The identities of the sites are
shown in Figure 3 and they are briefly described below:

Site 1: This antigenic site is constructed (Atassi and Lee, 1978a) by the side chains of the spatially adjacent five surface residues: Arg-125, Arg-5, Glu-7, Arg-14, Lys-13. The extended dimension of the site from Arg-125 to Lys-13 (C^{α}-to-C^{α}) is 30Å. These residues, which fall in an imaginary line circumscribing part of the surface topography of the protein, bind with antibody as if they are in direct peptide linkage. In fact the immunochemical reactivity of this site is fully satisfied by the surface-simulation synthetic peptide Arg-Gly-Gly-Arg-Gly-Glu-Gly-Arg-Lys, which does not exist in native lysozyme but mimics the arrangement of residues in this surface region. This concept, introduced by the author (Atassi et al., 1976b) has been termed 'surface-simulation' synthesis (Lee and Atassi, 1976). The surface-simulation synthetic site exhibits a directional preference (Arg-125 to Lys-13), which appears to be independent of the species of the immunized animal, at least with the rabbits and goats so far tested. The site has a restricted conformational freedom clearly evidenced by its sensitivity to variation of the spacing between its constituent residues in surface-simulation synthesis. The intactness of the disulfide bond 6-127 in native lysozyme is critical for the integrity of this site (Atassi et al., 1973a and 1976c).

Site 2: This antigenic site also consists (Atassi et al., 1976b; Lee and Atassi, 1977a) of spatially adjacent surface residues. These are: Trp-2, Lys-97, Lys-96, Asn-93, Thr-89, Asp-87. The extended dimension of the site from Trp-62 to Asp-87 (C^{α}-to-C^{α} distance) is 27.3Å. As with site 1, site 2 also describes an imaginary line which encircles part of the surface topography of the protein molecule. This line passes through the residues forming the site which behave functionally as if they are directly linked by peptide bonds. Thus, the surface-simulation synthetic peptide Phe-Gly-Lys-Lys-Asn-Thr-Asp, which does not exist in lysozyme but simulates a surface region of it, carries the full reactivity of the site (Atassi, et al., 1976b; Lee and Atassi, 1977a). With the antisera so far studied, the antigenic site exhibits a preferred directionality in surface-simulation synthesis (Trp-62 to Asp-87) towards the goat antisera and none towards the rabbit antisera. The antigenic site is subject to conformational restrictions indicated by requirement for appropriate spacing between the constituent residues (Lee and Atassi, 1977a). The intactness of the disulfide bonds 64-80 and 76-94 is essential to bring together the various constituent residues of the site (Atassi et al., 1976a). This antigenic site overlaps with the enzymic active site because they both share Trp-62 (Lee and Atassi, 1975; Atassi et al., 1976a).

Site 3: Like sites 1 and 2, this site is also constructed by spatially adjacent surface residues. The antigenic site comprises the five residues: Lys-116, Asn-113, Arg-114, Phe-34, Lys-33 and in its extended form has a C^{α}-to-C^{α} dimension (from Lys-116 to Lys-33) of 21Å (Lee and Atassi, 1977b). These residues describe an imaginary line which circumscribes part of the surface of the molecule and act functionally towards the antibody as if they are in direct peptide bond linkage. In fact, the surface-simulation synthetic peptide having the structure Lys-Asn-Arg-Gly-Phe-Lys (which does not exist in lysozyme) carries the full immunochemical reactivity of the site (Lee and Atassi, 1977b). With the two rabbit and two goat antisera so far studied the synthetic antigenic site exhibited a preferred directionality (Lys-116 to Lys-33), since the reverse surface-simulation synthetic sequence was immunochemically inefficient. The intactness of the disulfide bond 30-115 is critical for the integrity of this antigenic site in lysozyme (Atassi et al., 1973a). Antigenic site 3 overlaps with the hexasaccharide substrate binding site at the carbonyl group of Phe-34 and the side chain of Arg-114 (Lee and Atassi, 1977b).

Summary of the Antigenic Structure of Serum Albumin

The antigenic structure of serum albumin has been the subject of considerable interest for over two decades. Recent studies from this laboratory on bovine serum albumin have enabled an extensive understanding of the antigenicity of this protein. The location of five major antigenic sites have been determined in bovine serum albumin and the delineation has been confirmed by synthesis (Atassi et al., 1979). The five antigenic sites that have so far been delineated in bovine serum albumin are shown in Figure 4.

```
              137                                    146
   Site 1: Tyr-Leu-Tyr-Glu-Ile-Ala-Arg-Arg-His-Pro


              328                                    337
   Site 2: Phe-Leu-Tyr-Glu-Tyr-Ser-Arg-Arg-His-Pro


              525                                    534
   Site 3: Ala-Leu-Val-Glu-Leu-Leu-Lys-His-Lys-Pro


              308        ⟶          ┌314 359┐  ⟶    362
   Site 5: Ala-Glu-Asp-Lys-Asp-Val╀Cys  Cys╀Ala-Lys-Asp
                                    │    │
                                    S────S


              558        ⟶          ┌564 555┐  ⟵    552
   Site 6: Ala-Asp-Asp-Lys-Glu-Ala╀Cys  Cys╀Lys-Asp-Val
                                    │    │
                                    S────S
```

FIGURE 4. Structure and location of five regions found to carry antigenic sites of bovine serum albumin and have been verified by synthesis. The arrows show the directions of the peptide bonds. It is not implied that the antigenic sites comprise the entire size of the predicted regions but rather that they fall within these regions. (From Atassi et al., 1979)

Comparison of the Antigenic Structures of Myoglobin, Lysozyme and Serum Albumin

Determination of the antigenic structures of Mb and lysozyme has permitted the definition in precise molecular terms of the antibody recognition of protein antigens. Many of the general conclusions relating to antigenic structures of proteins which were derived from our precise definition of the entire antigenic structure of Mb (Atassi, 1972, 1975 and 1977b), are applicable to lysozyme equally as well. These include: The small size and sharp boundaries of the antigenic sites, their presence only in a limited number, their surface location, their sensitivity to changes in the conformation and to changes in the environment of the site (e.g. amino acid substitution), the variation of their immunodominancy with the antiserum and many other features. (For discussion of these general conclusions, see Atassi, 1972, 1975 and 1977b).

The sizes of the lysozyme antigenic sites in their extended forms are 30, 27 and 21Å respectively. These resemble the dimensions of the extended antigenic sites of sperm-whale myoglobin (Atassi, 1975, 1977b) which range between 19 and 23Å. Since the antigenic sites of a protein are not in the extended form, the actual dimensions of the sites in their folded shapes will be smaller than the values given. Nevertheless, the sizes of the antibody combining sites needed for binding with antigenic sites on either of the two proteins will have to be somewhat larger than the combining sites found for haptens by X-ray crystallography (Amzel et al., 1974; Padlan et al., 1976; Ely et al., 1973; Schiffer et al., 1973).

Significantly, both rabbits and goats make antibodies to native lysozyme with identical specificities for the same three antigenic sites. Also, antibodies produced in rabbit, goat, pig, cat, mouse (outbred) and chicken to sperm-whale myoglobin recognized the same antigenic sites on myoglobin (Atassi, 1975, 1977b; Twining et al., 1980).

Examination of the antigenic sites of lysozyme reveals that they are very rich in basic amino acids. This was also seen in Mb, but we caution against premature generalizations. Obviously, interactions with antibody are predominantly polar in nature (as to be expected from the surface location of protein antigenic sites) with considerable stabilizing effects being contributed by hydrophobic interactions and some hydrogen bonding. However, it should be emphasized that the basicity of the lysozyme antigenic sites cannot be the only underlying factor for their antigenic expression. It is well to caution here that the sequence and three-dimensional features that confer immunogenicity on given parts or surface areas of a protein molecule are still not too clear (Atassi, 1975). Undue speculation is inadvisable at this stage. Hopefully, a rationalization will become possible with the precise determination of the antigenic structures of several other proteins.

In spite of the aforementioned points of resemblance between the antigenic structure of Mb and lysozyme, the antigenic sites of these two proteins are radically different in structural terms. The five antigenic sites of Mb are each made up of residues that are directly linked to one another by peptide bonds. In contrast, in lysozyme each of the three antigenic sites constitutes spatially adjacent surface residues that are mostly distant in sequence (Atassi et al., 1976a; Lee and Atassi, 1976, 1977a, b; Atassi and Lee, 1978a; Atassi, 1978) reacting with antibody as if they are in direct peptide linkage. An important question here is what are the factors which determine the type of the site? Since the full antigenic structures of only two proteins are now determined, an unequivocal answer to this question cannot be formulated at this stage. Perhaps it can be tentatively concluded that an important factor in determining the type of the antigenic site may be dependent to a great extent on the stabilization or otherwise of the structure by internal disulfide crosslinks (Lee and Atassi, 1976). A more definitive understanding of this subject must await knowledge of the antigenic structures of several proteins.

Even though we had previously suggested (Atassi and Saplin, 1968) the existence of protein antigenic sites made up of spatially adjacent surface residues that are distant in sequence, their identification and precise definition in lysozyme (Atassi et al., 1976b; Lee and Atassi, 1976, 1977a, b; Atassi and Lee, 1978a) is the first such example in protein immunochemistry. A common feature to these two types of antigenic sites is that they occupy exposed regions on the surface topography of the respective protein (Atassi et al., 1976b), and this will most likely be the situation with all antigenic sites in native proteins. It should be stressed that the antigenic sites both in myoglobin and in lysozyme are sensitive to conformational changes in the respective protein, with those of lysozyme showing, as expected, a much higher sensitivity. Accordingly, it is totally inadequate to identify the antigenic sites of myoglobin by the terms "linear", "sequential", or "primary", or some such terms, while identifying the antigenic sites of lysozyme by the terms "spatial" "conformational", etc. We have proposed (Atassi, 1978; Atassi and Smith, 1978) that antigenic sites of the type seen in myoglobin (Atassi, 1975) and hemoglobin (Kazim and Atassi, 1977b) be named "continuous" antigenic sites which implies that they consist of conformationally distinct continuous surface portions of the polypeptide chain. For antigenic sites of the type seen in lysozyme (Atassi, 1978), the term "discontinuous" antigenic sites will be appropriate. A "discontinuous site" is made up of conformationally (or spatially) contiguous surface residues that are totally or partially not in direct peptide bond linkage.

The antigenic sites of serum albumin have not yet been narrowed down to their precise boundaries. The peptide regions shown in Figure 4 are not intended to imply that the entire region constitutes an antigenic site, but rather that the site falls within that region. Nevertheless, it can be readily seen that the antigenic sites of serum albumin exhibit the expected characteristics of having discrete boundaries and being: limited in number, sensitive to conformational and environmental changes, variable in immunodominancy with the serum. However, their status of exposure is not known. Unfortunately, the three-dimensional structure of a serum albumin has not yet been determined. Therefore, it is not possible to correlate the locations of the antigenic sites with the shape of the protein molecule. Three of the antigenic sites (sites 1, 2 and 3 in Figure 4) occupy continuous portions of the polypeptide chain of albumin and are, therefore, "continuous" antigenic sites. The other two antigenic sites (sites 5 and 6) are each localized around a disulfide bond and belong to the type termed "discontinuous" antigenic sites. However, by analogy with myoglobin (Atassi, 1975), lysozyme (Atassi, 1978) and hemoglobin (Kazim and Atassi, 1977b), it would be expected that the antigenic sites of albumin also occupy exposed structural locations. The predominance of polar and hydrophilic amino acids in the albumin antigenic sites (Figure 4) would tend to support this expectation.

FACTORS WHICH DETERMINE AND REGULATE THE ANTIGENICITY OF THE SITE

The Antigenic Sites are Inherent in the Three-Dimensional Structure

Until recently, it has been widely believed that the antigenic sites on a protein antigen are located at regions which differ in sequence from the corresponding homologous protein in the immunized host. Having determined the precise antigenic structures of Mb and lysozyme and most of the antigenic structure of albumin, we proceeded to investigate some of the factors responsible for the antigenicity of the sites. Initially, the antigenic structure of Mb was determined with antisera raised in rabbits and goats (Atassi, 1975).

Recently, we extended these studies to antisera that were raised in chicken, cat, pig and mouse (Twining et al., 1980). We have found that the same five antigenic sites on sperm-whale Mb are recognized by rabbit and goat antisera (Atassi, 1975, 1977b) and by chicken, cat, pig and mouse antisera (Twining et al. 1980). Also, both rabbits and goats make antibodies to native hen lysozyme with identical specificities for the same three antigenic sites (Atassi, 1978). This suggested to us (Kazim and Atassi, 1978) that the antigenicity of the sites is inherent in their three-dimensional location and is independent of any sequence identities between the injected protein antigen and the homologous protein of the immunized host. Other studies from our laboratory have strongly confirmed this conclusion. These will be summarized below together with their implications to immune recognition and in particular to autoimmune responses.

The realization that protein antigenic sites are "structurally-inherent" (for review, see Atassi and Kazim, 1978) enabled us to predict and verify by synthesis the location of two antigenic sites (Figure 5) of human hemoglobin (one each on the α and β chains) by extrapolation of the three-dimensional location of an antigenic site of sperm-whale Mb (Kazim and Atassi, 1977b).

Residue Location:	A_{13}	A_{14}	A_{15}	A_{16}	AB_1	B_1	B_2	B_3	B_4	B_5
Site 1 of Mb:	15 Ala	Lys	Val	Glu	Ala	Asp	Val	22 Ala		
Hb α (15-23):	15 Gly	Lys	Val	Gly	Ala	His	Ala	Gly	23 Glu	
Hb β (16-23):	16 Gly	Lys	Val	Asn	...	...	Val	Asp	Glu	23 Val

FIGURE 5. Diagram showing the sequence and structural location of antigenic site 1 of sperm whale Mb and the corresponding extrapolated regions of the adult human Hb α and β chains and whose activity was confirmed by synthesis. (From Kazim, A.L. and Atassi, M.Z., Biochem. J., 167, 275, 1977. With permission).

Our concept of "structurally-inherent" antigenic sites was further supported by the finding that even the antigenic sites of soybean leghemoglobin, a very distant member of this family of heme proteins, fall within the expected structural locations obtained by extrapolation of the Mb antigenic sites (Hurrell et al., 1978). Moreover, our recent findings on bovine and human serum albumins (Atassi et al., 1979; Sakata and Atassi, 1980a) show that their antigenic sites are located at equivalent structural locations.

The aforementioned findings strongly confirm that the conformational uniqueness of certain parts of a protein molecule plays a most critical role in the antigenic expression of the protein (Kazim and Atassi, 1978).

Implication of "Structurally-Inherent" Antigenic Site in Autoimmune Recognition

Comparison of the primary structures of sperm-whale and rabbit myoglobins, which have identical chain lengths, showed that only 5 out of 22 replacements fall within the boundaries of the antigenic sites (Figure 6)

```
SITE 1 of          15                                            22
   Sperm-Whale Mb  Ala   Lys   Val   Glu   Ala   Asp   Val   Ala
   Rabbit Mb       Gly   Lys   Val   Glu   Ala   Asp   Leu   Ala

SITE 2 of          56                            62
   Sperm-Whale Mb  Lys   Ala   Ser   Glu   Asp   Leu   Lys
   Rabbit Mb       Lys   Ala   Ser   Glu   Asp   Leu   Lys

SITE 3 of          94                      99
   Sperm-Whale Mb  Ala   Thr   Lys   His   Lys   Ile
   Rabbit Mb       Ala   Thr   Lys   His   Lys   Ile

SITE 4 of          113                          119
   Sperm-Whale Mb  His   Val   Leu   His   Ser   Arg   His
   Rabbit Mb       His   Val   Leu   His   Ser   Lys   His

SITE 5 of          145                          151
   Sperm-Whale Mb  Lys   Tyr   Lys   Glu   Leu   Gly   Tyr
   Rabbit Mb       Gln   Tyr   Lys   Glu   Leu   Gly   Phe
```

FIGURE 6. A diagram showing the primary structures of the five antigenic sites of sperm whale Mb and the corresponding regions of rabbit Mb. The sequences shown occupy identical positions in the respective protein chains. Identical positions having different amino acids in the two chains are indicated by blocks. (From Kazim, A.L., and Atassi, M.Z., Biochim. Biophys. Acta, 494, 277, 1977. With permission).

Two regions, corresponding to sites 2 (sequence 56-62) and 3 (sequence 94-99) in sperm-whale Mb were identical in the two proteins. Two other sites (sites 1 and 4) had only conservative substitutions. Thus in site 1, rabbit Mb has the substitutions Ala-15→Gly and Val-21→Leu and in site 4 the replacement Arg-118→Lys occurs. In the region corresponding to site 5, rabbit Mb has the replacements Lys-145→Gln and Tyr-151→Phe. At any rate, at least two antigenic sites in sperm-whale Mb were identical in sequence to the corresponding regions in rabbit Mb. Clearly, rabbits reacted by making antibodies to parts of sperm-whale Mb that were identical in sequence to rabbit's own Mb. In other words, sequence differences are not pre-requisite for antigenicity of the sites. Indeed it was found that rabbit antisera to sperm-whale Mb show considerable immunochemical cross-reactions with rabbit Mb

(Kazim and Atassi, 1977a). For more detail, this reference should be consulted.
Recently, we have extended these observations to show that this is a general
phenomenon quite independent of the immunized species. Thus, goat antisera to
sperm-whale Mb showed autoreactivity with goat Mb, and similarly chicken antisera reacted with chicken Mb, pig antisera with pig Mb and mouse antisera with
mouse Mb (Table 1) (Twining et al., 1980).

TABLE 1.   AUTOREACTIVITY OF SPERM-WHALE MB
ANTISERA WITH THE ANIMAL'S OWN MYOGLOBIN

%Antibodies Bound Relative to Binding by Sperm-Whale Mb as 100%*

A.	Goat Antisera:	G3	G4		
	Goat Mb	39.0	28.8		
B.	Rabbit Antisera:	77	80	M8	M9
	Rabbit Mb	40.3	28.8	37.7	41.9
C.	Chicken Antisera:	Ck1	Ck2		
	Chicken Mb	20.4	23.8		
D.	Mouse Antisera:	MS2	MS3	MS5	
	Mouse Mb	33.5	21.8	30.4	

*Plateau binding values of ^{125}I-labelled antibodies by immunoadsorbent ti-
tration studies. (Data from Twining, et al., 1980)

More recently, we have shown (Sakata and Atassi, 1980b) that rabbit antisera
against bovine or human serum albumin cross-reacted with rabbit albumin.

Our findings that the antigenicity of the Mb sites is not dependent on
sequence differences between the injected Mb and the Mb of the immunized host
led us to the reasoning that immunization of rabbits with rabbit Mb should
generate autoantibodies against this protein (Kazim and Atassi, 1978). Such
autoantibodies to rabbit Mb were in fact readily obtained (Figure 7) (Kazim
and Atassi, 1978).

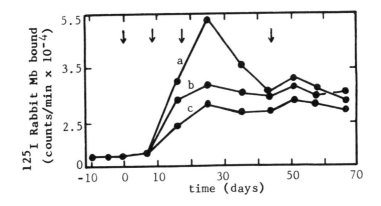

FIGURE 7. Screening of ^{125}I-rabbit Mb binding by antisera obtained from serial bleedings of three rabbits (RM1, RM2, and RM3) immunized with rabbit Mb. Arrows indicate times of immunization. (From Kazim, A.L. and Atassi, M.Z., Immunochemistry, 15, 67, 1978. With permission).

More recently, we have shown that rabbits immunized with their own serum albumin and mice immunized with mouse albumin each produced autoantibodies against their respective self-serum albumin (Sakata and Atassi, 1980b). This is highly significant in view of the fact that serum albumin is a normal and abundant constituent of serum. Clearly then, the potential for autorecognition is a natural and general phenomenon and strongly refutes the hypothesis that the antigenicity of protein antigenic sites is dependent on sequence differences between the injected antigen and the equivalent protein in the host animal. This erroneous concept overlooks basic functions of the immune system in immune surveillance, regulation, autoimmunity and tolerance.

Effects of Amino Acid Substitutions on Antigenic Sites

The binding of a protein antigenic site with its specific antibodies was repeatedly shown, during the course of our studies on the antigenic structure of Mb and lysozyme, to be highly dependent on the chemical characteristics of the residues constituting the site and on the conformational integrity of the site. Thus, alterations in the chemical nature of a side chain within a site (e.g. reversal or removal of a charge, creation of a new charge, elimination of a hydrogen bond, etc.) brought about either through chemical modification (e.g. Atassi, 1967a, 1968; Atassi and Thomas, 1969) or its evolutionary replacement in a homologous protein (Atassi, 1970; Atassi et al., 1970a, b) would cause a reduction or even complete elimination of the reactivity of the site (for review, see Atassi, 1975, 1977a, b). The presence and extent of reduction will depend on the nature of the chemical change to a site residue (Atassi and Habeeb, 1969; Atassi et al., 1971), on the location within the site of the residue being substituted or modified (Atassi et al., 1973b, 1975; Lee et al., 1975) and on its contribution to the overall binding energy of the site.

Apart from substitutions within the sites, whose effect is perhaps readily perceived, substitutions involving residues outside the antigenic sites would also be expected to exert considerable effects. It is relevant to note that the antibody response to native protein antigens is directed against their native three-dimensional structure (Atassi, 1967b; Atassi and Thomas, 1969). A substitution, even when distant from a site may cause a conformational readjustment and it is well documented that alterations in the conformation of an antigenic site will influence its reactivity (Atassi, 1967b, 1970; Atassi et al., 1970a, b; Andres and Atassi, 1970).

The chemical and conformational factors which contribute to and maintain the reactivity of an antigenic site are not, however, limited to only those which are localized within the site (Atassi, 1968; Atassi and Thomas, 1969). It must be remembered that protein antigenic sites exist as integral portions of the entire native protein molecule and are, therefore, also subject to chemical and conformational influences exerted from regions outside the antigenic sites and which are transmitted to the site through mutual interactions. Indeed, we have recently described antigenic sites as being in a certain electronic and steric equilibrium with the remainder of the protein molecule (Atassi and Kazim, 1980). An example of transmitted conformational effects may be taken from our early studies on myoglobin and hemoglobin which showed that conformational changes intentionally imposed on these two proteins by chemical modification clearly outside the antigenic sites lead in each protein to a reduction in its antigenic reactivity (Atassi, 1967b; Atassi and Skalski, 1969; Andres and Atassi, 1970). More recently, for lysozyme, we have demonstrated that a chemical change outside of an antigenic site but within interaction distance from an essential site residue (without detectable accompanying conformational changes) creates an electrostatic inductive effect which exerts a detrimental effect on the reactivity of that site (Lee and Atassi, 1977b).

These findings prompted us to undertake an analysis of the residues which comprise the environment of the antigenic sites of Mb and lysozyme and which, when altered, may be expected to influence their reactivity. Recently, we presented a description of the residues which constitute the environment of the antigenic sites of lysozyme, together with a somewhat detailed discussion of the general nature of protein binding sites and the forces affecting them (Atassi and Kazim, 1980). This was followed (Kazim and Atassi, 1980b) by identification of the nearest neighbor residues making up the immediate environment for each residue in the five antigenic sites of Mb (Atassi, 1975). Because of the expected rapid decay of the field of influence with increasing distance between a site residue and a nearest neighbor, we have considered that the effects will become negligible in most cases when the distance is greater than 7Å. Therefore, we have limited our analysis to those residues which fall within a 7Å radius of the antigenic site residues.

Knowledge of the precise locations of the antigenic sites of Mb and lysozyme and of the environmental residues around each site residue has enabled the evaluation of the effects of substitutions in the antigenic sites, in the residues close to these sites and in locations elsewhere in the molecule (Atassi and Kazim, 1980; Kazim and Atassi, 1980b). Recently, the immunochemical cross- reactions of 15 myoglobins were studied (Twining et al., 1980) and the findings have shown that the immunochemical cross-reactions can be reasonably rationalized on the basis of amino acid substitutions occurring in the residues of the antigenic sites and in the environmental (nearest-neighbor) residues surrounding the sites. Furthermore, conformational readjustments can frequently alter the binding energy of an antigenic site and consequently determine the proportion of antibodies with which it binds (Twining et al., 1980).

From the foregoing, it is clear that the structural and immunochemical effects of mutations is quite complex. A penetrating analysis of the immunochemical data from a given set of mutants can be achieved only with the knowledge of the antigenic structure of one of these homologous proteins which can then be used as a reference antigen. It is well to suggest here that caution should be exercised in the interpretation of the immunochemical cross-reactions of protein mutants to derive the unknown locations of the antigenic sites on these mutants. Other independent approaches (see Atassi, 1972, 1975) should be applied in the determination of protein antigenic structures.

Genetic Control of the Immune Response

Immune responses to various antigens are controlled by genes (Ir genes) coded within the H-2 (major histocompatibility) complex (Shreffler and David, 1975). Most studies of Ir gene control of immune responses have employed synthetic polymers of a few amino acids. Only recently, these studies were extended to include natural protein antigens (Melchers et al., 1973; Lozner et al., 1974; Keck, 1975). This information has added a new dimension to the understanding of the mechanism of T-cell recognition and antibody production.

Extensive studies on the genetic control of immune response to Mb and lysozyme and their respective antigenic sites have been initiated in our laboratories. The study of Mb and lysozyme offers a major advantage over other proteins because their entire antigenic structures have been determined (Atassi, 1975, 1978). We have also studied the genetic control of the immune response to human hemoglobin whose antigenic structure is now being determined in this laboratory. These studies have employed congenic strains of mice expressing the indepent haplotypes as well as selected recombinant strains and F_1 crosses.

Studies with Mb revealed that T-lymphocyte proliferative response to intact Mb was under H-2-linked Ir-gene control (Okuda et al., 1978). We identified at least two genes mapping in I-A and I-C subregions. In the case of lysozyme, we have found that the antibody and T-lymphocyte proliferative responses are also genetically controlled in mice (Okuda et al., 1979a). Both responses are controlled by two H-2I region loci, one being in the I-A and the other may be in the I-C subregions. More recently, we have undertaken studies with hemoglobin to probe the genetic control of the immune response to an oligomeric protein and the role of the individual subunits in the expression and regulation of the response. Such investigations have not been done on an oligomeric protein composed of non-identical subunits. Our recent findings (Krco et al., 1980) have shown that the immune response to Hb is also under genetic control and it is determined by two H-2 loci, one being in the K-A interval and the second in the D end. From in vitro challenge with each of the α and β subunits of Hb, it was found that the response to α-chain was controlled by a locus in the K end while control of the response to the β-chain was associated with the H-2D end (Table 2). It was postulated that the D region may play a regulatory influence in the response to Hb.

TABLE 2. SUMMARY OF Ir GENE MAPPING OF IMMUNE RESPONSIVENESS TO MB, LYSOZYME, HEMOGLOBIN AND THE α- AND β-SUBUNITS OF HEMOGLOBIN

Protein	MHC subregions regulating responsiveness		
Mb (sperm-whale)[1]	A	C	
Lysozyme (hen egg-white)[2]	A	C	
Hemoglobin (adult human)[3]	K-A		D
Hemoglobin α-chain[3]	K-A		
Hemoglobin β-chain[3]			D

Data from: [1]Okuda et al., 1978; [2]Okuda et al., 1979a; [3]Krco et al., 1980.

We have also carried out studies on the genetic control of the immune response in mice to the synthetic antigenic sites of sperm-whale Mb (Okuda et al., 1979b). These studies have revealed that individual antigenic sites in a molecule are controlled by unique Ir genes (i.e. the response to each antigenic site is under separate genetic control, see Figure 8).

For the determination of the complete antigenic structure of a protein, we would like to recommend that this should be done with outbred animals. If antisera are raised in a given congenic strain only some of the potential antigenic sites will be detected while the other sites, the response to which is genetically excluded, will go undetected.

Heterogeneity of the Response

The response to each antigenic site is heterogeneous, in that a variety of antibodies are produced to each antigenic site. This is not unusual nor unexpected since it is well known that even small haptenic determinant groups

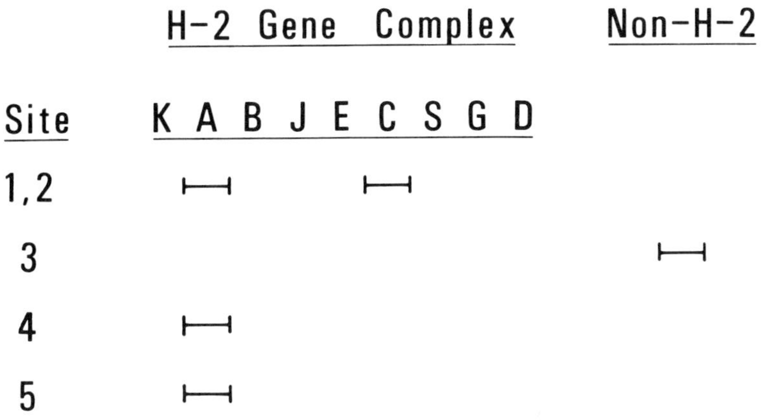

H-2 Gene Complex   Non-H-2

<u>Site</u>   K A B J E C S G D

1,2   ⊢—⊣   ⊢—⊣

3   ⊢—⊣

4   ⊢—⊣

5   ⊢—⊣

FIGURE 8. Ir gene mapping for individual antigenic sites of sperm whale myo-globin. (From Okuda, Twining, David and Atassi, J. Imm. <u>123</u>, 182, 1979. With permission).

(e.g. dinitrophenyl) generate a heterogeneous antibody response. What is the basis of this heterogeneity?

(a) It is well established that a variety of antibody molecules having identical specificities can be generated by appropriate conservative substi-tutions in the hypervariable regions. For example, the following amino acid substitutions in the combining site will generate antibodies of similar specificity:

Glu	Lys	Val
Asp	Lys	Val
Glu	Arg	Val
Asp	Arg	Val
Asp	Lys	Leu
	etc., etc.	

But even though these antibodies possess similar binding specificity, they will exhibit different binding energies with the antigenic site. Thus the source of heterogeneity is the presence of a variety of antibody molecules exhibiting the same specificity but having different affinities.

(b) In the process of the delineation of the antigenic sites of myoglobin and lysozyme to their precise boundaries, we have found that quite frequently (but not always) a portion of an antigenic site can bind some (but not all) of the antibodies to the whole site (Atassi and Saplin, 1968; Atassi, 1972; Koketsu and Atassi, 1973, 1974a, b). The extent of the binding ability of a portion of an antigenic site will depend on its size, on location of the

scission (i.e. which residues are missing from it) and on the stabilizing effect of any extra non-reactive segment of the peptide attached to the reactive
residues (Atassi, 1972). To explain these findings, we had proposed (Atassi,
1972) that "the small reactivity of a portion of an antigenic site can best
be explained if, in antibody response to an antigenic site antibodies are made
against various parts of the site. Maximal effective response, which is the
resultant average, will be directed against the center of the site". However,
it should be pointed out that reactivity of a portion of a site can also be
explained by the presence of antibodies having identical specificities but
differing in affinities (as in a above). Thus, whereas low affinity antibodies
are unable to bind with a portion of an antigenic site, because of insufficient
energy, higher affinity antibodies may well be able to do so.

It is possible to distinguish between the two alternatives by analysis of
the appropriate binding and inhibition curves. Our studies show that both
factors (a and b) contribute to the heterogeneity of the antibody response.
It is relevant, to caution, in view of the present widespread interest in
the preparation of monoclonal antibodies to a variety of antigens including
influenza and other viruses, that the ability to prepare a large number of
monoclonal antibodies does not mean that these antibodies possess a vast
spectrum of specificities. As seen above, a large number of antibodies can
be generated with binding specificity to a single antigenic site.

ANTIBODY COMBINING SITES CAN BE MIMICKED SYNTHETICALLY

From the foregoing short treatment, it is quite obvious that surface-
simulation synthesis constituted a conceptual breakthrough without which the
precise definition of the entire antigenic structure of lysozyme would have
been totally unattainable. However, as we have already pointed out (Atassi
et al., 1976b; Lee and Atassi, 1976; Atassi and Lee, 1978b), the remarkable
power of this unorthodox concept should not in any way be confined to the
determination of protein antigenic structures. The potential applications
of the concept have recently been discussed elsewhere (Atassi and Lee,
1978b; Atassi, 1978, 1979b). These can be summarized here by stating that
the concept can be used to synthetically mimic any type of protein binding
sites involving the interaction of a protein with other proteins or with
non-protein molecules.

The most intriguing question is whether an antibody combining site can
be mimicked by surface-simulation synthesis. Ability to perform this task
will obviously have far-reaching implications in immunology. Recent findings

from our laboratory (described in the next section) indicate that this has in-deed been accomplished. Thus, by mimicking the antibody combining site, at least in terms of binding function, the surface-simulation concept has scored a climax in protein immunochemistry. Although the concept came into being as a by-product of our determination of the antigenic structure of lysozyme, it should present a powerful new asset in protein chemistry.

Surface-Simulation Synthesis of the Immunoglobin New Combining Site to the γ-Hydroxyl Derivative of Vitamin K_1

Following our introduction and development of the concept of surface-simulation synthesis during the determination of the antigenic structure of hen egg-white lysozyme, we have examined whether an antibody-combining site can be reconstructed by surface-simulation synthesis. For our first attempt to test the feasibility of this idea, we have chosen the myeloma protein IgG New, which binds a hydroxyl derivative of vitamin K_1 (Vit. K_1 OH) (Amzel et al., 1974; Saul et al., 1978). The combining site residues (Ile-100 H, Ala-101 H, Asn-30 L, Tyr-90 L, Ser-93 L, Leu-94 L, Arg-95 L, Trp-47 H, Tyr-50 H, Tyr-33 H) were directly linked by peptide bonds, with appropriate intervening spacers (Twining and Atassi, 1978). Two peptides were synthesized (Figure 9) which mimicked the combining site but differed in the absence (peptide A) or presence (peptide B) of a spacer between Tyr-90 L and Ser-93 L. Also, a control peptide was synthesized having exactly the same amino acids as peptide B but which were in a different random sequence.

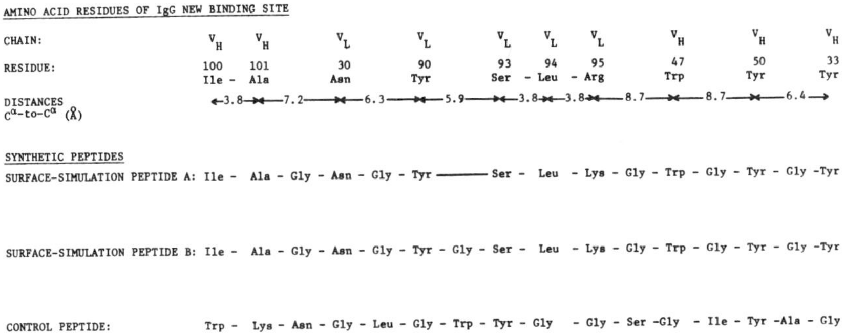

AMINO ACID RESIDUES OF IgG NEW BINDING SITE

CHAIN:	V_H	V_H	V_L	V_L	V_L	V_L	V_L	V_H	V_H	V_H
RESIDUE:	100 Ile	101 Ala	30 Asn	90 Tyr	93 Ser	94 Leu	95 Arg	47 Trp	50 Tyr	33 Tyr
DISTANCES C^α-to-C^α (Å)	←3.8→	—7.2—	—6.3—	—5.9—	—3.8→	←3.8—	—8.7—	—8.7—	—6.4→	

SYNTHETIC PEPTIDES

SURFACE-SIMULATION PEPTIDE A: Ile - Ala - Gly - Asn - Gly - Tyr ——— Ser - Leu - Lys - Gly - Trp - Gly - Tyr - Gly -Tyr

SURFACE-SIMULATION PEPTIDE B: Ile - Ala - Gly - Asn - Gly - Tyr - Gly - Ser - Leu - Lys - Gly - Trp - Gly - Tyr - Gly -Tyr

CONTROL PEPTIDE: Trp - Lys - Asn - Gly - Leu - Gly - Trp - Tyr - Gly - Gly - Ser -Gly - Ile - Tyr -Ala - Gly

FIGURE 9. A diagram showing the amino residues, and their numerical position in the sequence, which make close contact with Vit. K_1OH in the hypervariable region of IgG New. The diagram also gives the distances (in C^α-to-C^α) between

(continued on following page)

the constituent residues of the combining site as well as the total "extended" dimension of the site and the synthetic peptides. It should be emphasized that this is not intended to imply that the site is an extended surface. It is in fact a cavity. (From Twining, S.S. and Atassi, M.Z., J. Biol. Chem. 253, 5259, 1978).

Peptides A and B showed remarkable binding activity towards Vit. K_1OH while the control peptide exhibited no binding activity (Twining and Atassi, 1978). Peptide B, approximating more closely the correct spatial separation between the side chains, had a higher binding activity than peptide A. Inhibition studies confirmed the specificity of the binding between Vit. K_1OH and peptides A or B. The results clearly showed that a complex binding site, that of an antibody-combining site, can be successfully mimicked by surface-simulation synthesis (Twining and Atassi, 1978). Antibodies to peptide B have now been raised in rabbits after coupling it to rabbit serum albumin and studies are under way to determine whether the combining site and the idiotypic determinant of the myeloma protein coincide.

Surface-Simulation Synthesis of the Phosphorylcholine Combining Site of the Myeloma Protein M-603

More recently, the concept of "surface-simulation" synthesis has been applied (Kazim and Atassi, 1980a) to the combining site of the myeloma protein M-603. The X-ray co-ordinates of the binding site are known to a 3.1Å resolution (Segal et al., 1974; Padlan et al., 1976). We have been able to synthetically mimic the phosphorylcholine (PC) binding characteristics of M-603 in the surface-simulation peptide: Ser-Tyr-Gly-Gly-Arg-Tyr-Gly-Glu-Trp-Val (Figure 10).

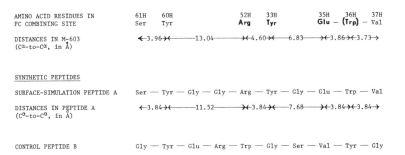

FIGURE 10. A diagram showing the amino acid residues in the phosphorylcholine binding site of M-603 and the structure of the synthetic surface-simulation peptide A designed to mimic it. The synthetic control peptide B, having the same composition but a scrambled sequence relative to peptide A, is also shown. Amino acid residues in M-603 which have been implicated in phosphorylcholine binding (Segal et al., 1974; Padlan et al., 1976) are shown in heavy type.

(continued on following page)

Parentheses around Trp 35 H indicate that it replaces Trp 104 aH for reasons
outlined in the text. The C^α-to-C^α distances in M-603 were calculated from
the C^α atomic coordinates (Feldman, 1976). The distances in peptide A were
calculated assuming a C^α-to-C^α distance of each peptide bond to be 3.84Å.
(From Kazim and Atassi, Biochem. J. 1980, in press).

In a solid phase radiometric assay, this peptide was found to bind to PC-
Sepharose. In contrast, a control peptide which had the same amino acid
composition but a different sequence (see Figure 11) showed little or no
binding activity. The specificity of binding to PC-Sepharose by the surface-
simulation peptide was further demonstrated by the inability of the control
peptide to significantly inhibit the binding of M-603, while the surface simulation peptide inhibited by more than 90% in the concentration range examined
(Kazim and Atassi, 1980a). Antibodies to the surface-simulation peptide have
also been raised.

These findings suggest that surface-simulation synthesis can be effectively employed to synthetically mimic antibody combining sites and may in the
future be a valuable tool with which to examine idiotypic specificities of
antibodies and to manipulate the immune response to clinically important
antigens. These avenues of investigation are being pursued in this laboratory.

The Possible Surface-Simulation Synthesis of Antibody-Combining Sites to
Lysozyme Antigenic Sites

The remarkable success of the surface-simulation synthesis concept in
reconstructing antigenic sites of spatially adjacent surface residues and of
combining sites of myeloma proteins has suggested to us its usefulness to investigate the feasibility of mimicking the antibody-combining sites to lysozyme antigenic sites (Atassi and Zablocki, 1977). It is evident from the
preceding sections that the proper application of surface-simulation synthesis
requires the detailed knowledge of the three-dimensional structure of the
protein under study and the unequivocal chemical identification of the residues
constituting a binding site as well as their accurate conformational spacing
and directional requirements. Obviously, none of these parameters is known
for the antibody-combining sites directed against lysozyme. However, we
reasoned (Atassi and Zablocki, 1977) that the situation is not entirely hope-
less since, in all likelihood, the antibody-combining site will be expected
to comprise residues that are not necessarily directly linked by peptide bonds
and that are complementary to those in the corresponding antigenic sites.
Furthermore, the directionality of the antigenic site and the spacings between its constituent residues and the corresponding parameters of the

antibody-combining site must be equivalent or comparable in order for appropriate binding to take place. Thus, by the precise knowledge of all the parameters of an antigenic site, it should be possible to create a reasonable design of its complementary antibody-combining site. At the time of writing, this had been done (Atassi and Zablocki, 1977) for two antigenic sites in native lysozyme.

Two peptides CS-2 and CS-3 (Figure 11) were designed (Atassi and Zablocki, 1977) on the basis of complementarity to antigenic sites 2 and 3, respectively, in ionic, hydrophobic, hydrophilic and side-chain length of the constituent amino acids.

ANTIGENIC SITE 2 AND THE PREDICTED COMPLEMENTARY SITE

CONSTITUANT RESIDUES OF THE ANTIGENIC SITE:	62 TRP	97 LYS	96 LYS	93 ASN	89 THR	87 ASP

DISTANCES:
(αC-to-αC, in nm)
|←——0.71——→|←0.41→|←0.56→|←0.51→|←0.54→|
|←——————————— 2.73 ———————————→|

THE SYNTHETIC ANTIGENIC SITE: PHE — GLY — LYS — LYS — ASN — THR — ASP

DISTANCES:
(αC-to-αC, in nm)
|←——————————— 2.16 ———————————→|

THE COMPLEMENTARY SITE (CS-2):   LEU — GLY — ASP — ASP — GLN — SER — LYS

ANTIGENIC SITE 3 AND THE PREDICTED COMPLEMENTARY SITE

CONSTITUANT RESIDUES OF THE ANTIGENIC SITE:	116 LYS	113 ASN —	114 ARG	34 PHE	33 LYS

DISTANCES:
(αC-to-αC, in nm)
|←0.5→|←0.4→|←——— 0.8 ———→|←0.4→|
|←——————————— 2.1 ———————————→|

THE SYNTHETIC ANTIGENIC SITE: LYS — ASN — ARG — GLY — PHE — LYS

DISTANCES:
(αC-to-αC, in nm)
|←——————————— 1.8 ———————————→|

THE COMPLEMENTARY SITE (CS-3):   ASP — GLN — ASP — GLY — LEU — ASP

FIGURE 11. A diagram showing antigenic sites 2 and 3 of hen egg white lysozyme and their predicted complementary antibody-combining sites. The spatially contiguous surface residues constituting each antigenic site and the numerical positions of these residues in the primary structure of lysozyme are shown. The distances (in nm) separating the consecutive residues and the overall dimension of each site are given, together with the dimension of the respective surface-simulation synthetic antigenic site. Below each antigenic site is given the structure of the respective complementary surface-simulation peptide which was predicted to mimic the antibody-combining site directed against that antigenic site. (From Atassi, M.Z., and Zablocki, W., J. Biol. Chem., 252, 8784, 1977. With permission).

Each of the two complementary peptides exhibited an appreciable inhibitory activity towards the reaction of lysozyme with its antisera which compared favorably with the activity of the respective antigenic sites and the inhibitory activities of the two peptides were additive. Peptide immunoadsorbents bound only lysozyme and not antibody or myoglobin. Neither of the two peptides had any immunochemical activity in the myoglobin or bovine serum albumin immune systems. Furthermore, control synthetic peptides of similar charge but different sequence, had no inhibitory effect on the lysozyme immune reaction (Atassi and Zablocki, 1977). The evidence indicated that the antibody-combining sites against antigenic sites 2 and 3 of native lysozyme were successfully mimicked synthetically, at least in terms of binding function.

We have stressed (Atassi and Zablocki, 1977) that the residues deduced in peptides CS-2 and CS-3 are in no way implied to be the actual residues brought together in the binding sites of the antibodies by the three-dimensional folding of the latter. This is difficult to know. Also, it was emphasized that the functional success of these two peptides does not imply a unique antibody site to a given lysozyme antigenic site. Other complementary amino acids may serve equally as well in the antibody-combining site. For example, the role of leucine may be satisfied by isoleucine, valine, phenylalanine, etc., but we have not tested that yet. By employing related alternatives to each residue, it will not be difficult to rationalize heterogeneity and differences in affinity of the antibody-combining site.

At the time these complementary sites were synthesized (Atassi and Zablocki, 1977) only antigenic sites 2 and 3 of lysozyme had been precisely defined (Lee and Atassi, 1977 a, b). However, to test whether or not our success with this complementarity approach represents a special situation, we are now studying synthetic peptides that are complementary to antigenic site 1 of lysozyme (Atassi and Lee, 1978a) as well as the 5 antigenic sites of myoglobin (Atassi, 1975).

The finding that two synthetic peptides (CS-2 and CS-3) which were designed to be complementary to antigenic sites 2 and 3 of lysozyme possessed antibody-like binding activity against their respective antigenic sites (Atassi and Zablocki, 1977) made it possible to investigate a very important question. Since each of these peptides mimics an antibody-combining site in

terms of binding function to a lysozyme antigenic site, would antibodies to
such a peptide then react with antisera to lysozyme? If the antibody-combining
site is truly mimicked in peptides CS-2 and CS-3, it would be extremely important to determine whether antibodies to these peptides would react with anti-
lysozyme antibodies. The achievement of this would obviously open up many
hitherto untapped avenues in immunology, in particular those pertaining to regulation and manipulation of the immune response by anti-combining site antibodies.

In recent work (Atassi and Sakata, 1980), antibodies were raised against
one of these peptides (CS-3) which is complementary to antigenic site 3 of
lysozyme to determine whether antibodies to this peptide will react with anti-
lysozyme antibodies. Radioiodinated anti-peptide antibodies were in fact
bound by immunoadsorbents carrying immune IgG fractions of two goat anti-
lysozyme antisera. Inhibition studies confirmed the specificity of the
binding. The results clearly showed that antibodies to a peptide, which was
designed to be complementary to a lysozyme antigenic site, have been found
to react with anti-lysozyme antibodies. This indicated that the complementary
peptide must have resembled closely the antibody combining sites in two lysozyme antisera, with regards to the spacing, the directional requirements for
surface-simulation synthesis and the nature of the residues, presumably in the
hypervariable regions on the heavy and light chains, of the anti-lysozyme
antibodies. Thus, by precise knowledge of a protein antigenic site, a complementary peptide can potentially be designed to mimic the arrangement of residues in the combining-sites of antibodies to that antigenic site. The success of the design can be tested by immunochemical studies on the complementary peptide and finally by the ability of its antibodies to react with anti-
protein antisera. To test whether or not the success of the present studies
represents a special case, we are now studying antibodies against complementary peptides to antigenic site 1 of lysozyme, complementary peptides
to the myoglobin antigenic sites (Atassi, 1975), and the surface-simulation
synthetic sites of myeloma proteins (Twining and Atassi, 1978; Kazim and
Atassi, 1980a).

IMPLICATIONS OF PRECISE DETERMINATION OF ANTIGENIC SITES
TO PROTEIN FUNCTION AND VIRUS RESEARCH

Our precise determination of protein antigenic sites has charted a strategy not only for determining such sites for other proteins but also for
delineating and synthesizing other types of protein binding sites and thus
has opened up a new dimension in studies on protein activities. We have
already shown the strategy and concepts developed during our determination of
the antigenic structures of myoglobin and lysozyme also enabled us to mimic

synthetically antibody combining sites. These are the only protein binding sites of any type that have so far been systematically delineated and synthetically mimicked. Binding sites representing other protein activities are now being mimicked in our laboratory by the concept of surface-simulation synthesis.

The strategy initially worked out with model proteins (myoglobin, lysozyme, serum albumin) should be extremely useful in developing immunological therapeutic approaches to viral infection. Such immunological approaches in principle offer the distinct advantage that they effect prevention of entry of the virus into the host cell. This is quite distinct from methods which depend on attacking the virus after it had entered the host cell (e.g. anti-viral drugs, inhibition of viral enzymes). Vaccines have been developed against a variety of viruses including influenza virus. However, the rapid mutation of the coat proteins (e.g. the hemagglutinin HA molecule in the influenza virus) has restricted the usefulness of these vaccines. As seen previously, substitutions inside or even outside a given antigenic site can destroy the binding activity of a site. The effect of substitutions outside the site is due to conformational changes in the protein antigen or to detrimental environmental effects in the neighborhood of the site. The systematic localization and then synthesis of the antigenic sites on virus proteins (e.g. HA molecule of influenza) should afford synthetic peptides that can be employed in the preparation of vaccines against appropriately prepared synthetic antigens. These synthetic vaccines can be made specifically to one (or more) antigenic sites which may overcome some of the foregoing problems and others seemingly encountered with cross-reactions between proteins of certain viruses and host cell proteins.

Another immunological approach which could be achieved in the more distant future would rely on the identification of the antibody combining site of selected monoclonal antibodies to the virus. The antibody combining site can then be chemically synthesized by the concept of surface-simulation synthesis. The synthetic peptides, suitably designed, can in principle be used to permanently neutralize the virus particle. The chemical strategies, already worked out in this laboratory with model systems, have removed any intellectual barriers that may face these approaches.

Acknowledgements

The work was supported by grants AM 18920 and AI 13181 from the National Institute of Arthritis and Metabolic Diseases and the National Institute of Allergy and Infectious Diseases, National Institutes of Health, U.S. Public Health Service.

REFERENCES

Atassi, M.Z. (1967a) Biochem. J. 102, 478-487.
Atassi, M.Z. (1967b) Biochem. J. 103, 29-35.
Atassi, M.Z. (1968) Biochemistry 7, 3078-3085.
Atassi, M.Z. (1970) Biochim. Biophys. Acta 221, 612-622.
Atassi, M.Z. (1972) in Specific Receptors of Antibodies, Antigens and Cells, 3rd Int. Convocation on Immunol., pp. 118-135, Karyer, Basel.
Atassi, M.Z. (1975) Immunochemistry 12, 423-438.
Atassi, M.Z. (1977a) in Immunochemistry of Proteins (Atassi, M.Z., Ed.) Vol. 1, pp. 1-161, Plenum, New York.
Atassi, M.Z. (1977b) in Immunochemistry of Proteins (Atassi, M.Z., Ed.) Vol. 2, pp. 77-176, Plenum, New York.
Atassi, M.Z. (1978) Immunochemistry 15, 909-936.
Atassi, M.Z. (1979a) Crit. Revs. Biochem. 6, 337-369.
Atassi, M.Z. (1979b) Crit. Revs. Biochem. 6, 371-400.
Andres, S.F. and Atassi, M.Z. (1970) Biochemistry 9, 2268-2275.
Atassi, M.Z. and Habeeb, A.F.S.A. (1969) Biochemistry 8, 1385-1393.
Atassi, M.Z. and Kazim, A.L. (1980) Biochem. J., in press.
Atassi, M.Z. and Kazim, A.L. in Immunobiology of Proteins and Peptides (Atassi, M.Z. and Stavitsky, A.B. Eds.) Vol. 1, pp. 19-40, Plenum, New York.
Atassi, M.Z. and Koketsu, J. (1975) Immunochemistry 12, 741-744.
Atassi, M.Z. and Lee, C.-L. (1978a) 171, 419-427.
Atassi, M.Z. and Lee, C.-L. (1978b) 171, 429-434.
Atassi, M.Z. and Pai, R.-C. (1975) Immunochemistry 12, 735-740.
Atassi, M.Z. and Sakata, S. (1980) Biochim. Biophys. Acta, in press.
Atassi, M.Z. and Saplin, B.J. (1968) Biochemistry 7, 688-698.
Atassi, M.Z. and Skalski, D.J. (1969) Immunochemistry.
Atassi, M.Z. and Smith, J.A. (1978) Immunochemistry 15, 609-610.
Atassi, M.Z. and Thomas, A.V. (1969) Biochemistry 8, 3385-3394.
Atassi, M.Z. and Zablocki, W. (1977) J. Biol. Chem. 252, 8784-8787.
Amzel, L.M., Poljak, R.J., Saul, F., Varya, J.M. and Richard, F.F. (1974) Proc. Nat. Acad. Sci. U.S.A. 71, 1427-1430.
Atassi, M.Z., Habeeb, A.F.S.A. and Ando, K. (1973a) Biochim. Biophys. Acta 303, 203-209.
Atassi, M.Z., Habeeb, A.F.S.A. and Rydstedt, L. (1970b) Biochim. Biophys. Acta 200, 184-187.
Atassi, M.Z., Koketsu, J. and Habeeb, A.F.S.A. (1976c) Biochim. Biophys. Acta 420, 358-375.
Atassi, M.Z., Lee, C.-L. and Habeeb, A.F.S.A. (1976a) Immunochemistry 13, 7-14.
Atassi, M.Z., Lee, C.-L. and Pai, R.-C. (1976b) Biochim. Biophys. Acta 427, 745-751.
Atassi, M.Z., Litowich, M.T. and Andres, S.F. (1975) Immunochemistry 12, 727-733.
Atassi, M.Z., Perlstein, M.T. and Habeeb, A.F.S.A. (1971) J. Biol. Chem. 246, 3291-3296.
Atassi, M.Z., Perlstein, M.T. and Staub, D.J. (1973b) Biochim. Biophys. Acta 328, 278-288.
Atassi, M.Z., Sakata, S. and Kazim, A.L. (1979) Biochem. J. 179, 327-331.
Atassi, M.Z., Tarlowski, D.P. and Paull, J.H. (1970a) Biochim. Biophys. Acta 221, 623-635.
Ely, K.R., Girling, R.L., Schiffer, M., Cunningham, D.E. and Edmundson, A.B. (1973) Biochemistry 12, 4233.
Habeeb, A.F.S.A. and Atassi, M.Z. (1970) Biochemistry 9, 4939-4944.
Hurrell, J.G.R., Smith, J.A. and Leach, S.J. (1978) Immunochemistry 15, 297-302.

Keck, K. (1975) <u>Nature</u>, London, <u>254</u>, 78-79.

Kazim, A.L. and Atassi, M.Z. (1977a) <u>Biochim. Biophys. Acta</u> <u>494</u>, 277-282.

Kazim, A.L. and Atassi, M.Z. (1977b) <u>Biochem. J.</u> <u>167</u>, 275-278.

Kazim, A.L. and Atassi, M.Z. (1978) <u>Immunochemistry</u> <u>15</u>, 67-70.

Kazim, A.L. and Atassi, M.Z. (1980a) <u>Biochem. J.</u>, in press.

Kazim, A.L. and Atassi, M.Z. (1980b) <u>Biochem. J.</u>, in press.

Koketsu, J. and Atassi, M.Z. (1973) <u>Biochim. Biophys. Acta</u> <u>328</u>, 289-302.

Koketsu, J. and Atassi, M.Z. (1974a) <u>Immunochemistry</u> <u>11</u>, 1-8.

Koketsu, J. and Atassi, M.Z. (1974b) <u>Biochim. Biophys. Acta</u> <u>342</u>, 21-29.

Krco, C., Kazim, A.L., David, C.S. and Atassi, M.Z. (1980) <u>Mol. Immunol.</u>, in press.

Lee, C.-L. and Atassi, M.Z. (1975) <u>Biochim. Biophys. Acta</u> <u>405</u>, 464-474.

Lee, C.-L. and Atassi, M.Z. (1976) <u>Biochem. J.</u> <u>159</u>, 89-93.

Lee, C.-L. and Atassi, M.Z. (1977a) <u>Biochim. Biophys. Acta</u> <u>495</u>, 354-368.

Lee, C.-L. and Atassi, M.Z. (1977b) <u>Biochem. J.</u> <u>167</u>, 571-581.

Lee, C.-L., Atassi, M.Z. and Habeeb, A.F.S.A. (1975) <u>Biochim. Biophys. Acta</u> <u>400</u>, 423-432.

Lozner, E.C., Sachs, D.H. and Shearer, G.M. (1974) <u>J. Exp. Med.</u> <u>139</u>, 1204-1214.

Melcher, I.K., Rajewsky, K. and Shreffler, D.C. (1973) <u>Europ. J. Immunol.</u> <u>3</u>, 754-761.

Okuda, K., Christadoss, P., Twining, S.S., Atassi, M.Z. and David, C.S. (1978) <u>J. Immunol.</u> <u>121</u>, 866-868.

Okuda, K., Sakata, S., Atassi, M.Z. and David, C.S. (1979a) <u>J. Immunogen.</u>, in press.

Okuda, K., Twining, S.S., David, C.S. and Atassi, M.Z. (1979b) <u>J. Immunol.</u> <u>123</u>, 182-188.

Padlan, E.A., Davies, D.R., Rudikoff, S. and Porter, M. (1976) <u>Immunochemistry</u> <u>13</u>, 945-949.

Sakata, S. and Atassi, M.Z. (1980a) <u>Molecular Immunol.</u> <u>17</u>, in press.

Sakata, S. and Atassi, M.Z. (1980b) <u>Fed. Proc.</u> <u>39</u>, in press.

Shreffler, D.C. and David, C.S. (1975) <u>Adv. Immunol.</u> 20, 125-195.

Saul, F.A., Amzel, L.M. and Poljak, P.J. (1978) <u>J. Biol. Chem.</u> <u>253</u>, 585-597.

Schiffer, M., Girling, R.L., Ely, K.R. and Edmundson, A.B. (1973) <u>Biochemistry</u> <u>12</u>, 4620.

Segal, D.M., Padlan, E.A., Cohen, G.H., Rudikoff, S., Potter, M. and Davies, D.R. (1974) <u>Proc. Nat. Acad. Sci. U.S.</u> <u>71</u>, 4298-4302.

Twining, S.S. and Atassi, M.Z. (1978) <u>J. Biol. Chem.</u> <u>253</u>, 5259-5262.

Twining, S.S. and Atassi, M.Z. (1979) <u>J. Immunol. Methods</u> 30, 139-151.

Twining, S.S., Lehmann, H. and Atassi, M.Z. (1980) <u>Biochem. J.</u>, submitted.

(See DISCUSSION on following page)

272

DISCUSSION

Cummings: Have you compared your synthetic peptides with Eli
    Sercarz's monoclonal antibodies to lysozyme?

Atassi: No, but I have other monoclonal antibodies which can be
    separated into three groups with specificity for the three
    sites.

Laver: Have you looked for suppressor peptides?

Atassi: The antigenic sites can have a regulating effect on
    each other, but we have not looked for suppressing effects.

AN EXPERIMENTAL APPROACH TO DEFINE THE ANTIGENIC STRUCTURES OF THE
HEMAGGLUTININ MOLECULE OF A/PR/8/34

WALTER GERHARD[+], JONATHAN YEWDELL AND MARK FRANKEL
[+]The Wistar Institute, Philadelphia, Pennsylvania 19104

INTRODUCTION

The antigenicity of a protein is defined as the protein structure with
which immunological effector mechanisms (humoral and/or cellular) interact in
a specific way. A major problem faced in the accurate delineation of the
antigenicity of a protein is the fact that these immunological effector
mechanisms are, in general, highly heterogeneous. Standard antisera, for
instance, are likely to contain a multitude of antibody populations that
are directed against an unknown number of antigenic sites of the protein under
study. Such antisera delineate, therefore, the overall antigenicity of a protein rather than its individual antigenic sites.

There are, in principle, two ways in which a complex antigen-antiserum
interaction can be reduced into components that correspond to the interaction
of antibodies with individual antigenic sites. First, the protein can be dissected into individual fragments that retain antigenic properties of the native
protein. This approach has the advantage of providing a direct correlation
between antigenicity and protein structure but it may not be applicable to the
fine dissection of conformational antigenic sites of the protein [1,2]. An
alternative approach, which was followed here, is to dissect the antiserum
into individual components that are likely to be specific for individual antigenic sites of the protein. The logical and, at present, most feasible way to
achieve this is to produce first a diverse panel of monoclonal antibodies
against the protein under study and, second, to group these antibodies
according to various criteria into families of antibodies that exhibit similar
properties and may be assumed, therefore, to delineate individual antigenic
sites of the protein. Consequently, these families of antibodies can then be
applied to study the structural correlates of the operationally defined
antigenic sites of the protein.

Since the characterization of the antigenicity, at a functional or a structural level, must be regarded in the context of the immunological effector mechanisms as well as the assay system used to define the antigenicity of a protein, it is important to discuss briefly the materials and methods from which the present analysis of the antigenicity of the hemagglutinin (HA) molecule of influenza virus A/PR/8/34 derives.

First, the present analysis is based on 40 monoclonal anti-HA antibodies produced from B cells of PR8-immunized BALB/c mice by the method of somatic cell hybridization [3,4]. It is clear from previous studies of the anti-PR8 response performed at the level of single B cell clones, that these 40 monoclonal antibodies represent only a fraction of the total anti-HA(PR8) repertoire of the BALB/c mouse [5,6]. We have attempted, therefore, to maximize the variety of antibody specificities by using different immunization schedules and fusion protocols in the generation of these hybridomas [7,8] . However, even if the present panel of hybridoma antibodies represents an unbiased cross-section of the BALB/c anti-HA(PR8) repertoire, the following definition of the antigenicity of the HA molecule remains relative to the BALB/c immune system.

Second, we have used two assays to measure the antigen-antibody interaction. The hemagglutinin-inhibition (HI) test was performed according to standard procedures. The second assay used in this analysis is an indirect radioimmunoassay (RIA) in which the amount of antibody binding to a solid-phase viral immunoadsorbent is measured by means of a radio-iodinated rabbit-anti-mouse-$F(ab')_2$-antibody preparation. The lower limit of antibody avidity detected in the RIA [9] is in the range of $10^6 M^{-1}$.

Another point that should be considered in this context is the determination of the anti-HA specificity. This was done by testing the antibody binding capacity in the RIA to a panel of recombinant viruses of known genotype (kindly provided by Drs. P. Palese and J. Shulman, Mt. Sinai Hospital, NY). Briefly, the antibodies were first tested in the RIA for binding to the parental viruses PR8 and Hong Kong of the recombinant panel. Second, all antibodies that bound to PR8 but not to HK were further tested for binding to the panel of recombinant viruses. Accordingly, antibodies that bound only to the recombinants that contain the HA-gene of PR8 were regarded as anti-HA antibodies. This method does not allow one, however, to determine the specificity of antibodies that bind to both parental viruses and, consequently, may miss anti-HA antibodies directed against highly conserved antigenic sites of the HA molecule.

The present report gives first a brief outline of the methods used to
construct an operational antigenic map of the HA molecule of A/PR/8/34 which
will be reported in detail elsewhere (manuscript in preparation). Second,
preliminary evidence for the structural correlates of the operational
antigenic map is presented.

THE CONSTRUCTION OF AN OPERATIONAL ANTIGENIC MAP BY MEANS OF MONOCLONAL ANTIBODIES

1. Definition of the antigenic site(s) by the hemagglutination
inhibition (HI) test. In order to evaluate the HI-activity of the various
hybridomas, ascitic fluids from hybridoma bearing mice were tested for their
HI-titer and antibody concentration against PR8 in the standard HI-test and
RIA respectively. The determination of the antibody concentration in the RIA
was based on the comparison of the binding observed with appropriate dilutions
of the test sample to the binding observed with affinity-purified BALB/c
anti-PR8 antiserum of known antibody concentration [9]. The HI-activity of each
antibody was then expressed as HI-titer exhibited by an antibody concentration
of 1 µg/ml.

As shown in Table 1, the antibodies covered a wide spectrum of HI-activities
ranging from less than 0.1 to 2500. The only grouping into distinct antibody
families that seemed justified under these conditions was according to the
presence or absence of HI-activity at the highest antibody concentration tested
which corresponded in the case of the three HI-negative antibodies to 10,
12 and 130 µg/ml. The antigenic site(s) delineated by the latter antibodies
was designated Y.

Table 1

Grouping of Antibodies on the Basis of their HI-Activity

Number of Antibodies (Isotype)	HI-Activity[a] (Range)	Antibody Group	Designation of Antigenic Site(s)
7 (IgM)	9-2500	HI-Pos.	
30 (IgG)	3-570	HI-Pos.	
3 (IgG)	< 0.1	HI-Neg.	Y

a) The HI-titer of hybridoma ascitic fluids was determined in the standard
HI-test against 4 agglutinating doses of PR8 using chicken red blood cells. The
HI-activity represents the HI-titer observed at an antibody concentration
(as determined in the RIA) of 1 µg/ml.

2. Definition of antigenic sites by means of virus mutants. In order to investigate the relationship between the antigenic determinants delineated by the HI-pos. anti-HA antibodies, we have adopted an approach that has been used extensively in the past to localize antigenic structures on a variety of proteins (for review see 2,11-13). The principle of the method is to introduce small antigenic modifications into the antigenic background of the parental protein and to use these modified proteins in comparative antigenic analyses as markers for given antigenic structures of the protein. The terminology used here for the description of the data is as follows. The antigenic structure with which the combining site (viz. paratope [14]) of an individual antibody interacts will be called epitope [14]. The term antigenic site will be used to designate an antigenic structure (usually corresponding to a group of overlapping epitopes) which is, at least on an operational basis distinct from and non-overlapping with neighboring antigenic sites.

A panel of 22 distinct antigenic markers has been generated in the form of mutant viruses derived from the parental virus PR8. Such mutant viruses could be selected readily by passage of the cloned parental virus in the presence of an "overneutralizing" dose of a monoclonal anti-HA antibody [10,15,16]. The HA molecule exhibited by the virus variants selected in this way can be characterized as follows. First, they seem to represent, in general, single point mutants of the parental HA molecule as evidenced, a) by the high frequency of occurrence (in the average of $10^{-5.5}$ single epitope mutants per infectious unit of parental virus) in cloned virus preparations [8,15,16], and b) by comparative analysis of peptide maps and amino acid composition of the HA polypeptides of parental and variant virus [16,17]. Second, each mutation induced an antigenic change that is at least partially encompassed by the HA-epitope delineated by the antibody used for the selection of the mutant. Third, although the mutation decreased, often to non-detectable levels, the capacity of the selecting antibody to bind to the homologous mutants, it did not modify detectably, the overall antigenicity of the HA molecule. Thus, the large majority of monoclonal anti-HA antibodies interacted to the same extent with parental and mutant viruses [10]. Similarly, anti-HA antisera were unable to differentiate between parental and mutant viruses [10]. In conclusion, the various mutants represent fine antigenic markers that encompass the HA-epitope delineated by the selecting antibody and that are localized in the antigenic structure of the HA molecule in which attachment of antibody mediates virus-neutralization.

Accordingly, we have used these mutants in antigenic analyses to determine
the relationship among the HA-epitopes delineated by the various HI-pos.
monoclonal anti-HA antibodies. In the present study, a linkage among HA-epitopes
was demonstrated if the antigenic change on a mutant-HA molecule prevented the
corresponding antibodies from binding to the variant virus in the RIA. On
this basis, the various HI-pos. antibodies could be grouped into 5 families.
As shown in Table 2, four of these antibody families were each characterized
by the fact that their corresponding epitopes were modified by one or several
of a given set of mutations but not by mutations that modified the epitopes
delineated by any of the other antibody families. Furthermore, a fifth
antibody family delineates an epitope group that was not modified by any of
the mutations selected in the present study. Thus, each antibody family appears
to delineate an epitope-group of the HA-molecule of PR8 that is able to
mutate independently from the other epitope groups. On this operational basis,
these epitope-groups seem to correspond to non-overlapping antigenic sites of
the HA molecule which have been designated B, PC, DN, LA and X.

Table 2

Grouping of HI-Pos. Antibodies by Mutant Analysis

Number of Hybridoma Antibodies	Binding of Antibodies in RIA to Mutant Group				Designation of Antigenic Site Delineated
	B (6)	PC (9)	DN (4)	LA (3)	
4	-	+	+	+	B
12	+	-	+	+	PC
4	+	+	-	+	DN
8	+	+	+	-	LA
6	+	+	+	+	X

Replicate samples of the antibodies were tested in the RIA for their binding
capacity to 20 HA-units of parental virus and the various mutant viruses.
a) Number of antigenically distinct virus mutants per mutant group. b) Negative
(-) indicates that the individual antibodies of the given antibody family exhibit, compared to the parental virus, decreased or non-detectable binding
to one, several or all mutant viruses of the given mutant group. Positive
(+) indicates that the antibodies bind to the same extent to the parental virus
and all virus mutants within the given mutant group.

The present antigenic map must be regarded as preliminary, however, since it is based on a limited number of mutants and antibodies. For instance, the possibility can not be excluded that some or all of these antigenic sites have in common structures of the HA molecule in which no antigenic change happened to be localized. The HA-mutant as well as the antibody panel is therefore currently being expanded with the hope that one could derive in this way a more accurate antigenic map.

RELATIONSHIP BETWEEN THE OPERATIONAL ANTIGENIC MAP AND THE STRUCTURE OF THE HA MOLECULE

The production of a panel of mutant viruses and their use in the organization of antibodies into reactivity families is merely the first phase in the analysis of the HA molecule. In the next phase of this approach the relationship of antigenic sites to structural or functional characteristics of the HA would be studied. An example of the type of studies that can be performed is the following comparison of antibody reactivities to purified virus treated under different conditions.

Electron microscopic observations indicate that the HA-spikes form a dense array of surface projections on the intact virion [18]. In order to test whether various parts on the HA molecule have different accessibility, the various antibody families were compared for extent of binding to "wet" and "dried" viral immunoadsorbent. The PR8 virus used in these experiments was freshly banded (velocity) in a linear sucrose gradient, the visible virus band was collected and sucrose was removed by dialysis against phosphate buffered saline (PBS). The two types of viral immunoadsorbents were then prepared as follows: 25 µl samples of virus (diluted in PBS to give 2 HA-units of virus per sample) were added to wells of polyvinyl plastic plates and i) dried overnight at 37°C ("dried"), or ii) incubated overnight at room temperature without allowing evaporation to occur ("wet"). It was hoped that the latter procedure would help to preserve the native spatial arrangement of the HA spikes.

Table 3

Binding of Antibodies to Wet or Dried Viral Immunoadsorbent

Number of Antibodies Tested	Antigenic Site	Difference in Binding Capacity of Antibodies to Wet Versus Dried Viral Immunoadsorbent Fraction: Average	SD [a]		HI-Activity[b]
3	Y	− 0.66 ±	0.10		< 0.1
7 [c]	LA	− 0.20 ±	0.14		3 − 65
5 [c]	X	− 0.19 ±	0.12		
2	B	+ 0.28 ±	0.07		
4	DN	+ 0.40 ±	0.06		140 − 570
5 (2)	PC	+ 0.40 ±	0.11	(+ 1.61)	

a) In order to compare the various antibodies independent of the actual cpm observed (which may vary depending on antibody avidity and isotype) the difference in binding to wet versus dried immunoadsorbent was expressed as a fraction according to the formula:

$$(cpm(wet) - cpm(dried))/cpm(dried)$$

b) HI-titer observed at antibody concentration of 1 µg/ml

c) One antibody in each of the indicated families exhibited an atypical reactivity in this assay and, awaiting a reassessment of their clonality and specificity, have not been included in the Table.

The various antibodies were then tested at or close to saturating conditions (excess antibody compared to available antigenic sites) for binding in the RIA to "wet" and "dried" PR8 immunoadsorbent (Table 3).

With 4 exceptions (2 antibodies in the PC group, data shown in brackets, and one antibody in the LA and X group respectively, see also Legend of Table 3) antibodies that belong to the same family exhibit a similar reactivity pattern in this assay. The families of PC, B and DN appear similar with respect to their binding to these virus preparations in that they bind better to the "wet" than to the "dried" virus while the family Y binds better to "dried" than to "wet" viral immunoadsorbent. The antibody families LA and X exhibit a reactivity intermediate to the above groups. Finally, Table 3 shows that grouping the families in this manner correlates well with grouping them with respect to HI-activity.

These observations clearly indicate that drying affects the antibody binding capacity of the viral immunoadsorbents. This may result from a different spatial arrangement among HA spikes or from a different degree of denaturation of the various sites during the process of drying. However, in conjunction with the HI-activity, these observations are compatible with the interpretation of different accessibilities of various antigenic sites on the HA spike. We may speculate that antigenic sites may be localized on the HA spike at three levels. The top level (closest to the tip of the spike) may be occupied by the sites B, DN and PC, the intermediate level by the site LA and X and the bottom level (toward base of spike) by the site Y. Electron microscopic analyses, using monoclonal antibodies, as performed previously by Wrigley et al. [19], may allow us to verify the different location of these antigenic sites on the HA spike.

The use of HI-activity and the reactivity of antibody families against "wet" versus "dried" viral immunoadsorbent are preliminary attempts to study the correlation between the operational antigenic map and the structure of the HA molecule. One may easily envisage numerous other studies in which the effect of detergent treatment, subunit purification, reduction and alkylation and enzymatic cleavage is analyzed in relation to the antigenicity of the various antigenic sites of the HA molecule. Furthermore, functional characterization of the antibody families with assays such as neuraminidase inhibition, virus neutralization, complement fixation or antibody dependent cell-mediated lysis can be used to characterize individual antigenic sites. Therefore, the use of monoclonal antibodies should provide a large body of coordinated information on the structure-function relationship of the separate antigenic sites which compose the antigenicity of the HA molecule of the influenza virus PR8.

ACKNOWLEDGEMENT

This work was supported by Grant No. AI-13989 and by Grant No. NS11036 (NINCDS) from the National Institutes of Health.

REFERENCES

1. Crumpton, M.J. (1974) in The Antigens, M. Sela, ed, Academic Press, NY, 2, 1-78.
2. Reichlin, M.(1975) Adv. Immunology 20,71-123.
3. Kohler, G., and Milstein, C. (1975) Nature, 256,495-497.
4. Koprowski, G., W. Gerhard and C.M. Croce (1977) Proc. Natl. Acad. Sci. (USA) 74, 2985-2988.
5. Cancro, M.P., W. Gerhard and N.R. Klinman (1978) J. Exp. Med. 147,776-787.
6. Gerhard, W. (1978) in Topics in Infectious Diseases, W.G. Laver, H. Bachmayer and R. Weil, eds, Springer-Verlag, 3,15-23.
7. Gerhard, W., C.M. Croce, D. Lopes and H. Koprowski (1978) Proc. Natl. Acad. Sci. (USA) 75, 1510-1514.
8. Gerhard, W., J. Yewdell, M.E. Frankel, D. Lopes, and L. Staudt. (1980, in press) in Monoclonal Antibodies, R. Kennett, and T. McKearn, eds, Plenum Press.
9. Frankel, M.E., and W. Gerhard. (1979) Molecular Immunology 16, 101-106.
10. Gerhard, W., and R.G. Webster (1978) J. Exp. Med. 148,383-392.
11. Atassi, M.Z. (1975) Immunochemistry, 12, 423-438.
12. Urbanshi, G.J. and E. Margoliash (1977) J. of Immunology, 110,1170-1180.
13. Van Regennoitel, M.H.V. (1967) Virology 31,467-480.
14. Jerne, N.K. (1960) Ann. Rev. Microbiology, 14, 341-358.
15. Yewdell, J., R.G. Webster and W. Gerhard (1979) Nature, 279,246-248.
16. Laver, W.G., G.M. Air, R.G. Webster, W. Gerhard, C.W. Ward and T.A.A. Dopheide (1979) Virology, 98,226-237.
17. Laver, W.G., W. Gerhard, R.G. Webster, M.E. Frankel and G.M. Air (1979) Proc. Natl. Acad. Sci. 76, 1425-1429.
18. Wrigley, N.G. (1979) Brit. Med. Bull. 35, 35-38.
19. Wrigley,N.G., W.G. Laver, and J.C. Downie (1977) J. Mol. Biol. 109, 405-421.

(See DISCUSSION on following page)

DISCUSSION

Atassi: Could your results be due to different affinity constants of your
  monoclonal antibodies?

Gerhard: I think it is unlikely. When we compare avidity, the ones we have
  looked at are similar.

Lai: Is the wet vs dry test a way to test for binding energy?

Gerhard: No it isn't. It is probably a reflection of accessibility of sites.

Ertl: Did you ever test your antibodies in a cellular immuno-assay and were
  there any differences to the solid phase assay?

Gerhard: Antibodies directed to antigenic site Y did not bind to virus-infected
  cells - all the others did.

Underwood: How many monoclonal antibodies did you use in the selection
  experiments, and what were your criteria for using those particular ones?

Gerhard: So far, we have used seven antibodies to select mutants, using in turn
  antibodies in which binding was not affected by the changes incuded by other
  antibodies.

Rott: Do any monoclonal antibodies have no HI activity but do neutralize virus?

Palese: We have something which is non-HI but neutralizing.

Underwood: How many of the variants could be distinguished by heterogeneous
  antisera?

Gerhard: In these variants, none.

ANTIGENIC DRIFT IN HONG KONG (H3N2) INFLUENZA VIRUSES:
SELECTION OF VARIANTS WITH POTENTIAL EPIDEMIOLOGICAL
SIGNIFICANCE USING MONOCLONAL ANTIBODIES.

ROBERT G. WEBSTER[+] AND WILLIAM G. LAVER[++]
[+]St. Jude Children's Research Hospital, P.O. Box 318, Memphis, Tennessee,
USA; [++]John Curtin School of Medical Research, Australian National
University, Canberra ACT 2601, Australia

INTRODUCTION

Antigenic drift in influenza A viruses is believed to occur by selection
of variants with altered hemagglutinin and neuraminidase molecules that are
imperfectly neutralized by the host's immune system.[1,2] Naturally occurring
antigenic variants of A/Hong Kong/1/68 (H3N2) influenza virus have multiple
changes in the amino acid sequence of the large polypeptide chain of the
hemagglutinin molecule (HA1); which of these changes is associated with
antigenic changes is not known.[3,4,5] Antigenic variants of A/Mem/1/71
(H3N2) influenza virus selected with monoclonal antibodies, on the other
hand, show single amino acid substitutions in the sequence of the HA1 polypeptide.[6] These changes in sequence must be responsible for the change in
antigenic reactivity; for the monoclonal antibodies used in the selection no
longer react with the altered hemagglutinin molecules.

Since none of the antigenic variants of influenza viruses thus far
selected with monoclonal antibodies in a single step procedure have been
shown to be distinguishable from wild-type virus with heterogeneous
antisera,[6,7] it is difficult to see how variants survive in nature. The
frequency of variants in cloned wild type virus with changes in a single
antigenic site on the hemagglutinin molecule is approximately 1 in 10^5 when
estimated with a single monoclonal antibody[6,8] and is 1 in 10^{10} when two
different monoclonal antibodies are used in combination. This suggests that
simultaneous multiple mutations occur with a low frequency and would be an
unlikely explanation for the many different antigenic variants detected
recently in field strains of H1N1 virus with monoclonal antibodies.[9]

The aims of the present studies were to determine the number of non-
overlapping antigenic determinants on the HA molecule and whether some
viruses with single point mutation in the HA gene have potential epidemiological significance. The results show that there are at least three non-
overlapping antigenic determinants on the HA molecule of A/Mem/1/71 (H3N2),

and that although many point mutants affected in antigenic areas of the molecule were isolated, only very few variants had changes that might have epidemiological potential.

MATERIALS AND METHODS

Viruses and serological assay

The recombinant influenza virus, A/Memphis/ 1/71 (H3) - Bel/42 (N1) - abbreviated to Mem-Bel - and naturally occurring variants of the Hong Kong (H3N2) subtype, identified in the text were grown in chick embryos and purified.[10] In addition, a series of antigenic variants of Mem-Bel were selected with monoclonal antibodies (see below). Hemagglutination (HA) titrations and hemagglutination-inhibition (HI) tests were done as described.[11]

Monoclonal antibodies

Hybrid cell lines forming antibodies to the HA of Mem-Bel were selected following fusion of myeloma cells P3/X-63-Ag8 with immune spleen cells according to the method of Kohler and Milstein.[12,13]

Selection of antigenic variants

The selection of single step antigenic variants was done as described.[14] Antigenic variants with multiple alterations were selected by growing the cloned single step antigenic variants in a second monoclonal antibody to a different antigenic site on the hemagglutinin molecule. The resulting antigenic variants were cloned twice at limit dilution and another antigenic variant was selected in the presence of a third monoclonal antibody; these viruses will be referred to as "sequential" variants. The antigenic variants were all given trivial names so that they could be identified easily in the text, and a "monoclonal" variant will be defined as an antigenic variant selected with monoclonal antibody.

Preparation of antibodies to specific antigenic sites on the hemagglutinin molecule by adsorption

Hyperimmune antisera to the isolated hemagglutinin of the antigenic variants were made in rabbits[15] and after adsorption with parental Mem-Bel virus all HI antibodies to the parental strain were removed. The remaining antibodies were specific for the antigenic variants.

RESULTS

Reactivity patterns of antigenic variants of Mem-Bel selected with monoclonal antibodies

Previous studies have shown that monoclonal variants of Mem-Bel have
single amino acid substitutions in the HA1 polypeptide[6] and that they failed
to react with the antibody used for the selection. A panel of monoclonal
antibodies to the hemagglutinin of Mem-Bel were tested by HI to determine if
their reactivities with the variants formed a pattern (Table 1). It is
apparent from Table 1 that the monoclonal antibodies fell into three groups
and that one monoclonal antibody (Mem 4/5) could not be grouped. It is also
apparent from Table 1 that variation at one site in the HA molecule can
occasionally cause an increased reactivity with a monoclonal antibody to a
different area of the molecule. Thus, an antigenic variant selected with
monoclonal antibody Mem 212/2 (Sue) reacts to higher titers with monoclone
H14/A2 than with the parental virus.

TABLE 1

REACTIVITY PATTERNS OF ANTIGENIC VARIANTS OF MEM/1/71-BEL SELECTED WITH
MONOCLONAL ANTIBODIES[a].

DIFFERENCES IN HI ANTIBODY TITERS BETWEEN WILD-TYPE VIRUS AND ANTIGENIC
VARIANTS (TRIVIAL NAME OF VARIANTS IN PARENTHESES)[b]

Group	Monoclonal antibodies	H14/A2 (Carol)	H14/A20 (Fred)	Mem 212/2 (Sue)	Mem 123/4 (Meg)	Mem 29/1 (Flo)	HK 30/2 (Ian)	Mem 200/2 (Fran)
I	H14/A2	<	+1.8	+3.6	0	0	0	-1.3
II	H14/A20	0	<	<	<	0	0	-2.3
	212/2	0	0	<	<	+1.2	+1.1	-3.0
	138/1	0	0	0	-2.5	0	0	0
III	196/5	0	0	0	0	<	-3.1	<
	181/3	0	0	0	0	<	0	<
?	4/5	0	0	0	0	0	0	-1.7

[a]Over thirty different monoclonal antibody preparations were used in this
study and only seven are illustrated in the table.
[b]Figures give the differences in HI titers between the homologous virus and
variants in $\log_2$ units.
< = HI titers of variants at least 32-fold less than homologous titer.
[c]Monoclonal antibody used for selection of variants.

The only discrepancy with the subdivision of monoclonal antibodies into three groups was found with a variant selected with monoclonal antibody 200/2 (Fran). This variant was inhibited by monoclonal antibodies in each of the three groups. The major differences in reactivity of Fran with the panel of monoclonal antibodies occurred in the group of variants that include Flo and Ian, but some differences were detected in the other two groups. This again suggests that substitution in one area of the molecule can influence the antigenicity in another area, presumably by effecting conformational changes.

These results suggest that there are at least three non-overlapping antigenic areas on the hemagglutinin molecule. An alternate explanation - from the results with Fran - that could be considered is that the groupings given above are artifacts and that the antigenic area is actually one region consisting of overlapping determinants.

Detailed analysis of antigenic variants of Mem/1/71 selected with monoclonal antibodies from group II

Since all the field strains of the H3N2 viruses studied to date have shown amino acid substitutions at residue 144 of the HA1 polypeptide,[5] additional antigenic variants were selected in this region of the molecule. Twelve antigenic variants selected with monoclonal antibodies from group II have been analyzed serologically. (Table 2).

The adsorbed sera clearly distinguished the variants designated Jack, Jill and Joe from Bob, Ann and Bev (Table 2). The HI antibody titer to Jack, Jill and Jim was 10-fold higher than to Bob, Ann and Bev. The other variants (Mary and Sue) could similarly be distinguished from each other. The adsorbed sera did not inhibit other variants (Meg and Fred) that showed amino acid substitutions in an adjacent region of the molecule. These results show that adsorbed sera could clearly distinguish between these "monoclonal" variants and the following paper by Laver et al., will show that these variants have a single amino acid substitution at residue 143.

Reaction of monoclonal variants with heterogeneous ferret and rabbit sera to the parental Mem/1/71 virus

Previous studies with antigenic variants of A/PR/8/34 (HON1) or Mem/1/71 (H3N2) selected with monoclonal antibodies have shown that none of the variants could be differentiated from wild-type virus with heterogeneous sera.[6,14] This suggests that single step mutants selected in this way would have no survival advantage in nature. We, therefore, examined the above series of antigenic variants in HI tests with post-infection ferret sera to

TABLE 2

ANTIGENIC ANALYSIS OF ANTIGENIC VARIANTS OF MEM-BEL SELECTED WITH MONOCLONAL
ANTIBODIES FROM GROUP II

Monoclonal Antibodies to MEM HA Used for Selection of Variants	Antigenic Variant (Trivial Name)		HI Antibody Titer with[a] Specific Antisera to "Jack"
None	Mem-Bel (Parent)		<10
H14/A20	V1	Fred	<10[b]
	V2	Bob	120[b]
	V3	Mary	450
Mem/212/2	V1	Ann	120
	V2	Ken	30
	V3	Sue	450
	V7	Joe	2,000
Mem 27/2	V5	Bev	120
	V9	Kay	50
Mem 123/4	V1	Jack	2,000
	V3	Jill	2,000
	V10	Meg	<10

[a]Antiserum to the isolated hemagglutinin molecule of Jack adsorbed with
Mem-Bel (see Materials and Methods).
[b]The figures give the reciprocal of the dilution inhibiting 3 out of 4 HA
units of virus.

determine if any of them could be distinguished from wild-type virus. The
only antigenic variant that could be distinguished in this way was Meg -
selected with monoclone Mem 123/4 - this variant gave 10-fold lower titers
with post-infection ferret serum than the parental virus (results not
shown). In addition, double immunodiffusion tests with hyperimmune rabbit
antisera to the isloated HA of Mem/1/71 showed a distinct spur between the
parental virus and the variant designated Meg, again indicating that this
variant can be differentiated from the parental virus with heterogeneous
antibodies.

Since this variant resulted from a single amino acid change from glycine
to aspartic acid at residue 144, we can conclude that some single amino acid
substitutions can produce variants that might have a selective advantage in
nature.

Selection of sequential antigenic variants with monoclonal antibodies

Antigenic variants with substitutions in each antigenic area on the HA molecule might be expected to show antigenic differences from the parental virus with heterogeneous antisera. Variants were, therefore, selected by sequential passage of virus in monoclonal antibodies to the three different areas of the HA molecule (Table 3).

TABLE 3

ANTIGENIC ANALYSIS OF ANTIGENIC VARIANTS OF MEM/1/71-BEL SELECTED SEQUEN-
TIALLY WITH MONOCLONAL ANTIBODIES

Sequential antigenic variants	HI antibody titers with the following monoclonal antibodies and ferret sera				Ferret anti-[b]
	H14/A2	H14/A21	H14/A20	Mem 4/5	HK/1/68
Mem/1/71	200	44,000	88,000	5,000	1,500
↓(H14/A2)[a]					
"Eric"	<10	40,000	93,000	5,000	1,600
↓(H14/A21)					
"Ray"	<10	<10	65,000	5,000	1,100
↓(H14/A20)					
"Wog"	<10	<10	<10	5,000	250
"Martha"	<10	<10	<10	5,000	150

[a]Monoclonal antibody used for selection (see Materials and Methods for details).
[b]Mean HI titers with 3 post-infection ferret sera.
The figures are the reciprocal of the dilution inhibiting 3 out of 4 HA units of virus.

After each sequential selection with a different monoclonal antibody, the resulting variants failed to react with the monoclone used in selection. The antigenic changes were additive and by the third sequential selection, antigenic differences were detected with monoclones to the three distinguishable areas of the HA molecule. The sequential variants still reacted with monoclone 4/5 showing that changes had not occurred in the area of the molecule recognized by this monoclonal antibody. Antigenic analysis of the sequential variants with post-infection ferret sera showed that after two sequential selections the variants could not be distinguished from the parent virus but that the third sequential variants (Wog and Martha, Table 3) had approximately 10-fold lower HI titers than the parent strain.

These data show that antigenic variants that are distinguishable from the parental virus with post-infection ferret sera can be selected sequentially with monoclonal antibodies, but it is not clear how heterogeneous antibodies would permit sequential selection of variants in nature.

Antigenic analysis of naturally occurring variants of H3N2 strains with monoclonal antibodies

Field strains of epidemiologically important H3N2 viruses were examined with monoclonal antibodies to determine if they also showed changes in the regions of the HA1 molecule arbitrarily defined by the monoclonal antibodies given in Table 1. The region of the molecule where antigenic variations first occurred in nature was in the area defined by the antibodies in group II (Table 4). Subsequent variations occurred in group III with the emergence of A/Port Chalmers/1/73 and Mem/102/72. The area of the HA1 molecule recognized by group I monoclonal antibodies was the most conserved, minor variants occurring in 1973 with the appearance of A/Port Chalmers/1/73, but significant variation did not occur until 1977 with the appearance of A/Texas/1/77. These serological findings are in accord with the sequence changes described in the naturally occurring variants of H3N2 viruses.[5] It is apparent from Table 4 that there were two antigenic variants of H3N2 viruses co-circulating in 1968; Hong Kong/1/68 being distinguishable from Aichi/2/68 in at least one of the reactivity groups.

TABLE 4

REACTIVITY PATTERNS OF MONOCLONAL ANTIBODIES TO A/MEM/1/71 HEMAGGLUTININ WITH NATURALLY OCCURRING H3N2 VARIANTS[a]

DIFFERENCES IN HI ANTIBODY TITERS WITH THE FOLLOWING VIRUSES

Reactivity Group	Monoclonal Antibody	Hong Kong/1/68	Aichi/2/68	Eng/878/69	Eng/187/70	Eng/42/72	Mem/102/72	P.C./1/73	Scot/840/74	Tx/1/77
I	H14/A2	0	0	0	0	0	0	-2.0	0	<
II	27/3	-3.5	0	<	<	-3.6	-3.6	<	<	<
	80/1	<	0	<	<	<	<	<	<	<
III	196/5	-1.6	0	0	-1.7	0	-2.9	<	<	<
	29/1	-1.4	0	0	-1.4	0	0	<	<	-3.1

[a]Over thirty monoclonal antibodies were used in this analysis and the results from only five are given.
[b]Figures give the differences in HI titers between the homologous virus (Mem/ 1/71) and the naturally occurring variants in $\log_2$ units.
< = HI titer of variants at least 32-fold less than homologous titer.

DISCUSSION

Preliminary reports suggested that there may be at least four non-overlapping areas[8] on the hemagglutinin molecule. The present studies show that monoclonal antibodies to the HA molecule of Mem/1/71 (H3N2) allow the identification of at least three antigenic areas on the hemagglutinin molecule. Changes at one antigenic site can influence the ability of antibody to combine at a second site, the antibodies to the second site can increase or decrease in reactivity. The difficulty with this kind of analysis is that the panel of monoclonal antibodies is incomplete and may not represent all antigenic determinants on the HA molecule so that there is a minimal number of non-overlapping determinants. An alternate explanation for these results is that the antigenic area on the hemagglutinin molecule is a continuum and is not subdivided.

None of the antigenic variants of influenza viruses selected previously with monoclonal antibodies could be distinguished with heterogeneous antisera,[6,14] suggesting that these variants would not have a selective advantage in nature. In the above studies at least one single step variant (Meg) could be distinguished from parental virus with post-infection ferret sera and with hyperimmune antisera to the parent hemagglutinin. This variant showed a single amino acid substitution of glycine to aspartic acid at residue 144 in the HA1 polypeptide (see Laver et al this volume). It is not known with certainty that this is the only substitution occurring in the HA1 molecule but it is significant that changes at residue 144 were also detected in field strains that became epidemiologically important.[5]

An alternative method of generating antigenic variants that could be distinguished from the parental strain with heterogeneous sera was by sequential selection. In the above studies, a variant (Wog or Martha) derived by three sequential passages in different monoclonal antibodies was distinguishable from parental virus with post-infection ferret sera. Whether sequential variants could be generated in nature is not known; it is possible that some people may have restricted antibody populations, especially at long intervals after infection with earlier variants when the antibody titers had declined.

At this time, it is not known where the changes in the HA1 polypeptide of the hemagglutinin are located in the three-dimensional structure of this molecule. The single amino acid substitution in variants selected with monoclonal antibody could occur in the antigenic sites or at residues remote from the site and induce conformational changes in the antigenic sites.[6]

Studies on chemical modifications of the substituted amino acids and x-ray crystallography may, in the future, answer these questions.

Studies on naturally occurring variants of the H3N2 subtype with monoclonal antibodies to Mem/1/71 show that there were two different antigenic variants co-circulating in 1968. A/Aichi/2/68 that was isolated from Japan in November, 1968[16] being distinguishable from the prototype virus isolated from Hong Kong in July, 1968.[17] It is possible that the Aichi/2/68 strain spread to USA and that the Hong Kong/1/68 strain spread to England, for the earliest variants from England are similar to the Hong Kong/1/68 strain.

SUMMARY

Monoclonal antibodies provided evidence for at least three antigenic areas on the hemagglutinin molecule of A/Mem/1/71 (H3N2) influenza virus. Antigenic analysis showed that most of the variants selected with monoclonal antibody could not be distinguished from parental viruses with heterogeneous sera, suggesting that they are probably epidemiologically irrelevant. One variant, however, could be distinguished from parental virus with heterogeneous sera and this variant had a change in the sequence at residue 144 of the HA1 polypeptide; from glycine in the parent to aspartic acid in the variant. Similar amino acid changes have been found in naturally occurring variants at this residue. These studies suggest that some amino acid substitutions are more important than others for producing viruses with epidemiological potential.

Antigenic analysis of naturally occurring H3N2 strains with monoclonal antibodies showed changes in the regions of the molecule arbitrarily defined by the monoclonal antibodies and established that two distinct variants co-circulated in 1968; Hong Kong/1/68 being distinguishable from Aichi/2/68 in at least two antigenic areas. It would appear that there may have been two separate lineages of H3N2 viruses, Hong Kong/1/68 giving rise to variants in England and Aichi/2/68 to variants in USA and Australia.

ACKNOWLEDGMENTS

This work was supported by Grants AI-15345 and AI-08831 from the National Institute of Allergy and Infectious Diseases, and by ALSAC.

REFERENCES
1. Dowdle, W.R., Coleman, M.T. and Gregg, M.B. (1974) Prog. Med. Virol. 17, 91-135.

2. Webster, R.G. and Laver, W.G. (1975) in The Influenza Viruses and Influenza, Kilbourne, E.D. ed., Academic Press, New York, pp. 269-314.

3. Ward, C.W. and Dopheide, T.A.A. (1979) Brit. Med. Bull. 35, 51-56.

4. Waterfield, M.D., Espelie, K., Elder, K. and Skehel, J.J. (1979) Brit. Med. Bull. 35, 57-63.

5. Laver, W.G., Air, G.M., Webster, R.G., Gerhard, W., Ward, C.W. and Dopheide, T.A.A. (1979) Proc. Royal Soc. (in press).

6. Laver, W.G., Air, G.M., Webster, R.G., Gerhard, W., Ward, C.M. and Dopheide, T.A.A. (1979) Virology 98, 226-237.

7. Gerhard, W. (1977) Top. Infect. Dis. 3, 15-24.

8. Yewdell, J.W., Webster, R.G. and Gerhard, W. (1979) Nature (London) 279, 246-248.

9. Webster, R.G., Kendal, A.P. and Gerhard, W. (1979) Virology 96, 258-264.

10. Laver, W.G. (1969) in Fundamental Techniques in Virology, Habel, K. and Salzman, N.P., eds., Academic Press, New York, pp. 82-86.

11. Fazekas de St. Groth, S. and Webster, R.G. (1966) J. Exp. Med. 124, 331-345.

12. Kohler, G. and Milstein, C. (1976) Eur. J. Immunol. 6, 511-519.

13. Koprowski, H., Gerhard, W. and Croce, C.M. (1977) Proc. Natl. Acad. Sci. USA 74, 2985-2988.

14. Gerhard, W. and Webster, R.G. (1978) J. Exp. Med. 148, 383-392.

15. Laver, W.G., Downie, J.C. and Webster, R.G. (1974) Virology 59, 230-244.

16. Fukumi, H. (1969) Bull. Wld. Hlth. Org. 41, 353-359.

17. Chang, W.K. (1969) Bull. Wld. Hlth. Org. 41, 349-351.

DISCUSSION

Krug: Does the residual activity after the successive passages mean there is another site?

Webster: That is very likely.

Salser: In the sequential variant was the last change the only one which was significant for the difference with heterogeneous antibody.

Webster: That's quite likely.

Salser: You chose ferret serum to discriminate the variants - would the variant showing a change have been detected using human antiserum?

Webster: The ferret is the most discriminatory; human would not be better. Rabbit also discriminated.

White: The data you and Walter have presented can be interpreted in another way: We can assume there is only one critical antigenic site consisting of, say, six amino acids. This site will elicit a whole series of monoclones binding with varying degrees of goodness of fit, affinity and avidity. If one amino acid is substituted, some monoclones will bind and some won't. In an extreme case, none of the monoclones will bind.

Webster: The data do not fit with this. Are you saying that there is only one antigenic site?

White: I'm saying we should keep an open mind. Perhaps all the amino acid substitutions you see are affecting only one site.

Webster: How many antigenic sites would Dr. Atassi expect on a molecule the size of the HA?

Atassi: It's hard to say. We know that one replacement within a site does not necessarily wipe it out.

Salser: It seems to be that your data is incompatible with Dr. White's theory.

THE ANTIGENIC SITES ON INFLUENZA VIRUS HEMAGGLUTININ. STUDIES ON THEIR
STRUCTURE AND VARIATION

W.G. LAVER[+], G.M. AIR[+], R.G. WEBSTER[++], W. GERHARD[*], C.W. WARD[**] AND
T.A. DOPHEIDE[**].
[+]Department of Microbiology, John Curtin School of Medical Research, P.O. Box
334, Canberra City; [++]St. Jude Children's Research Hospital, P.O. Box 318,
Memphis, Tennessee, U.S.A.; [*]The Wistar Institute, Thirty-sixth Street at
Spruce, Philadelphia, U.S.A.: [**]C.S.I.R.O., Division of Protein Chemistry, 343
Royal Parade, Parkville, Victoria.

SUMMARY

A number of changes in amino acid sequence occur in the hemagglutinin of
variants of Hong Kong (H3N2) influenza virus isolated between 1968 and 1977 but
it is not known which of these sequence changes are responsible for the
antigenic differences between these natural variants.

We have therefore looked for sequence changes in Hong Kong (H3N2) variants
selected with monoclonal hybridoma antibodies. These presumably recognize and
bind to a single antigenic site out of many on the hemagglutinin molecule.
Variants selected with a particular monoclonal antibody show such dramatic
changes in the site recognized by that antibody that no binding between the
antibody and the variant can be detected. 23 variants, selected with various
monoclonal antibodies, have so far been examined. In 17 of these, a single
change was found in the amino acid sequence of the large hemagglutinin
polypeptide HA1. In four variants a change was found, but this could not be
precisely located, and in the other two variants the changes probably occurred
in two large insoluble peptides we were unable to analyse.

In 10 of the monoclonal variants the proline at position 143 in HA1 had
changed to serine, threonine, leucine or histidine. For some reason we do not
understand, it did not change in any of the field strains we examined, although
in the latter, amino acids close to proline 143 changed.

We have raised antibody to the new antigenic site on one of the variants and
used this to select variants of this variant. We found that the amino acid
which had changed in this variant (proline to histidine) did not revert or
change again in the second generation variants. Instead, in three of these, a
neighbouring glycine residue changed to aspartic acid.

Chemical modification of hemagglutinin molecules suggests that the amino
acids which changed in the monoclonal variants were not located in the
antigenic sites, but that the sequence changes occurred somewhere else in the
HA molecule and induced conformational changes which altered the sites.

INTRODUCTION

Antigenic variation in the hemagglutinin "spikes" of influenza virus is a major obstacle to the development of an effective vaccine against influenza. This variation is of two kinds, slow gradual antigenic drift, and sudden major antigenic shifts, which seem to occur by entirely different molecular mechanisms; for review see Webster and Laver, 1975[1]. This article will consider the mechanism of drift.

Antigenic drift is thought to be due to the selection, by an immune population, of mutant virus particles with altered antigenic determinants which possess a growth advantage in the presence of antibody.

The aim of the present work is to establish 1) the number of different antigenic sites on the hemagglutinin 2) the chemical structure of these sites and 3) the way in which the sites change during antigenic drift.

We have attempted to answer these questions be determining the changes occurring in the amino acid sequence of the hemagglutinin polypeptide during natural antigenic drift and in antigenic variants selected in vitro with monoclonal, hybridoma antibodies.

We have also examined the effect of chemical modification of amino acids in the hemagglutinin molecule on its antigenic activity.

RESULTS

Amino acid sequence changes in the hemagglutinin of natural variants (field strains) of A/Hong Kong (H3N2) influenza virus isolated between 1968 and 1977.

The following Hong Kong (H3N2) variants were examined: A/Aichi/2/68, A/England/878/69, A/England/187/70, A/Memphis/1/71, A/England/42/72, A/Memphis/102/72, A/Port Chalmers/1/73, A/Victoria/1/75 and A/Texas/1/77. These viruses were obtained from W.H.O. reference laboratories with the exception of the Memphis strains which were local isolates. The viruses were grown as recombinants with the neuraminidase from A/Bel/42 (HON1) and were cloned twice at limit dilution before analysis.

We have examined the hemagglutinins of these nine Hong Kong variants for amino acid sequence changes, by matching the compositions of their soluble tryptic peptides with the known amino acid sequence of the homologous peptides from the Hong Kong variant, A/Memphis/102/72 (Ward and Dopheide, this volume). Techniques for growth and purification of the viruses, isolation of the hemagglutinin molecules, separation of the HA1 and HA2 polypeptides, mapping of the soluble tryptic peptides and amino acid analysis have been described[2]. The results (Fig. 1) showed that at least 18 changes in amino acid sequence, 9 of which were located precisely, occurred in the soluble tryptic peptides of the large hemagglutinin polypeptide (HA1) of A/Hong Kong/68 (H3N2) influenza virus between 1968 and 1977 (Laver et al., in press). These peptides contained 262 residues (82% of the total HA1 sequence). In HA2, only two changes in 129 residues (58% of the total sequence of HA2) were detected. Sequential changes at a particular locus were not found; and as far as we can tell, once an amino acid changed, it did not change again in any subsequent variant examined. However, it is likely that some of these sequence changes are unrelated to the antigenic differences between the hemagglutinins, and this analysis of natural variants may not reflect the differences in antigenic determinants on the hemagglutinin molecule. By using monoclonal antibodies, we have been able to select and analyse variant viruses in which the changes in sequence of the hemagglutinin polypeptides have a better chance of being restricted to those affecting the determinant recognized by that particular monoclonal antibody, changing it in such a way that it can no longer "fit" the corresponding combining site on the antibody.

Sequence changes in the hemagglutinin polypeptides of Mem/71 variants selected with monoclonal hybridoma antibodies.

We have examined variants of Hong Kong virus (the A/Mem/1/71 strain was used) selected with monoclonal antibodies and determined the differences in amino acid sequence associated with the altered capacity of the hemagglutinin to combine with antibody. Preparation of these variants and their antigenic properties are described (Webster et al., this volume).

8 different monoclonal antibodies designated Mem/29/1, HK 30/2, H14/A2, H14/A21, H14/A20, Mem/212/1, Mem/27/2 and Mem/123/4 were used to select a total of 23 antigenic variants of Mem/71 virus. The hemagglutinin molecules were isolated from the variant viruses, the HA1 and HA2 polypeptides were separated and the HA1 polypeptides were examined for sequence changes by amino acid analysis. Changes in sequence of peptides from the antigenic variants could, in most cases, be deduced from composition data. In those cases in which this method gave ambiguous results, the peptide was sequenced directly.

The dramatic change in antigenic activity of the variants which enabled them to escape neutralization by the antibody used for their selection was, in most cases, found to be associated with a single change in sequence of the large polypeptide (HA1) of their hemagglutinin "spikes". The 17 variants in which the sequence change could be located precisely are listed in Table 1. Of the other 6 variants two (selected with H14/A21 antibody) showed a change in peptide 23 (residues 217-224), two (selected with HK 31/2 antibody) showed a change in peptide 4 (residues 157-201) and two showed no change at all in the soluble tryptic peptides. In these last two (selected with Mem 29/1 antibody) the change may have occurred in the two insoluble peptides (residues 110-140 and 230-255) we were unable to analyse.

Preparation of antibodies against the new antigenic determinants on the variants.

Attempts were made to raise antibody against the new antigenic sites on the hemagglutinin molecules from three of the variant viruses. We hoped to use this antibody to select second generation variants to see whether the amino acid which changed in the first selection changed again in the second selection.

The variants chosen were one of the four variants selected with H14/A2 monoclonal antibody, where the asparagine residue at position 54 in HA1 changed to lysine, the variant selected with H14/A21 monoclonal antibody where the serine at position 205 in HA1 changed to tyrosine, and the variant selected with Mem 123/4 antibody where the proline at position 143 in HA1 changed to histidine (Table 1). We thought it would be difficult to prepare monoclonal hybridoma antibodies which bound to the new site but which would not bind to any site on the wild-type hemagglutinin and we therefore instead immunized rabbits with the hemagglutinin molecules from each of these three groups of variants. The hyperimmune sera were then absorbed with purified concentrated wild-type virus until the hemagglutinin-inhibition titers of the sera for the wild-type virus reached undetectable levels. The absorbed sera were then tested, in HI tests, against the variant viruses.

The results showed that when sera raised against the variants selected with H14/A2 and H14/A21 monoclonal antibodies (where the sequence changes were asparagine 54 to lysine and serine 205 to tyrosine respectively) were absorbed with wild-type Mem/71 virus, no HI activity to the variants remained after total removal of all HI activity to the wild-type virus.

On the other hand, when sera raised against variants selected with Mem 123/4 monoclonal antibody was absorbed with wild-type Mem/71 virus, high levels of HI activity to the variant remained after all HI activity to the wild-type virus had been removed. This antibody to the variant was not removed after repeated absorption of the serum with wild-type virus. Variant 1 had a sequence change in HA1 of proline 143 to histidine and the antibody left after absorption was presumable directed against the single "new" antigenic site which formed on the hemagglutinin molecule as a result of this change in sequence. In this respect it behaved like monoclonal antibody.

Selection of second generation variants.

The antibody prepared against the new antigenic site on the proline 143 to histidine variant (Table 1) was used to select three further variants of this variant in the same way as described for the initial selection of variants with monoclonal antibodies.

The hemagglutinin molecules from the second generation variants were then examined for changes in amino acid sequence. None of the three second generation variants selected with the antibody prepared against the new antigenic site on the hemagglutinin had a sequence change which involved the "new" histidine residue at position 143. Instead, each of the variants showed a single sequence change of glycine to aspartic acid in peptide 17 of HA1. This peptide contains three glycine residues at positions 142, 144 and 146 (Fig. 1) and sequence determination on one of the variants showed that it was the glycine at position 144 which changed to aspartic acid.

Chemical modification of the hemagglutinin.

Hemagglutinin molecules from some of the variants were reacted with 1-fluoro 2-4-dinitrobenzene, tetranitromethane or diazotized sulphanilic acid.

The variants chosen were those in which the change in sequence associated with the appearance of a new antigenic site on the hemagglutinin was to an amino acid capable of reacting with one of these reagents to form a stable derivative. They were the variants selected with H14/A2 monoclonal antibody, where the asparagine at position 54 in HA1 was replaced by lysine, the variant selected with H14/A21 monoclonal antibody where the serine at position 105 changed to tyrosine and the variant selected with Mem/123/4 monoclonal antibody in which the proline at position 143 in HA1 was replaced by histidine. We thought that if these new amino acids formed part of the new antigenic sites they should be accessible and capable not only of binding antibody but also able to react with the small organic reagents. Furthermore, if these amino acids did form part of the antigenic site, their chemical modification should interfere with the binding of antibody directed against the new site.

Reactions with 1-fluoro 2-4-dinitrobenzene (FDNB)

When purified influenza virus particles were treated with FDNB, DNP-substituted hemagglutinin molecules could be isolated and the DNP-substituted HA1 and HA2 polypeptide separated and peptide mapped in the same way as the unreacted virus particles. The FDNB-treated HA of H14/A2 variant 1, reacted with FDNB at pH 8.4 and 37°C for 1½ hr, was unaltered in HA activity and, as far as we could tell, in antigenic properties. Under these conditions, the "new" lysine residue at position 54 did not react to form a DNP derivative, although other lysine residues in the molecule reacted to some extent and the lysine at position 307 was completely converted to ε-DNP lysine.

When the reaction with FDNB was done under more drastic conditions at pH 9 for 3-4 hrs at $37^{\circ}C$, approximately 47% of the total lysine in HA1 was converted to ε-DNP-lysine. About 60% of the "new" lysine residue at position 54 was converted to ε-DNP-lysine and lysine residues 290, 307 and 310 reacted 100%. Lysine residues which apparently did not react at all were at positions 92, 259, 264 and 326.

Reaction with tetranitromethane (TNM)

TNM specifically nitrates tyrosine residues at pH 8.0^{3}. Therefore hemagglutinin molecules from H14/A21 variant 1, which showed a sequence change at position 205 in HA1 of serine to tyrosine, were treated with TNM for 3-4 hrs at pH 8 and 25°. Since it was difficult to isolate the HA from TNM-treated virus, isolated hemagglutinin molecules were treated with TNM. The TNM-treated HA was unaltered in HA activity and, as far as we could tell, in antigenic properties.

Of the 10 tyrosine residues in the soluble tryptic peptides which we were able to examine, those at positions 161, 178, 195, 257, 205 and 302 did not react at all with tetranitromethane. The tyrosine at position 308 reacted completely and of the three tyrosines in peptide 7 (at positions 98, 100 and 105) one reacted completely and the other two not at all, or else each had been partly substituted. Sequencing of this peptide from TNM-treated HA has not been done.

The "new" tyrosine (position 205) in this variant HA did not react at all.

Reaction with diazotized sulphanilic acid.

Diazotized sulphanilic acid couples to histidine and tyrosine. Hemagglutinin molecules isolated from the variant selected with H14/A21 monoclonal antibody which had a change at position 143 in HA1 of proline to histidine were reacted with diazotized sulphanilic acid for 3-4 hr at 0°. Excess reagent remained of the end of the reaction.

Following reaction with diazotized sulphanilic acid, hemagglutinin activity disappeared completely, but the antigenic properties of the hemagglutinin (as measured in immuno-diffusion tests) did not differ from those of the untreated hemagglutinin. The HA1 and HA2 polypeptides were separated and their tryptic peptides were mapped and analysed. The "new" histidine at position 143 reacted 100% with diazotized sulphanilic acid under the conditions used. The two histidine residues at positions 183 and 184, and the histidine at position 56, did not react at all.

The tyrosine residues at positions 161, 178, 195, 257 and 302, which did not react with tetranitromethane, also did not react with diazotized sulphanilic acid under the conditions used. Of the three tyrosines in peptide 7 (at positions 98, 100 and 105), either one reacted 100% or each of the three reacted approximately 30%, as in the results with tetranitromethane. The tyrosine at position 308 did not react at all with diazotized sulphanilic acid under the conditions used. This was a surprise finding, because this tyrosine reacted 100% with tetranitromethane.

DISCUSSION

We have found that variants of A/Hong Kong/68 (H3N2) influenza virus selected with various monoclonal hybridoma antibodies show single changes in the amino acid sequence of the HA1 polypeptide.

These single sequence changes caused such a dramatic change in the antigenic site on the hemagglutinin, recognized by the particular monoclonal antibody used to select the variant, that no binding between the two occurred. Some variants selected with the same monoclonal antibody showed different sequence changes and some variants selected with different monoclonal antibodies showed the same sequence change.

Several variants showed a change in the proline residue at position 143 in HA1. In different variants, this proline changed to serine, threonine, leucine or histidine. These changes are all possible from single nucleotide changes in the RNA. The other two possible single nucleotide changes (proline to alanine or arginine) have not yet been found .

For some reason which we do not understand, the proline at position 143 in HA1 did not change in any of the natural variants of Hong Kong virus (field strains) isolated between 1968 and 1977. In the field strains, residues close to the proline at position 143 changed.

A possible explanation for this may be that substitution of the proline residue at position 143 in HA1 did not alter the antigenic properties of the hemagglutinin to such an extent that the variants resulting from the change were able to escape neutralization by the heterogeneous antisera in immune individuals. The first antigenic variant of Hong Kong influenza virus to appear in man (A/England/878/69)[4] showed a change of glycine to aspartic acid at position 144 in HA1. One monoclonal variant also showed a change in residue 144 of glycine to aspartic acid. This monoclonal variant differs antigenically from Eng/878/69 virus (Fig. 2), therefore, other sequence changes must have occurred in Eng/878/69 which are not in the soluble peptides and which therefore we so far have been unable to locate.

The change at position 144 of glycine to aspartic acid did, however, change the antigenic properties of the hemagglutinin to such an extent that this variant could be distinguished from the wild-type with heterogeneous antisera in immunodiffusion tests (Fig. 2) and in HI tests. Most of the other monoclonal variants showing single sequence changes could not be distinguished from wild-type virus using heterogeneous antisera, suggesting that some changes in sequence are much more influential in causing antigenic drift than others.

We do not know whether the amino acids which changed in the variants were located within the antigenic site recognized by the monoclonal antibody used to select that particular variant or if the sequence changes occurred in some region of the HA molecule remote from the antigenic site, changing the site by changing the conformation of the hemagglutinin.

We found that when one of the variants selected with H14/A2 monoclonal antibody (showing a change at position 54 in HA1 of asparagine to lysine) was treated with 2-4-dinitro fluoro benzene, the new lysine at position 54 reacted to form DNP derivative, but much more slowly than other lysine residues in the molecule. Treatment of the variant selected with H14/A21 monoclonal antibody (with a sequence change at position 205 of serine to tyrosine) with tetranitromethane did not lead to any nitration of the new tyrosine residue although some other tyrosine residues in the HA1 polypeptide were 100% nitrated by this reagent.

We are not sure at the moment of the significance of these findings. It would seem reasonable to assume that if a particular amino acid is accessible to antibody, then it would also be accessible to small reagents. However, the type of reagent may profoundly affect this "accessibility", as evidenced by the tyrosine at position 308 of HA1, which reacted 100% with tetranitromethane but not at all with diazotized sulphanilic acid. Hence a residue capable of reacting with some reagents (including antibody) may not react with others. However, the results may mean that the amino acids which changed in the variants were not located in the antigenic sites. Further support for this conclusion comes from the finding that while the new histidine at position 143 in the variant selected with Mem/123/4 monoclonal antibody, did react with diazotized sulphanilic acid, the substituted HA molecule still bound antibody prepared against the new antigenic site. It is hard to imagine how this histidine could be directly involved in antibody binding when such drastic substitution has so little effect.

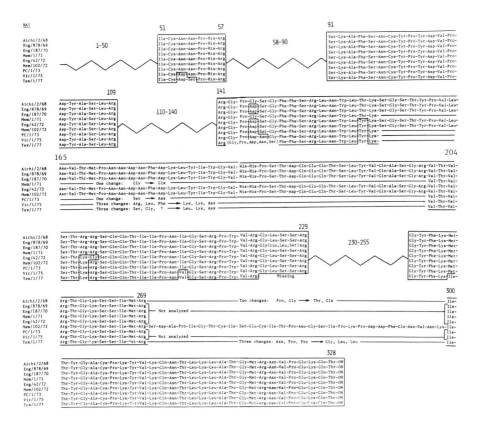

Fig. 1. Comparative partial amino acid sequences of the hemagglutinin heavy chains (HA1) from nine different Hong Kong influenza A variants isolated between 1968-1977. The amino acid sequences were determined for the A/Memphis/102/72 strain (Ward & Dopheide, this volume). Sequences for the other strains were deduced from the amino acid composition of their tryptic peptides. Boxed areas indicate regions of identical sequence and the residues which changed are indicated. It is not known which of the two GLY residues of Vic/75 peptide 17 changed to SER in TEXAS/77, nor how one of the two SER residues in AICHI/68 peptide 25 changed to GLN in ENG/187/70. The four zig-zag lines denote regions of sequence associated with two large soluble tryptic were not reliably analysed by single hydrolysis and with two large insoluble tryptic peptides which we were unable to separate and analyse.

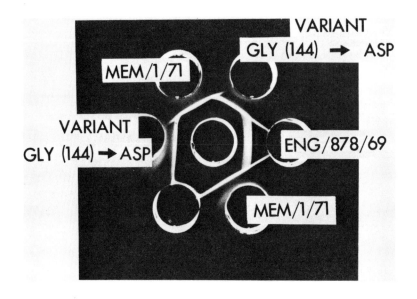

Fig. 2. Double immunodiffusion test showing cross-reactions between hemagglutinin molecules from wild-type A/Mem/1/71 virus, variant 10 selected with Mem 123/4 monoclonal antibody (which showed a change of glycine to aspartic acid at position 144 in HA1) and the first antigenic variant of Hong Kong virus to be isolated from man (A/Eng/878/69) which also showed a change of glycine to aspartic acid at position 144 in HA1.

Virus particles disrupted with SDS are in the peripheral wells and hyperimmune rabbit antiserum to isolated Mem/1/71 hemagglutinin is in the center.

TABLE 1

SEQUENCE CHANGES FOUND IN THE HA1 POLYPEPTIDE FROM ANTIGENIC VARIANTS OF
A/MEMPHIS/1/71 VIRUS SELECTED WITH THE MONOCLONAL ANTIBODIES LISTED.

Monoclonal Antibody	Variant	Sequence Change[1]
H14/A2	V1	Asparagine (54) → Lysine
	V2	Asparagine (54) → Lysine
	V3	Asparagine (54) → Lysine
	V4	Asparagine (54) → Lysine
H14/A21	V1	Serine (205) → Tyrosine
H14/A20	V1	Asparagine (133) → Lysine
	V2	Proline (143) → Serine
	V3	Proline (143) → Leucine
Mem/212/1	V1	Proline (143) → Serine
	V2	Proline (143) → Threonine
	V3	Proline (143) → Leucine
	V7	Proline (143) → Histidine
Mem 27/2	V5	Proline (143) → Serine
	V9	Proline (143) → Threonine
Mem 123/4	V1	Proline (143) → Histidine
	V3	Proline (143) → Histidine
	V10	Glycine (144) → Aspartic acid

(1) Numbers in brackets give the position of the amino acid in HA1.

ACKNOWLEDGEMENTS

Jean Clark, Donna Cameron, Sally Campbell and Martha Sugg provided excellent technical assistance. This collaborative project was greatly helped by international direct dialling telephone facilities provided by the Australian Overseas Telecommunications Commission. This work was supported in part by grants AI-15343 and AI-08831 from the National Institute of Allergy and Infectious Diseases, and by ALSAC.

REFERENCES

1. Webster, R.G. and Laver, W.G. (1975) in The Influenza Viruses and Influenza, Kilbourne, E.D. ed., Academic, New York, pp. 269-314.
2. Laver, W.G., Air, G.M., Webster, R.G., Gerhard, W., Ward, C.W. and Dopheide, T.A. (1979) Virology, 98, 226-237.
3. Sokolovsky, M., Riordan, J.F. and Vallee, B.L. (1976) Biochemistry, 5, 3582-3588.
4. Periera, M.S. and Schild, G.C. (1971) J. Hyg. Camb. 69, 99-103.

DISCUSSION

Salser: Have you found any changes in HA2?

Laver: We looked in a number of variants and never found any change in HA2, so we gave up looking.

Sambrook: Is the new site more antigenic?

Laver: When antisera to variants with the Asn (54) to Lys change, or the Ser (205) to Tyr change were absorbed with wild-type virus, no antibody was left. However, when antisera to the variant with the change PRO (143) to HIS were absorbed with wild-type virus (until all antibody to the wild-type was removed) antibody to the new antigenic site on the variant remained; so it is quite clear that some regions of the molecule are much more immunogenic than others.

White: Is it possible to modify lysines and thus protect unglycosylated HA against proteolysis for vaccine use?

Laver: We don't know that carbohydrate does block proteolysis.

White: Non-glycosylated HA is not as immunogenic and there is a lot of evidence that carbohydrate does protect.

Klenk: The proteolysis is strain-dependent. Some strains are completely resistant, in the non-glycosylated form, others are readily degraded.

Salser: Regarding the change in the field strains at position 155 in HA1 of Thr → Tyr (which requires two nucleotide changes) double base changes have been found rather frequently in the β-galactosidase repressor gene, which is surprising.

ANTIGENIC AND IMMUNOGENIC PROPERTIES OF INFLUENZA VIRUS
HEMAGGLUTININ FRAGMENTS

D.C. JACKSON[+], L.E. BROWN[+], R.J. RUSSELL[+], D.O. WHITE[+], T.A. DOPHEIDE[++]
AND C.W. WARD[++]
[+]Department of Microbiology, University of Melbourne, Parkville, Victoria, 3052,
Australia; [++]C.S.I.R.O., Division of Protein Chemistry, Royal Parade, Parkville,
Victoria, 3052, Australia.

The molecular basis of protein antigenicity and immunogenicity can be
investigated in two ways. One method involves a comparison of the antigenic,
and the immunogenic properties of chemically modified or naturally occurring
variants of the molecule. Changes in amino acid sequences arising through
mutation or chemical modification of specific residues would be expected to
modify the structure and therefore effect a change in the molecule's
immunological properties. Examination of the differences in properties and
amino acid sequences between such homologous proteins may be made allowing
correlation of an immunological property with a particular structural feature.
However, caution is required when interpreting results obtained in this way,
as changes in antigenicity or immunogenicity may result indirectly from amino
acid substitutions in areas of the molecule quite remote from any antigenic
determinant.

The second method involves the examination of fragments of the molecule for
their ability to bind to antibodies directed against the native protein and to
elicit antibodies capable of interacting with the parent molecule. The
limitation of this approach is that some fragments may not retain sufficient of
their original conformation to be representative of the region of the intact
molecule from which they were derived. Nevertheless, it is a simple and direct
way of discovering which part(s) of the molecule carry antigenic and immunogenic
activity.

The influenza virus hemagglutinin lends itself to both approaches because a
range of hemagglutinins are available from the large number of subtypes and
strains that exist. The sequence data, now available for several different
strains, is beginning to make possible a study, at the level of primary protein
structure, of the mechanisms underlying antigenic shift and drift.

Here, we describe the results of experiments in which the hemagglutinin (HA)
molecule of influenza A/Memphis/102/72 (H3) is cleaved by cyanogen bromide at
methionine residues and the resulting fragments examined for their antigenic
and immunogenic properties.

Hemagglutinin and its fragments. Purified HA obtained from the virus
influenza A/Memphis/102/72 (H3) - A/Bel/42 (N1), hereafter called Mem_H-Bel_N,
was incubated for 16 hr. with cyanogen bromide in 100 fold molar excess over
the number of methionine residues present[1]. The digest was fractionated[2] on a
column of Sephadex G-100 in 50% formic acid (Fig. 1a). Dansyl end-group
determinations and amino acid analyses were used to identify the components
of each peak.

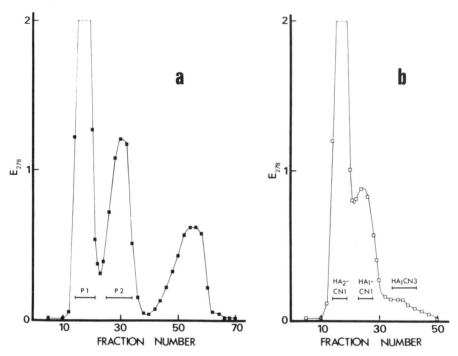

Fig. 1. Elution profile of cyanogen bromide fragments of influenza viral
hemagglutinin from Sephadex G-100. (a) Hemagglutinin was cleaved with
cyanogen bromide and introduced to a column (0.9 cm x 120 cm) of Sephadex
G-100 in 50% formic acid. Flow rate was 4.6 ml/hr and 30 min. fractions
collected. (b) Cyanogen bromide fraction P1 was reduced under nitrogen with
dithiothreitol and fractionated on G-100 as described above. (Modified from
Jackson et al. 1979, Virology 93, 458-465 with permission).

Fraction P1, which was eluted in the void volume, contained the following
cyanogen bromide polypeptides linked together by disulphide bridges: CN1
derived from the N-terminal end of the heavy chain (HA_1); CN3 also derived
from HA_1 and CN1 derived from the C-terminal end of the light chain (HA_2).
These polypeptides are designated HA_1CN1, HA_1CN3 and HA_2CN1 respectively.
Fraction P2 contained the 92-residue cyanogen bromide polypeptide CN2 from

HA$_1$ and the 98-residue polypeptide CN2 from HA$_2$ designated HA$_1$CN2 and HA$_2$CN2 respectively. Fractions 45-62 contained the two octapeptides from HA$_1$ and the seventeen and eighteen-residue peptides from HA$_2$. These peptides, HA$_1$CN4, HA$_1$CN5, HA$_2$CN4 and HA$_2$CN3 respectively, were separated from each other by high voltage paper electrophoresis.

The components of P1 were separated by reduction with dithiothreitol under denaturing conditions followed by gel filtration (Fig. 1b). Amino acid analyses and dansyl end-group determinations of the eluted species confirmed the identity of each peak; HA$_2$CN1 is eluted in the void volume reflecting its highly aggregated state, followed by HA$_1$CN1 and HA$_1$CN3. Each of these three polypeptide fragments was desalted over Sephadex G-25, diluted into nitrogen-saturated water and treated with diiodoethane to effect reformation of S-S bonds. The polypeptide fragment HA$_2$CN1 is extremely hydrophobic and insoluble and consequently not suitable for study in aqueous solution.

The heavy chain was isolated from purified HA according to the method of Laver[3] and digested with cyanogen bromide as described above. This preparation was not reduced and alkylated before cleavage with cyanogen bromide consequently the polypeptides obtained in this way are assumed to be in their oxidised form and are referred to as HA$_1$Pox.

A schematic representation of the hemagglutinin monomer of A/Memphis/102/72 and its cyanogen bromide cleavage products is shown in Figure 2.

Preparation of Antisera. Rabbits were inoculated intramuscularly and subcutaneously with purified virus or with HA fragments emulsified in Freund's complete adjuvant as previously described[4]. Immunoglobulin G was isolated from pre-immune and immune sera by affinity chromatography on protein A-Sepharose.

Animals inoculated with influenza virus grown in hen's eggs develop antibodies directed against the carbohydrate moiety of the hemagglutinin molecule[5]. To allow a study of the antigenic structure of the polypeptide portion of the molecule, these anti-carbohydrate antibodies must be removed. Because the carbohydrate moiety of viral glycoproteins is characteristic of the host cell-type in which the virus is propagated[6,7] adsorption of antisera with purified virus of an unrelated strain, but grown in hen's eggs, allows removal of anti-carbohydrate activity. In some cases, therefore, IgG preparations were adsorbed with A/Shearwater/E.Aust./1/72 (Hav 6)-A/Bel/42 (N1) virus, hereafter referred to as Shearwater$_H$-Bel$_N$. Antibodies directed against *polypeptide* determinants are not removed because H3 and Hav6 subtypes do not share any

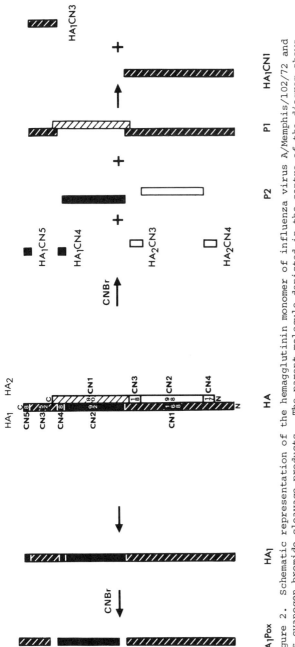

Figure 2. Schematic representation of the hemagglutinin monomer of influenza virus A/Memphis/102/72 and its cyanogen bromide cleavage products. The parent molecule depicted in the centre of the diagram shows the order within the HA_1 and HA_2 chains, of the fragments obtained by CNBr cleavage. The fragments are numbered in decreasing order of size, and the number of amino acid residues in each peptide is given, e.g. peptide CN3 derived from HA_1 (HA_1CN3) contains 52 amino acid residues. The HA_1 and fragments derived from it are represented by solid bars; HA_2 and its fragments by open bars. The orientation of the N- and C-terminal ends of the two chains with respect to one another is unknown. Cross-hatching indicates fragments containing carbohydrate side chains. These fragments also contain half-cystine residues which interconnect the light and heavy chains. Cyanogen bromide cleavage of separated HA_1 yields a mixture of the three major fragments in oxidized form (HA_1Pox), the two octapeptides being lost during dialysis. Cleavage of the whole HA monomer gives rise to three preparations. P2 is a mixture of HA_1CN2 and HA_2CN1. P1 is the disulphide-linked complex of HA_1CN1, HA_1CN3 and HA_2CN1, which can be reduced and reoxidized to yield HA_1CN1 and HA_1CN3 in soluble form. The two octapeptides from HA_2 (HA_1CN4, HA_1CN5, HA_2CN4 and HA_2CN3 respectively) are eluted together from G-100. They were subsequently separated by high voltage paper electrophoresis. (Modified from Jackson et al. (1979) J. Immunol. 123 with permission).

known determinants although the possibility cannot be dismissed that there are common determinants yet to be described.

Detection of antigenic activity. The position of antigenic determinants within intact proteins can be defined by examining the ability of fragments of the antigen to inhibit the reaction of the native protein with homologous antibody[8]. This approach was used in the present study but attempts to employ intact HA were unsuccessful due to its limited solubility. This problem was overcome by covalently coupling HA to activated Sepharose 4B and measuring the binding of radiolabeled IgG to this solid phase immunosorbent[9]. The method is simple, sensitive and specific. The interaction of antibody with immobilised HA can be inhibited by 70% with HA_1 (Table 1). These results indicate that the hemagglutinin heavy chain contains substantial antigenic activity, a finding consistent with previous reports[10,11].

TABLE 1

INHIBITION OF BINDING OF RADIOLABELED ANTI-MEM$_H$ IgG to SEPHAROSE-HA USING INTACT AND MODIFIED HA_1

Inhibitor	Percentage Inhibition of Binding	
	250 pmoles inhibitor	125 pmoles inhibitor
HA_1	72[a]	70
Reduced and alkylated HA_1	0	1
CNBr cleaved HA_1	5	0
CNBr cleaved, reduced and alkylated HA_1	0	2

[a]Results are expressed as the percentage inhibition of binding of anti-Mem$_H$ IgG to 2.5 pmoles A/Mem/102/72 HA covalently coupled to Sepharose. Anti-Mem$_H$ IgG was obtained from anti-(Mem$_H$-Bel$_N$) IgG by adsorption with Shearwater$_H$-Bel$_N$ virus. (Reproduced from Jackson et al. Virology 89, 199, with permission).

In contrast to the results with intact HA_1, neither reduced and alkylated HA_1 nor HA_1 cleaved with cyanogen bromide were able, even when present in a large molar excess, to inhibit the reaction between intact HA and labeled antibody. These results indicated that destruction of intrachain disulphide bonds by carboxyamidomethylation or cleavage of peptide bonds at methionine residues causes sufficient change in the conformation of antigenically active regions of the polypeptide either to prevent their interaction with antibody or to reduce their affinity of binding to the extent that it is not observed in a competitive inhibition assay. For this reason a *direct* binding assay was developed to test the ability of HA fragments to bind to antibody in the absence of competing HA.

Protein A from *Staphylococcus aureus,* which binds the Fc piece of IgG, lends itself to the isolation of IgG-antigen complexes in direct binding assays. These were carried out by incubation of radiolabeled fragments with antibody followed by addition of protein A covalently bound to Sepharose beads. After washing, any antigen-antibody complexes formed can be assayed by determining the radioactivity associated with the protein A-Sepharose[4].

Using this method reduced and alkylated HA_1 bound antibody to the same extent as unmodified HA_1, and heavy chain cleaved with cyanogen bromide was also appreciably antigenic[9]. These results demonstrated that the preparations had indeed retained sufficient conformational integrity to be bound by antibody or that the antibody was able to *induce* the necessary conformation for binding[8]. In the case of reduced and alkylated cyanogen bromide peptides derived from HA_1, little or no antigenic activity was detected, indicating that the disulphide bridges which link at least two of the five fragments derived from HA_1 (Dopheide and Ward, this volume) are necessary for the retention of conformational stability and hence antigenicity of HA_1 once this polypeptide has been cleaved at methionine residues. The fact that carboxyamidomethylated cyanogen bromide fragments are not bound by anti-viral antibody previously adsorbed with $Shearwater_H$-Bel_N provides additional evidence that anti-carbohydrate antibodies are satisfactorily removed by this adsorption protocol.

Antigenic activity of hemagglutinin fragments. A comparison of the ability of various radiolabeled fragments of Mem HA to react with IgG is shown in Table 2. All of the preparations which contain the HA_1CN1 region and only these, are capable of binding to anti-viral antibody even in the presence of host antigen or following adsorption of the IgG with heterologous virus to remove antibodies against the carbohydrate side chains on HA. The binding of HA_1 of A/Bel/42 (HON1) is abrogated by either of these procedures and is therefore mediated by interaction of anti-"host-antigen" antibodies with the carbohydrate side chains of HA_1. The polypeptide common to all of the antigenically active fragments of Mem HA is the cyanogen bromide peptide HA_1CN1 indicating that antigenic activity of Mem HA resides in the N-terminal 168 amino acid residues of hemagglutinin heavy chain.

TABLE 2

ANTIGENIC PROPERTIES OF HEMAGGLUTININ FRAGMENTS

Radiolabeled Fragment[a]	IgG			
	Anti-(Mem_H-Bel_N)	Anti-Mem_H[b]	Anti-(Mem_H-Bel_N) + Host Antigen[c]	Pre-Immune
HA_1	37.7[d]	30.7	32.3	3.3
HA_1 Pox	26.9	16.4	17.2	2.2
P1	44.4	31.3	32.5	2.3
P2	8.1	3.3	3.4	3.1
HA_1CN1	19.5	12.9	14.3	1.3
HA_1CN3	4.4	2.9	4.3	1.1
HA_1CN4,HA_1CN5,HA_2CN3,HA_2CN4	0	0	0	0
Bel HA_1	17.7	3.2	1.6	1.6

[a]Polypeptide fragments containing tyrosine were radioiodinated using the chloramine T method. Equimolar amounts (0.25 pmoles) were added to 5 μg IgG and held at ambient temperature for 18 hrs. Antigen-antibody complexes were then detected using protein A-Sepharose. Those peptides which do not contain tyrosine were radiolabeled with tritium and 3 nmoles treated with 200 μg IgG for 18 hrs. before addition of protein A-Sepharose.

[b]Anti-Mem_H IgG was prepared by adsorption of anti-(Mem_H-Bel_N) IgG with A/Shearwater/E.Aust./1/72 (Hav6)-A/Bel/42 (N1) to remove anti-neuraminidase and anti-carbohydrate antibodies.

[c]Host carbohydrate antigen was prepared from uninfected chorioallantoic membranes from hen's eggs by Dr. Graeme Laver.

[d]Results are expressed as the percentage of antigen bound.

Immunogenic activity of hemagglutinin fragments. An alternative way in which to investigate the regions of a protein to which antibodies will bind is to inoculate animals with isolated fragments of the molecule and determine if any antibodies produced are able to bind to the parent molecule. Following inoculation of cyanogen bromide fragments, IgG from rabbit sera were titrated against HA_1 from Mem and Bel viruses. The results, Fig. 3, demonstrate that each fragment examined elicits IgG antibodies which are capable of binding to Mem HA_1. However, the titer of the IgG preparations vary with P2 being the poorest immunogen.

Fragments containing HA_1CN1 also elicit antibody that cross-reacts with

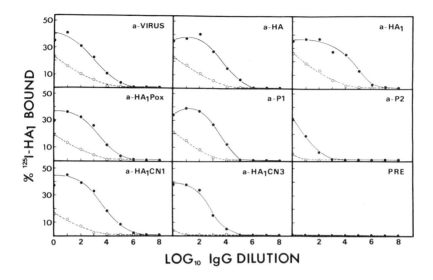

Fig. 3. Titration curves of IgG preparations against HA. Immunoglobulin G obtained from animals inoculated with Mem$_H$-Bel$_N$ virus, HA, HA fragments or from an unimmunised animal were titrated against 0.5 pmoles ^{125}I-HA$_1$ from Mem (●———●) or Bel (o----o) viruses. (Reproduced, with permission, from Jackson et al. (1979) J. Immunol., 123).

Bel HA$_1$. This cross-reactive antibody can be completely removed by adsorption with Shearwater$_H$-Bel$_N$ virus, without affecting binding to Mem HA$_1$ (Fig. 4). This finding suggests that the cross-reactivity is again due to anti-carbohydrate IgG. It will be noted that P2, which contains no carbohydrate[12], elicits no antibody capable of binding Bel HA$_1$ nor indeed does HA$_1$CN3 elicit anti-carbohydrate activity although this is a glycopeptide. Unlike HA$_1$CN1, however, HA$_1$CN3 carries carbohydrate of simple structure[13] suggesting that only carbohydrate of the complex type is immunogenic (see also Ward et al., this volume).

To determine the specificities of the antibodies produced, equimolar amounts of individual radiolabeled fragments were reacted with each of the anti-fragment preparations. The results of this experiment, (Table 3), show that the binding of each polypeptide to homologous antibody is, with the exception of P2, substantial. Antibodies elicited by HA$_1$CN1 bind only to the immunogen HA$_1$CN1 or to larger fragments of the HA molecule containing the HA$_1$CN1 region viz. HA$_1$, HA$_1$Pox and P1. Similarly, substantial binding occurs in cases where antibodies raised against larger fragments are reacted with smaller components of the immunogen. This is evident in the case of HA$_1$Pox

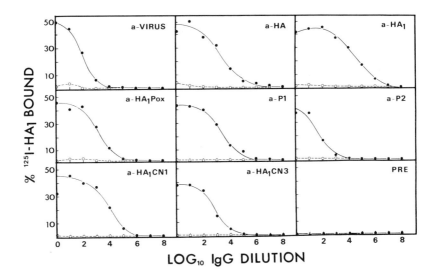

Fig. 4. Effect of removal of anti-carbohydrate antibodies on binding of IgG preparations to HA₁. Immunoglobulin G obtained from animals inoculated with Mem_H-Bel virus, HA, HA fragments or an unimmunised animal were adsorbed with Shearwater_H-Bel_N virus and titrated against 0.5 pmoles ^{125}I-HA₁ from Mem (●——●) or Bel (o----o) viruses. (Reproduced, with permission, from Jackson *et al.* (1979) J. Immunol. 123).

TABLE 3

BINDING OF IgG TO RADIOIODINATED HEMAGGLUTININ FRAGMENTS

IgG Preparation	Radioiodinated HA fragment					
	HA₁	HA₁Pox	P1	P2	HA₁CN1	HA₁CN3
anti-virus	51[a]	34	47	2	24	3
anti-HA	44	52	50	2	44	27
anti-HA₁	29	43	36	3	41	47
anti-HA₁Pox	44	44	45	5	42	17
anti-P1	48	49	51	3	45	6
anti-P2	6	5	5	6	5	1
anti-HA₁CN1	51	53	55	3	49	8
anti-HA₁CN3	45	12	29	2	10	24
prebleed	0	0	0	1	1	0

Note: The system contained 2 pmoles radiolabeled fragments and 25 µg IgG.

[a]Results are expressed as the percentage of the radiolabeled fragment which is bound by IgG. (Reproduced, with permission, from Jackson *et al.* (1979) J. Immunol. 123).

which contains both HA_1CN1 and HA_1CN3 and induces antibodies that react with each of these polypeptides. Antibodies raised against Pl bind to Pl, HA_1, HA_1Pox and HA_1CN1, each of which has stretches of polypeptide in common with the immunogen. The fragment HA_1CN3 appears to be less immunogenic when part of Pl than when inoculated alone.

The data in Table 3 also provide information about the accessibility of various regions of the HA molecule. Isolated HA fragments, when inoculated into a rabbit, elicit antibodies which react *in vitro* with HA_1CN1 and HA_1CN3, whereas intact virions elicit antibodies reacting only with HA_1CN1. This suggests that within whole virus, the region of the HA molecule represented by HA_1CN3 is not available to lymphocyte receptors but can be recognised when HA, released from the virus, is used as the immunogen. For similar reasons, it may be concluded that the HA_1CN2 and HA_2CN2 regions are not accessible to lymphocyte receptors even when presented in isolated HA.

The ability of anti-fragment antibodies to bind to intact virions was investigated by reaction of IgG with Mem_H-Bel_N virus biosynthetically labeled

TABLE 4

ANTI-VIRAL ACTIVITY OF IgG PREPARATIONS

IgG Preparation	Virus Bound[a]	HI Titer Against[b]:	
		Mem_H-Bel_N-	Bel
anti-virus	36	20,700	<80
anti-HA	54	64,000	160
anti-HA_1	46	1,600	256
anti-HA_1Pox	21	400	32
anti-Pl	18	400	32
anti-P2	4	25	10
anti-HA_1CN1	17	200	64
anti-HA_1CN3	4	50	10
preimmune	2	10	4

[a]Mem_H-Bel_N virus (10^4 HAU) biosynthetically labeled with ^{35}S-methionine was incubated with 25 µg IgG. After isolation of antigen-antibody complexes, the amount of radiolabel associated with protein A-Sepharose was determined and expressed as a percentage of the total.

[b]Results are expressed as the reciprocal of the dilution of IgG inhibiting, by 50%, 4HAU of virus. (Modified from Jackson *et al.* (1979) J. Immunol. 123 with permission).

with ^{35}S-methionine. The results (Table 4) provide additional evidence of the inaccessibility of the HA_1CN3 and P2 regions of HA within intact virus as IgG induced by these regions does not bind to whole virions. Antibodies elicited by each of the HA_1CN1-containing fragments, however, are capable of binding to virus.

In order to assess the biological relevance of these antibodies each of the IgG preparations was examined for its ability to inhibit hemagglutination, to neutralize virus infectivity and to lyse influenza-infected MDCK cells in the presence of complement. Each IgG preparation exhibited some degree of hemagglutination inhibitory activity against Mem_H-Bel_N although the titres of anti-P2 and anti-HA_1CN3 were insignificant (Table 4). Much lower hemagglutinating inhibitory activity was apparent when each antibody preparation was titrated against Bel virus suggesting that a small proportion of the inhibitory activity is due to anti-carbohydrate antibodies. When the ability to neutralise $10^{2.5}$ EID_{50} of Mem_H-Bel_N virus was tested, only those antibodies raised against whole virus or intact HA were capable of neutralization. Similarly, anti-fragment IgG was ineffective in lysing Mem_H-Bel_N infected MDCK cells whereas IgG against intact HA still showed significant lysis at a 10^{-4} dilution.

A range of fragmentation techniques and methods for chemically modifying specific amino acid residues within polypeptides has allowed the antigenic structures of two proteins to be determined completely[14,15]. More recent innovations have involved synthesis of short stretches of polypeptide followed by an examination of their immunological properties[15,16] and selection of antigenic variants by use of specific antibody followed by an examination of the differences in amino acid sequence between variant and the parent strain (Laver et al. this volume). Applied to influenza virus, each of these techniques is contributing to our overall knowledge of the regions of the hemagglutinin molecule recognised by antibody.

REFERENCES

1. Ward, C.W. and Dopheide, T.A. (1976) FEBS Lett. 65, 365-368.
2. Jackson, D.C., Dopheide, T.A., Russell, R.J., White, D.O. and Ward, C.W. (1979) Virology 93, 458-465.
3. Laver, W.G. (1971) Virology 45, 275-288.
4. Jackson, D.C., Brown, L.E., White, D.O., Dopheide, T.A. and Ward, C.W. (1979) J. Immunol. 123.

320

5.Gerhard, W., Braciale, T.J. and Klinman (1975) Eur. J. Immunol. 5, 720-725.

6.Etchison, J.R. and Holland, J.J. (1976) Proc. Natl. Acad. Sci. U.S.A. 71, 4011-4014.

7.Klenk, H.D., Schwartz, R.T., Schmidt, M.F.T. and Wollert, W. (1977) in Topics in Infectious Diseases, vol. 3. The Influenza Virus Hemagglutinin. Laver, W.G., Bachmayer, H. and Weil, R. eds., Springer verlag pp. 83-99.

8.Crumpton, M.J. (1974) in The Antigens, Sela, M. ed., Academic Press, New York. Vol. 11 pp 1-78.

9.Jackson, D.C., Russell, R.J., Ward, C.W. and Dopheide, T.A. (1978) Virology 89, 199-205.

10.Brand, C.M. and Skehel, J.J. (1972) Nature New Biol. 238, 145-147.

11.Eckert, E.A. (1973) J. Virol. 11, 183-192.

12.Ward, C.W. and Dopheide, T.A. (1979) Br. Med. Bull. 35, 51-56.

13.Dopheide, T.A. and Ward, C.W. (1978) Eur. J. Biochem. 85, 393-398.

14.Atassi, M.Z. (1977) in Immunochemistry of Proteins vol. 2 Atassi, M.Z. ed. Plenum Press New York and London. pp 77-176.

15.Atassi, M.Z. (1978) Immunochemistry 15, 909-936.

16.Langbeheim, H., Arnon, R. and Sela, M. (1976) Proc. Natl. Acad. Sci. U.S.A. 73, 4636-4640.

DISCUSSION

Webster: Have you measured the affinity of the antibodies to the fragments?

Jackson: No.

Laver: Did you check whether the viruses not neutralized by antibody raised against HA1 were variants?

Jackson: No.

IN VITRO STUDIES ON THE SPECIFICITY OF HELPER T CELLS

FOR INFLUENZA VIRUS HEMAGGLUTININ

E. MARGOT ANDERS, JACQUELINE M. KATZ, LORENA E. BROWN, DAVID C. JACKSON AND
DAVID O. WHITE
Department of Microbiology, University of Melbourne, Parkville, Victoria 3052,
Australia.

The antibody response of B lymphocytes to the hemagglutinin (HA) of influenza
virus is dependent on help from T lymphocytes. Congenitally athymic (nude) mice
inoculated with influenza virus produce no hemagglutination-inhibition (HI)
antibody[1] and immunization of adult thymectomized, X-irradiated, bone marrow-
reconstituted mice with purified HA shows a strong thymus-dependence of antibody
formation[2]. While much work is currently being directed towards identification
of the serologically defined antigenic determinants on HA (this volume), nothing
is known regarding the regions of HA that are antigenic for helper T (T_H) cells.
It is not known whether these are the same determinants as are recognised by
B cells, or whether they perhaps involve other areas of the HA molecule which
are possibly common to different subtypes. For some non-viral antigens, the
receptors on T and B lymphocytes have been found to bear similar idiotypes[3,4],
suggesting that they recognize the same determinants. However, data have also
been reported indicating that T_H cells may have a broader specificity than B
cells[5], or that T_H cells, though equally specific, do not recognize an identical
range of determinants[6]. Furthermore, considerable evidence exists that the
determinants reacting with T cells may be less conformation-dependent than
determinants reacting with antibody[7].

In this study, the specificity for HA of T_H cells raised in influenza virus-
primed mice has been examined using two different approaches. The first
involves measurement of the anti-HA antibody synthesized *in vitro* by influenza-
primed B cells receiving help from T cells primed to the homologous or heterologous strain of virus. The second approach has been to measure "non-specific"
helper activity resulting from the interaction of influenza virus-primed
T cells with purified HA prepared from the homologous or heterologous strains,
or with fragments of HA. Non-specific helper activity is assayed as help for
unprimed B cells undergoing a primary antibody response to sheep red blood
cells.

Viruses and HA. Influenza viruses were grown and purified by the method of
Laver[8]. The virus strains used were: Bel (A/Bel/42 (H0N1)), Port Chalmers

(A/Port Chalmers/73 (H3N2), and the recombinant viruses Aichi$_H$-Bel$_N$ (A/Aichi/68 (H3)-A/Bel/42 (N1)), Jap$_H$-Bel$_N$ (A/Japan/305/57 (H2)-A/Bel/42 (N1)) and Mem$_H$-Bel$_N$ (A/Memphis/102/72 (H3)-A/Bel/42 (N1)). Purified HA was prepared from SDS-disrupted preparations of virus by electrophoresis on cellulose acetate blocks, essentially by the method of Laver[9]. Polyacrylamide gel electrophoresis in SDS of each of the HA preparations yielded two protein bands corresponding in molecular weight to the heavy (HA$_1$) and light (HA$_2$) chains of HA, with no evidence of contaminating proteins.

<u>Mice and cells</u>. Inbred female BALB/c mice were used. Mice were immunized intraperitoneally with 200 HAU of live virus in allantoic fluid. Spleen cell suspensions were prepared and cultured, sometimes after selective depletion of T or B cells by methods previously described from this laboratory[10]. Briefly, spleen cell suspensions depleted of T cells were prepared by treatment of mice *in vivo* with antithymocyte serum 2 days before sacrifice, followed by treatment of the spleen cells *in vitro* with anti-mouse T cell serum plus complement. For use as a source of T$_H$ cells, spleen cell suspensions depleted of B cells were obtained by irradiating the mice (650R) prior to taking the spleens, and then passing the spleen cells through nylon wool columns.

<u>T cell help for the synthesis of secondary anti-HA antibody *in vitro*</u>. A strong secondary anti-HA response was obtained *in vitro* by culture of Port Chalmers virus-primed mouse spleen cell suspensions in Marbrook chambers in the presence of purified Port Chalmers virus (Fig. 1a). Anti-HA antibody in the culture supernatants was quantitated by a solid-phase radioimmunoassay with purified HA as substrate[10]. Depletion of T cells from the immune spleen population led to a greatly diminished response (Fig. 1b), which was restored by reconstitution of the cultures with T cells from mice primed to the homologous virus. The response was restored to a much lesser extent by the addition of unprimed T cells. It seemed feasible, therefore, to examine the specificity of the T$_H$ cells by attempting to reconstitute the antibody response with T cells primed to different virus strains. The system can be depicted thus:

Cells in culture		Antigen	Antibody against HA of strain 1
T$_1$	+ B$_1$	1	++++
T$_{unprimed}$	+ B$_1$	1	+
T$_2$	+ B$_1$	1	?

where 1 and 2 are different strains of influenza virus.

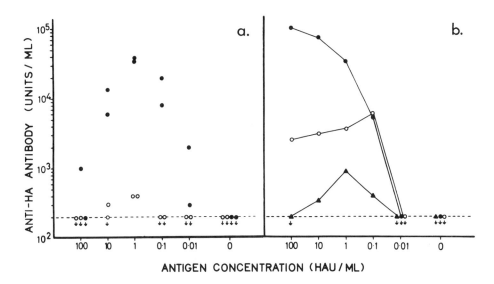

ANTIGEN CONCENTRATION (HAU / ML)

Fig. 1a. *In vitro* anti-HA antibody response of Port Chalmers-primed (●) or unprimed (O) mouse spleen cells cultured in the presence of purified Port Chalmers virus. Primed mice had been immunized with Port Chalmers virus three months previously. Ten million spleen cells in 1 ml of medium, were cultured with different concentrations of antigen in the inner section of Marbrook chambers. After 10 days' incubation, anti-HA antibody in the culture supernatants was quantitated by a solid-phase radioimmunoassay with purified Port Chalmers HA as substrate. Units of antibody are based on a reference Port Chalmers antiserum which has been defined as containing 10^6 units of anti-HA antibody per ml[10].

Fig. 1b. T cell-dependence of the secondary anti-HA antibody response *in vitro*. Port Chalmers-primed spleen cells were depleted of T cells and cultured in the presence of purified Port Chalmers virus either alone, or together with a source of Port Chalmers-primed or unprimed T cells. Mice used as the source of primed T cells had been immunized with Port Chalmers virus 12 days previously. Cultures contained: (▲) 1 x 10^7 Port Chalmers-primed B cells; (●) 5 x 10^6 Port Chalmers-primed B cells plus 5 x 10^6 Port Chalmers-primed T cells; (O) 5 x 10^6 Port Chalmers-primed B cells plus 5 x 10^6 unprimed T cells.
Modified from Anders *et al* (1979) J. Immunol. 123, 1356-1361, with permission.

In attempting to use this system to examine T_H cell specificity, however, a number of problems were encountered. The amount of antibody obtained in the presence of unprimed cells varied in different experiments, and could reach quite high levels, thereby reducing the sensitivity of the system for analysing the help given by T cells primed to a different virus. This problem probably relates to the generation of variable amounts of non-specific helper activity by unprimed T cells in response to constituents of the medium during the 10-day culture period, as has been observed by others[11,12]. Another disadvantage of

the system was that, since the same antigen was being used to stimulate both
the T and the B cells, it was not possible to carry out an independent antigen
dose-response study on the primed T cells alone. Furthermore, while purified
HA also gave a good antibody response, it would be impossible to determine
whether a negative response to small HA fragments were due to lack of an
antigenic determinant for B cells or for T cells. These difficulties have been
overcome by using an assay in which the help generated was measured in a system
unrelated to influenza.

Assay of non-specific helper activity generated by the interaction of
influenza virus-primed T cells with purified HA. Helper T cells help B cells
respond to antigen in two different ways. Interaction of T_H cells with antigen
leads to the release of both "antigen-specific"[13,14] and "non-specific"[15,16]
helper factors: the former provide help for B cells responding to determinants
on the same antigen molecule as stimulated the T_H cell; the latter help the
response of B cells to other antigens quite unrelated to that stimulating the
T_H cell. Antigen-specific help and non-specific help appear to be functions of
two distinct subpopulations of T_H cells[16].

In order to test for the production of non-specific helper factor in
response to purified HA, T cells prepared either from mice primed to $Aichi_H-Bel_N$
virus or from unprimed mice were cultured together with a source of normal
B cells and with SRBC, in the presence and absence of purified Aichi HA. The
culture method was that of Mishell and Dutton[17], and after 4 days' incubation
the cultures were assayed for direct (IgM) anti-SRBC plaque-forming cells (pfc)
using the Cunningham plaque assay[18] (Fig. 2). Control cultures lacking B cells
produced no plaques, and those lacking T cells produced very few. Culture of
T and B cells together in the absence of Aichi HA yielded a low background
number of plaques which was similar whether the T cells were primed or unprimed.
For unprimed T cells, the addition of Aichi HA to the cultures led to no
further increase in plaque numbers over the background level without antigen.
Cultures containing $Aichi_H-Bel_N$-primed T cells, on the other hand, gave significantly higher numbers of plaques in the presence of Aichi HA, the increase
being dependent on the dose of HA used. The assay was thus capable of detecting the interaction of virus-primed T cells with homologous HA.

When the response of $Aichi_H-Bel_N$-primed T cells to heterologous HAs was
tested, it was found that Mem HA gave a stronger response than did Aichi HA
itself; Jap HA also elicited a response, but not Bel HA. In reciprocal
experiments, T cells primed to Jap_H-Bel_N virus responded to Jap HA and to

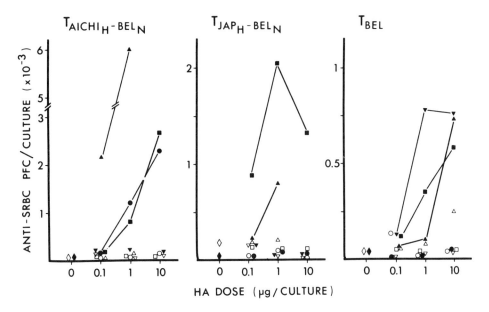

Fig. 2. Generation of non-specific helper activity by influenza virus-primed
T cells in response to HA purified from different strains. Mice were primed
with 200 HAU of live Aichi$_H$-Bel$_N$, Jap$_H$-Bel$_N$, or Bel virus, and 4 to 5 weeks
later the spleens were taken and depleted of B cells to provide a source of
virus-primed helper T cells. Mishell-Dutton-type cultures were set up containing 6×10^6 primed or unprimed T cells, 2.5×10^6 normal unprimed B cells,
2×10^6 SRBC and varying doses of different HA preparations in a total volume
of 0.5 ml. Direct (IgM) anti-SRBC plaque-forming cells (pfc) were enumerated
after 4 days of culture. Each point represents the mean number of plaques
obtained from triplicate (or sometimes duplicate) cultures. Control cultures
lacking B cells gave no detectable plaques (<5/culture). Control cultures
lacking T cells gave 5 to 30 plaques/culture. Closed symbols represent the
response of virus-primed T cells; open symbols represent unprimed T cells.
(●○) Aichi HA; (▲△) Mem HA; (■□) Jap HA; (▼▽) Bel HA; (◆◇) no antigen.

Mem HA, but not to Aichi HA or Bel HA. T cells primed to Bel virus responded
to Bel HA, Jap HA and Mem HA, but not to Aichi HA (Fig. 2).

The fact that T cells from mice primed to virus of any of three subtypes,
H0, H2 or H3, responded to both Mem HA (H3) and Jap HA (H2) suggests the
presence on the HA of viruses from different subtypes of determinants cross-
reactive for helper T cells. In general, the cross-reactions between subtypes
were weaker than the reaction with the homologous HA at the same antigen
concentration, the exception being the response of Aichi$_H$-Bel$_N$-primed T cells
to Jap HA which closely resembled the homologous response. Viruses of the
H2 subtype have been reported to be mitogenic for murine lymphocytes[19].

Reactivity to Jap HA in the helper T cell assay was not due to non-specific
mitogenic effects, however, since no response was obtained with unprimed
T cells; furthermore, we have not observed any evidence of mitogenesis using
purified HA (as opposed to H2 virus) as antigen, as judged by the number of
cells present at the end of the culture period.

In contrast to the results obtained with Mem HA and Jap HA, cross-reaction
between subtypes was not evident in experiments using purified Aichi HA and
Bel HA. The observation that T cells primed to Jap_H-Bel_N or Bel responded
to Mem (H3) but not to Aichi (H3) suggests the possibility that SDS denatures
the cross-reactive determinant in Aichi HA. There is a precedent for this in
the work of Dowdle *et al*[20] in which an asymmetric serologic cross-reaction
between the HAs of Aichi and Jap could be demonstrated using sera raised to
whole virus, but no cross-reaction was found with sera raised to purified
HA[20,21]. Furthermore, in the present work, the preparation of purified Mem HA
used stimulated a stronger response by $Aichi_H$-Bel_N-primed T cells than did
Aichi HA itself, and so the difference in the ability of the two HAs to
produce detectable cross-stimulation of Bel- or Jap_H-Bel_N-primed T cells may
be quantitative rather than qualitative.

The fact that some T cell cross-reaction between HAs of different subtypes
is observed is not altogether surprising. While the dominant serologic
responses to HA are subtype-specific and strain-specific, a serologic cross-
reaction has been demonstrated between the HAs of the H3 and H2 subtypes[20], and
of the H1 and HO subtypes[22], and subtle antigenic relationships have been
observed between other combinations of subtypes in serologic tests[23]. Cross-
recognition of different HA subtypes by T_H cells may contribute to the phenomenon of heterotypic immunity, in which prior experience of virus of one subtype can lead to an accelerated HI antibody response to a challenge virus of
different subtype and may even provide limited protection against the challenge
virus[24,25]. A similar role in heterotypic immunity has recently been suggested
for T_H cells primed to matrix protein[26]. Further experiments using a range of
other strains of influenza virus are required to determine the extent of the
T_H cell cross-reactivity to HA.

Response of helper T cells to fragments of HA. In order to determine the
location of the sites on HA that are recognized by T_H cells, we have commenced
a study using cyanogen bromide-derived fragments of HA as antigen in the assay
for generation of non-specific help. The use of such fragments has proved
valuable in delineating the regions of the HA molecule that are antigenic for

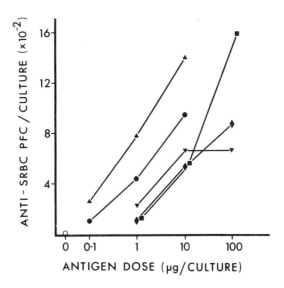

Fig. 3. Response of Aichi$_H$-Bel$_N$ virus-primed T cells to Mem HA$_1$ and to preparations of cyanogen bromide-cleaved Mem HA and Mem HA$_1$. Cultures were set up as described in the legend to Fig. 2. (●) Aichi HA; (▲) Mem HA; (■) Mem HA$_1$; (♦) cyanogen bromide-cleaved Mem HA; (▼) cyanogen bromide-cleaved Mem HA$_1$ (O) no antigen.

B cells, locating a major part of the antigenic activity of Mem HA on the N-terminal cyanogen bromide peptide of HA$_1$ (Jackson *et al.*, this volume). Fig. 3 shows the results of a preliminary experiment in which T cells primed to Aichi$_H$-Bel$_N$ virus were tested for their response to Mem HA$_1$ and cyanogen bromide-cleaved preparations of Mem HA and Mem HA$_1$, as well as to intact Mem HA and Aichi HA. Again, the response to Mem HA was greater than that to Aichi HA. Significant helper activity was also generated in response to intact Mem HA$_1$, and to the cleaved preparations of Mem HA and HA$_1$. It is hoped that extension of these studies using isolated cyanogen bromide-derived fragments and peptides generated by other methods will allow definition of the precise regions on HA recognized by helper T cells.

REFERENCES

1. Burns, W.H., Billups, L.C. and Notkins, A.L. (1975) Nature 256, 654-656.
2. Virelizier, J.L., Postlethwaite, R., Schild, G.C. and Allison, A.C. (1974) J. Exp. Med. 140, 1559-1570.
3. Binz, H. and Wigzell, H. (1975) J. Exp. Med. 142, 197-211.
4. Eichmann, K. and Rajewsky, K. (1975) Eur. J. Immunol. 5, 661-666.
5. Hoffmann, M. and Kappler, J.W. (1973) J. Exp. Med. 137, 721-739.
6. Isac, R. and Mozes, E. (1977) J. Immunol. 118, 584-588.

328

7. Arnon, R. and Geiger, B. (1977) in Immunochemistry: An Advanced Textbook, Glynn, L.E. and Steward, M.W. ed., John Wiley & Sons, Chichester, pp 307-363.
8. Laver, W.G. (1969) in Fundamental Techniques in Virology, Habel, K. and Salzman, N.P. ed., Academic Press, New York, pp. 82-86.
9. Laver, W.G. (1964) J. Mol. Biol. 9, 109-124.
10. Anders, E.M. Peppard, P.M., Burns, W.H. and White, D.O. (1979) J. Immunol. 123, 1356-1361.
11. Schreier, M.H. and Lefkovits, I. (1979) Immunology 36, 743-752.
12. Kindred, B., Bösing-Schneider, R. and Corley, R.B. (1979) J. Immunol. 122, 350-354.
13. Feldmann, M. and Basten, A. (1972) Nature New Biol. 237, 13-15.
14. Taussig, M.J. (1974) Nature 248, 234-236.
15. Schimpl, A. and Wecker, E. (1972) Nature New Biol. 237, 15-17.
16. Marrack, P.C. and Kappler, J.W. (1975) J. Immunol. 114, 1116-1125.
17. Mishell, R.I. and Dutton, R.W. (1967) J. Exp. Med. 126, 423-442.
18. Cunningham, A.J. and Szenberg, A. (1968) Immunology 14, 599-600.
19. Butchko, G.M., Armstrong, R.B., Martin, W.J. and Ennis, F.A. (1978) Nature 271, 66-67.
20. Dowdle, W.R., Marine, W.M., Coleman, M. and Knez, V. (1972) J. Gen. Virol. 16, 127-134.
21. Webster, R.G. and Laver, W.G. (1972) Virology 48, 433-444.
22. Baker, N., Stone, H.O. and Webster, R.G. (1973) J. Virol. 11, 137-140.
23. Schulman, J.L. (1975) in The Influenza Viruses and Influenza, Kilbourne, E.D. ed., Academic Press, New York, pp. 373-393.
24. Schulman, J.L. and Kilbourne, E.D. (1965) J. Bacteriol. 89, 170-174.
25. McLaren, C. and Potter, C.W. (1974) J. Hyg. 72, 91-100.
26. Russell, S.M. and Liew, F.Y. (1979) Nature 280, 147-148.

DISCUSSION

Atassi: Did you try more than one strain of mice? You could have a strain which responds to only some sites, for instance.

Anders: No.

Ertl: Have you tested your T-cell preparations with anti-B cell serum?

Anders: No, but these preparations produce no influenza antibody at all?

ANTIGENIC DRIFT IN THE HAEMAGGLUTININ FROM VARIOUS STRAINS OF INFLUENZA
VIRUS A/HONG KONG/68 (H3N2)

B.A. MOSS[+], P.A. UNDERWOOD[+], V.J. BENDER[+] and R.G. WHITTAKER[++]
+C.S.I.R.O., Molecular and Cellular Biology Unit, P.O. Box 184, North Ryde,
N.S.W. 2113, Australia, and ++School of Biochemistry, University of New
South Wales, P.O. Box 1, Kensington, N.S.W., 2033, Australia.

INTRODUCTION

The type A viruses of influenza are mutable pathogens whose surface proteins,
haemagglutinin and neuraminidase, undergo antigenic evolution by a process of
mutation and selection. Although mutations occur randomly, it is believed that
natural selection by antibody pressure, as a function of exponentially increasing "herd-immunity", screens changes in the antigenic determinants of these
proteins and imposes an orderly evolutionary pattern.

Our objective is to chemically define the nature of the antigenic site(s) of
haemagglutinin[1,2]. Although analyses of natural variants do detect a number of
chemical changes[3,4], many may be unrelated to the antigenic differences between
the various haemagglutinins. Moreover, the genealogy of field strains is
obscure. A theoretical approach to overcome these problems is to select in the
laboratory a series of antigenic mutants whose members are serologically
equivalent to natural variants, but unhindered by the other types of mutation
expected in field strains[5]. To this end, Fazekas de St. Groth selected
antigenic mutants of the Hong Kong field strain, A/NT/60/68 (H3N2), which would
grow in the presence of the most avid fraction of homologous antisera[5,6]. By
this method it was hoped that changes in the viral surface proteins,
particularly in the antigenically more important haemagglutinin molecule, would
have a better chance of being restricted to the antigenic sites.

Haemagglutinins from a number of laboratory mutants and field strains of
the Hong Kong (H3) subtype have been used to correlate serological properties
with chemical changes in the molecule during antigenic drift.

MATERIALS AND METHODS

Virus Strains

Antigenic mutants were derived by Fazekas de St. Groth and Hannoun from a
prototype Hong Kong strain, A/NT/60/68[5,6] and their genealogy and relationship
to field strains reported. NT60, 29C, 30D, 34C and 375/14 were grown for us
in the laboratory of Dr. Fazekas de St. Groth, and haemagglutinin was subsequently isolated for chemical evaluation[1]. Strains of the same nomenclature

were also grown by us from inocula kindly provided by Dr. C. Hannoun.

We have also grown and purified the following recombinant field strains: X-31 (A/Aichi/68 [H3] - A/PR/8/34); Qld/70 (A/Queensland/7/70 [H3] - A/Bellamy/ 42 [NI]); Mem/72-Bel (A/Memphis/102/72 [H3] - A/Bellamy/42 [NI]); Mem/72-PR8 (A/Memphis/102/72 [H3] - A/PR/8/34). X-31 was from the Commonwealth Serum Laboratories, while the other recombinant viruses were gifts from Dr. W.G. Laver, Australian National University.

Immunological Tests of Viruses

Hyperimmune sera against 15 different laboratory derived mutants were pre-pared in rabbits by described methods[7]. A panel of 24 monoclonal hybridoma antibodies to A/Memphis/1/71 [H3] haemagglutinin was used to help classify the mutant viruses. These haemagglutinin specific antibodies were generously supplied by Drs. R.G. Webster and W. Gerhard[8].

Haemagglutination and haemagglutination-inhibition titres were determined as described by Fazekas de St. Groth and Webster[9].

Preparation of Haemagglutinin

The procedures for the preparation of the SCM-haemagglutinin subunits, HA1 and HA2, were described previously[1] except that gel filtration was on a Bio-Gel P300 column. In addition, HA1 was prepared by a solvent extraction procedure[10] and further purified by fractionation on Bio-Gel P300.

Micropeptide Maps

Micromethods were essential because of the poor growth characteristics of the laboratory mutants[5], and low yields of haemagglutinins. Comparative two-dimensional micropeptide maps of tryptic or combined tryptic-thermolytic peptides were prepared from 0.5 - 2 nanomoles of haemagglutinin and variant peptides analysed as described[3,11].

RESULTS

Immunological Titrations

Although the hyperimmune rabbit sera were broadly cross-reactive, antigenic differences between variants and parental virus could be distinguished. As shown in Table 1 the antisera exhibit variable cross-reactions with the laboratory mutants tested. For example, 34C is reactive with all antisera, whereas 30D shows considerably reduced activity with all antisera except the homologous. Other strains show intermediate reactivities, each profile being unique.

Clearly the mutant strains are antigenically different from each other, although their order shows some departure from the original sequence of selection.[5,6] This may be due to mutations occurring during growth of the laboratory strains in the absence of antiserum.

The field strains, X-31, Qld/70, Mem/72-Bel and Mem/72-PR8, were also
antigenically distinguishable with the battery of antisera (unpublished data).

Table 1   Cross Reactions of Laboratory Mutants

	Antisera Against				
Virus	34C	375/14	NT60	29C	30D
34C	100	115	129	126	219*
375/14	65*	100	110	102	166*
NT60	55*	55*	100	87	209*
29C	66	42*	78	100	234*
30D	19*	9*	19*	21*	100

The titres are normalised to the homologous reaction (100%). Each represents
the mean of 9 antisera per antigen and is given as a percentage of the
homologous reaction. *Values are significantly different from 100 at the 5%
level of significance.

Since whole animal sera are heterogeneous, containing antibodies of differing specificity and affinity, we examined antigenic relationships between the
virus strains with the more specific monoclonal anti-haemagglutinin antibodies.

For comparison of mutant strains obtained from NT60, the titres of the panel
of monoclonal antibodies against NT60 were used to derive a baseline in con-
structing relative neutralisation profiles (Fig.1).

Included in Fig.1 is field strain Qld/70, which had been shown previously to
have an identical mutation with 29C [2].

The data reflect the trend observed with the whole antisera titres and substantiate that the laboratory strains are discrete antigenic identities.
Mutant 29C is clearly different from NT60, a fact which was not obvious from
the antisera data, thus emphasising the sensitivity of monoclonal antibody
titrations. A decreasing order of mutant virus – antibody interaction is
apparent with 34C > 375/14 > NT60 > 29C > 30D.

The panel of monoclonal antibodies has been grouped on the basis of their
reported reactivities with selected antigenic mutants[8]. A,B and H are
respectively the monoclonal antibodies H14/A2, H14/A20 and H14/A21 used to
select these authors' mutants. Antibodies C-G distinguish mutants selected by
H14/A20; antibodies I-M distinguish mutants selected by H14/A21, while N-X
failed to distinguish the mutants from the parent strain A/Memphis/1/71(Mem/71).
By comparison, all 24 monoclonal antibodies showed variable cross reactions
with our laboratory mutants (Fig.1).

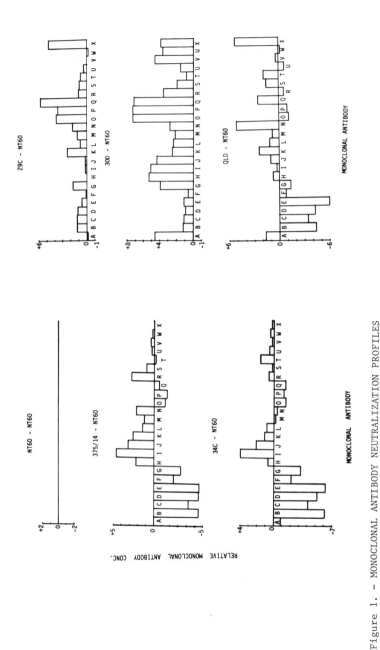

Figure 1. - MONOCLONAL ANTIBODY NEUTRALIZATION PROFILES

Each virus was titrated with 24 monoclonal antibodies (abscissa) and the amount of each required for neutralization was plotted as a function of the amount required to neutralize the parental virus strain NT60 (ordinate - relative concentration in $\log_2$ units). Any mutant requiring more of a particular antibody for neutralization than an equivalent amount of NT60 has a positive value while more easily neutralized strains have negative values. Nomenclature:- A – H14/A2 (Gerhard nomenclature)[8] B–H14/A20, C–126/2, D–123/4, E–212/1, F–93/1, G–27/2, H–H14/A21, I–25/1, J–196/4, K–B18, L–HK30/2, M–200/2, N–4/3, O–138/2, P–74/6, Q–181/1, R–61/1, S–110/3, T–179/2, U–29/1, V–197/6, W–72/1, X–3/1.

Changes have occurred in our mutants that alter reactivity with certain antibodies without apparently affecting others, e.g. B-F in 29C and 30D is basically unchanged while the responses of G-J differ markedly between the two strains. On the other hand, other antibodies exhibit variable interaction with the mutants, e.g. relatively less antibody O,P,Q is required to neutralise 34C and 375/14 than NT60, but increasingly more is required for 29C and 30D indicating some sharing or overlapping of antigenic determinants.

Micropeptide Maps of Haemagglutinin

Comparative tryptic peptide maps of NT60, 375/14, 29C and 30D HA1 were remarkably alike with only a few variable peptides evident (Fig.2). Comparative tryptic-thermolytic maps were also run on all strains. These failed to detect additional changes in 29C and Q1d/70. An extra difference was detected in 30D (Fig.3). Tryptic-thermolytic maps also revealed that the missing tryptic peptide 2 of 375/14 (Fig.2) and 34C was itself unchanged. It was subsequently found by nucleotide sequencing[13] that the arginine residue preceding the peptide was replaced by glycine in 34C so that the missing peptide remained uncleaved from a much larger 45 residue tryptic peptide. The change in 375/14 has not yet been determined.

The identity of variant peptides are summarised in Table 2 and aligned with the known sequence in Table 3.

TABLE 2   LOCATION OF PEPTIDES IN THE PRIMARY STRUCTURE OF HAEMAGGLUTININ

A. TRYPTIC PEPTIDE	POSITION	IDENTITY
1*	141-150	ARG-GLY-PRO-ASP-SER-GLY-PHE-PHE-SER-ARG
1a*		ARG-GLY-PRO-GLY-SER-GLY-PHE-PHE-SER-ARG
1b		GLY-PRO-GLY-SER-GLY-PHE-PHE-SER-ARG
2	202-207	VAL-THR-VAL-SER-THR-ARG
3 *	217-224	ILE-GLY-SER-ARG-PRO-TRP-VAL-ARG
3a#		ILE-GLY-SER-ILE-PRO-TRP-VAL-ARG
4*	225-229	GLY-LEU-SER-SER-ARG
4a*		GLY-GLN-SER-SER-ARG
B. TRYPTIC-THERMOLYTIC PEPTIDE		
1	182-193	VAL-HIS-HIS-PRO-SER-THR-ASN-GLN-GLU-GLN-THR-SER
1a		ILE-THR-ASN-GLN-GLU-GLN-THR-SER
1b		VAL-HIS-HIS-PRO
2		Probably ILE-PRO-TRP-VAL-ARG of tryptic peptide 3a

* Confirmed by nucleotide sequencing[13]
# Identified by nucleotide sequencing[13]

334

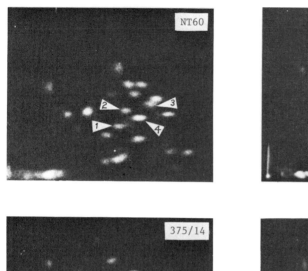

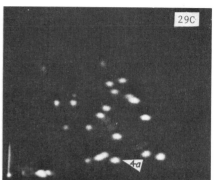

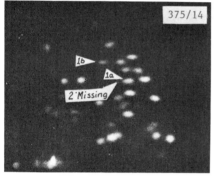

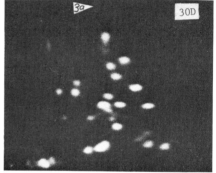

Figure2. Tryptic Micropeptide Maps
of NT60,375/14,29C,30D and Q1d/70 HA1.

Peptides are resolved by electrophoresis at pH3.5 in the 1st
dimension (horizontal) and by ascend-
ing chromatography in - butanol:
pyridine: acetic acid: water (150:
100:3:100) in the 2nd. Peptides were
visualised with Fluorescamine[14].
Sequences of the parental peptides
(1 to 4) and variants (1a to 4A) are
given in Table 2. Mutant 34C gives
a pattern identical with 375/14.
NT60 always contains traces of
peptide 1a and 1b. Q1d/70 (and
other strains) may also differ in

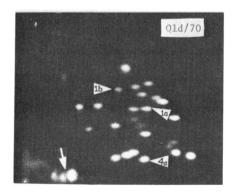

the large tryptic peptides near the origin (marked by blank arrow), one
of which is a glycopeptide[15].

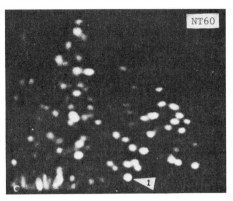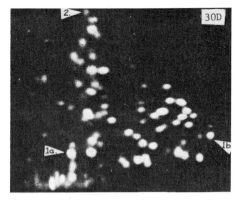

Figure 3. Tryptic-thermolytic micropeptide maps of NT60 and 30D HA1. The sequences of the variant peptides are given in Table 2.

TABLE 3. LOCATION OF CHANGES IN ANTIGENICALLY DIFFERENT STRAINS

ANTIGENIC CHANGES

STRAIN					
NT60	N-term -49- KICNNPHR -82- KRGPDSGFFSR -30- GVHHPS TNQEQTSL YVQASGR VTVSTRR -8- NIGSR PWVRGLSSR -99- C-term				
29C					GQSSR
34C		GPGSGFFSR		GVTVSTRR	
375/14		GPGSGFFSR		‹MISSING› (as 34C?)	
30D			VHHPITNQEQTS		IGSIPWVR
QLD		GPGSGFFSR			GQSSR

Laver et al. 1979	K (A2-VI to 4)	S or L (A20-V2 and V3 resp)		Y (A21-V1)	← MISSING → (A21-V2,V3)

N.B. NT60 sequence shown differs from that determined by nucleotide sequencing [13] (a) Asp for Gly at position 144 - see text (b) Arg for Gln at position 327, this change was not indicated by peptide mapping.

We have found no distinguishable differences between peptide maps of bromelain released HA2 subunits from any of our mutants[1-3]. Nucleotide sequence analyses of the entire HA2 gene fragment from NT60 and 29C were identical and only three amino acid changes were deduced between NT60 and Mem/72-PR8 [12,13]. Laver et al. also found little or no differences between the soluble tryptic peptides of HA2 from experimentally selected and naturally occurring variants [4,8].

DISCUSSION

Our studies have revealed that amino acid changes in the laboratory mutants are limited both in number and location in the HA1 molecule. They are not restricted to a unique locus, a result consistent with our interpretation of the monoclonal antibody titrations. Indeed some of the mutants (34C, 375/14, 30D) have undergone changes in at least two loci relative to the parent strain NT 60.

We find that the peptides which vary in these antigenic mutants also vary (among others) in field strains[3,4]. Changes in some peptides are identical, e.g. the leu→gln mutation in residue 226 of 29C, Qld/70 and Mem/72-PR8[3], and the asp→gly mutation in residue 144 of 34C, 375/14, Qld/70 and X-31. The other changes in the mutants have not yet shown correspondence with any seen in field strains but data on the latter is incomplete[4]. Nevertheless, all these changes help to identify those regions of the haemagglutinin molecule which are antigenically relevant.

From the monoclonal antibody neutralization profiles of the viral strains (Fig.1) it should be possible to infer the nature of some amino acid changes. For example, any strain that gives the distinctive profile with antibodies B-G (as found with 375/14, 34C and Qld/70) would predictably have the glycine for aspartic acid substitution in residue 144 of HA1. This was demonstrated in field strain X-31 which gave the distinctive B-G profile and the substitution was later detected by peptide mapping (unpublished data). Mem/71, which reportedly has glycine[4], also has this profile. A comparable response seems to occur with antibody X and involves the leu→gln change in residue 226 of 29C and Qld/70 (also Mem/72-PR8, but not Mem/72-Bel., which retains leucine; unpublished). However, the same antibody responds similarly in 30D to a different change, perhaps the arg→ile substitution in residue 220, only six amino acids away.

Although 29C and Qld/70 have the glutamine change in common, the monoclonal antibody titrations indicate that other changes in them, such as the asp→gly substitution, must have a strong bearing on the antigenic reactivity. The identification of these changes is in progress[13]. It is expected that as more mutants are examined the ability to predict the changes will improve, especially for the antibody group H-M which shows a range of responses to the changes in 34C, 375/14 and 30D. These changes are relatively close in the primary sequence, occurring in residue 201 of 34C and 375/14 and in residues 186 and 220 of 30D.

The gly→asp change in residue 144 seems significant in that it is one of first to appear in field strains[4] and may affect a strategic antigenic site[8]. Interestingly, we find that NT60 preparations are persistently dimorphic, with the aspartic acid form predominating. (In all our work at the protein level, antibody titrations and peptide mapping, the glycine form did not appear to exceed 10%. However, the preparation of NT60 for nucleic acid studies proved peculiar in that only glycine was revealed by nucleotide sequencing[13]). Such dimorphism displayed by NT60 might be due to the stable co-existence of two allelic antigenic strains[16]. Strains 375/14 and 34C are entirely in the glycine form, whereas the aspartic acid form is conserved in 29C and 30D. The nature of the other mutations in these strains may dictate whether the glycine or aspartic acid form is successful following selection with homologous anti-serum suppressive to the parent virus. It is also worth noting here that selection of recombinant strains of A/Memphis/102/72 has resulted in two anti-genically distinguishable variants, Mem/72-Bel and Mem/72-PR8 (leu→gln at position 226) indicating that caution should be exercised in the use of genetic recombinants.

The changes detected by us (Tables 2 and 3) and by Laver and co-workers[8] all represent significant alterations in the charge and/or size of the amino acid side chains. Four of the seven detected involve charge changes [asn→lys at 54, asp→gly at 144, arg→gly at 201 and arg→ile at 220] with the remaining three being changes in size and hydrophobicity [pro→ser or leu at 143, ser→ile at 186, ser→tyr at 205]. Each change could be expected to influence directly the binding of the antibody molecule or alternatively to have major effects on other residues in their immediate environment thereby exerting a secondary effect on antibody binding. Of particular interest is that one of the changes occurs at a prolyl residue[8] (at 143), while three others occur immediately adjacent to prolyl residues (at 144, 186, 220) which suggests an association of antigenicity with bends in the haemagglutinin molecule. Two of the five antigenic regions of myoglobin also occur in bends of that molecule, adjacent to prolyl residues[17], perhaps implicating a similar mode of antibody-antigen interaction for haemagglutinin.

ACKNOWLEDGEMENTS

We are grateful to Mrs. Jann Harrison, Mrs. Shana Lennox and Mr. John Rawlinson for their competent and enthusiastic technical assistance. We also acknowledge that Influenza virus is a manifestation of Proteus, the mythical Greek sea god, whose greatest power was his ability to change his shape and identity instantly. He was also noted for his wisdon and knowledge of future events. Anyone who wanted Proteus to answer a question had to catch him and hold him fast in spite of all his changing forms. Only then would he answer ......or would he?

REFERENCES

1. Moss, B.A. and Underwood, P.A. (1978) in "Topics in Infectious Diseases" (W.G. Laver, Bachmayer and R. Weil Eds)Vol. 3, pp 145-166 Springer-Verlag, Vienna
2. Whittaker, R.G., Moss, B.A. and Underwood, P.A. (1979) Proc. Aust. Biochem. Soc. 12, 18
3. Whittaker, R.G., et al. Manuscript in preparation
4. Laver, W.G., Air, G.M., Dopheide, T.A.A. and Ward, C.W. (1979) Nature (Lond.), in press
5. Fazekas de St. Groth, S. (1978) in "Topics in Infectious Disease (W.G. Laver, H. Bachmayer and R. Weil, Eds) Vol. 3, pp 25-48, Springer-Verlag, Vienna
6. Fazekas de St. Groth, S. and Hannoun, C. (1973) Compte Rendu Acad. Sci., Paris 276, 1917-1920 (series D)
7. Underwood, P.A., Infection and Immunity, in press
8. Laver, W.G., Air, G.M., Webster, R.G., Gerhard, W., Ward, C.W. and Dopheide, T.A.A. (1979) Virology, 98, 226-237
9. Fazekas de St. Groth, S. and Webster, R.G. (1966) J. Exp. Med. 124, 331-345
10. Eckert, E.A. (1973) J. Virol 11, 183-192
11. Whittaker, R.G., Moss, B.A. and Appleby, C.A. (1979) Biochem. Biophys. Res. Commun 89, 552-558
12. Sleigh, M.J., Both, G.W., Brownlee, G.G., Bender, V.J. and Moss, B.A. This volume
13. Both, G.W., Sleigh, M.J., Bender, V.J. and Moss, B.A. This volume
14. Vandekerckhove, J. and Van Montagu, M. (1974) Eur. J. Biochem. 44, 279-288
15. Bender, V.J., and Moss, B.A. (1979) Proc. Aust. Biochem. Soc. 12, 15
16. Kilbourne, E.D. (1978) Proc. Natl. Acad. Sci. U.S.A. 75, 6258-6262
17. Attassi, M.Z. (1975) Immunochem. 12, 423-438

DISCUSSION

Webster: Is the variant with a change at position 144 in HA1 distinguishable with heterogenerous antisera?

Moss: Yes, and it can be distinguished with antisera to the other mutants.

STRUCTURAL STUDIES ON THE HAEMAGGLUTININ GLYCOPROTEIN OF INFLUENZA VIRUS

IAN A. WILSON[+], JOHN J. SKEHEL[++] AND DON C. WILEY[+]
[+]Gibbs Laboratory, Dept. Biochemistry and Molecular Biology, Harvard University,
12 Oxford St., Cambridge, MA 02138, USA: [++]Division of Virology, National
Institute for Medical Research, Mill Hill, London, NW7 1AA, England.

SUMMARY

X-ray crystallographic investigation of the haemagglutinin glycoprotein
of influenza virus has produced a three-dimensional image of the trimeric
molecule at 3Å resolution. A single isomorphous derivative, mercury phenyl
glyoxal, was used in the phase determination. The non-crystallographic three-
fold axis was determined from the solution of the difference Patterson at 3Å
resolution. Three-fold averaging of the electron density map indicates the
monomer and molecular boundaries. Interpretation of the map awaits improvement
of the phases by non-crystallographic symmetry averaging.[1]

INTRODUCTION

The major surface glycoprotein of influenza virus, the haemagglutinin,
has been crystallized[2] and its three-dimensional structure is being determined
to 3Å resolution by X-ray crystallographic methods. The haemagglutinin is a
trimer composed of two disulphide-linked polypeptide chains, HA_1 and HA_2,
including 19% by weight of carbohydrate. The protein can be cleaved from the
viral membrane by bromelain, leaving a C-terminal polypeptide "tail" (5000
daltons) embedded in the lipid.[3] Preliminary electron density maps have
revealed one bromelain released trimer (about 197,000 daltons) per asymmetric
unit of the crystal. Amino acid sequence determination of the complete monomer
is well advanced[4] and will greatly facilitate the interpretation of the electron
density map. The solution of a mercury phenyl glyoxal difference Patterson and
the calculation of a preliminary electron density map using single isomorphous
phases and non-crystallographic symmetry averaging[1] is presented.

MATERIALS AND METHODS

Native and derivative crystals. The haemagglutinin glycoprotein of the
Hong Kong strain of influenza virus (H3N2),[5] when released by bromelain from
the membrane,[3] has been crystallized by microdialysis (50 microlitre) against
1.2-1.45M sodium citrate, 0.1% sodium azide, pH 7.5.[2] Large single octahedral
crystals (up to 1mm[3]) are formed with tetragonal space group $P4_1$ or $P4_3$, cell

dimensions a = 163.2Å, c = 177.4Å and one molecule per asymmetric unit (see results for discussion of this observation). A mercury phenyl glyoxal derivative was prepared by placing a preformed crystal into a suspension of 10^{-2}M mercury phenyl glyoxal[6] in the mother liquor of 1.45M sodium citrate, 0.1% sodium azide, pH7.5 for at least 15 hours. A second mercury iodide derivative has been prepared by soaking crystals in 1mM mercury iodide in mother liquor for at least 24 hours at room temperature. Data collection of this second derivative is in progress and no measurements from these crystals have been included in the present structure analysis.

DATA COLLECTION

X-ray diffraction intensities were recorded photographically (Ilford Industrial-G film, Eliot GX-6, 100µM focus, 39kV, 19mA, Franks focusing optics[7] at 4° C). At least two 1° oscillation photographs (exposure time 12 hours per degree) can be recorded from each crystal before X-ray damage is evident in the diffraction pattern. From 14 to 20° of oscillation data can be collected from some large crystals by translating the crystal to expose a fresh volume to X-rays every 24 hours. The crystals diffract to 3Å resolution with considerable loss in intensity with smaller spacings.

Data processing. Seventy-eight native and sixty-two derivative films were collected on an automated Supper oscillation camera and processed on an Optronics scanner (50µ raster).[8] Intensities from first and second films for each degree were merged by Fox and Holmes[9] scaling. Different films were scaled together by scaling the Wilson plots for the fully recorded intensities of each film to an average Wilson plot of the fully recorded intensities of the best measured films. Partially recorded intensities ($\geq$50% recorded) were scaled to the fully recorded measurements by post-refinement methods.[10,11] Data processing statistics are shown in Table 1.

RESULTS

Difference Patterson. The location of six mercury atoms per asymmetric unit (two per monomer of the HA trimer) was determined from the difference Patterson at 3Å resolution. Inspection of the two Harker sections (Figure 1) at 5.5Å and 3Å illustrates the difficulty encountered in a Patterson of an 800,000 dalton asymmetric unit (200,000 dalton protein, 600,000 daltons solvent). Only two atoms (1 and 2 in Figure 2) have strong self Harker vectors. The four other solutions have at least one self Harker vector which is less significant than many other vectors on the Harker sections. Possible single

TABLE 1

DATA PROCESSING STATISTICS

Data set	No. films	Total reflections measured	Unique reflections	R_{sym}[1][2]	R_{whole}[3]	R_{asym}[4]
Native	78	408,672	83,015	.12	.11	.18
Derivative	62	338,738	78,077	.13	.13	.20

[1]$R = \Sigma |s_i I_{hi} - \bar{I}_h| / \Sigma \bar{I}_n$

s_i = scale factor for crystal i

I_{hi} = intensity of reflection h of crystal i

$\bar{I}_h$ = average intensity of reflection

[2]R_{sym} --for symmetry related reflections on the same film

[3]R_{whole}--for fully recorded reflections from different films

[4]R_{asym} --for all reflections ($\geq 50\%$ recorded) on different films, final scaling

TABLE 2

HEAVY ATOM PARAMETERS USED IN PHASE DETERMINATION

atom site	x	y	z (Å)	occupancy[1]	B(Å^2)[2]
1	31.0	53.4	0.0[3]	0.47	22.7
2	25.1	54.0	21.8	0.61	19.9
3	0.4	42.9	-16.5	0.34	23.8
4	3.9	57.7	38.6	0.39	24.0
5	13.0	41.6	7.3	0.44	25.0
6	41.7	78.5	0.9	0.34	24.8

[1] relative fractional occupancies (not absolute)
[2] isotropic temperature factor
[3] atom 1 z fixed at 0.0

Atoms 1, 2, 5 form one trimer and atoms 3, 4, 6 the second trimer. The Kraut R was 0.14, phasing power 1.36 for the 42,299 reflections used in the refinement with a figure of merit of 0.34.

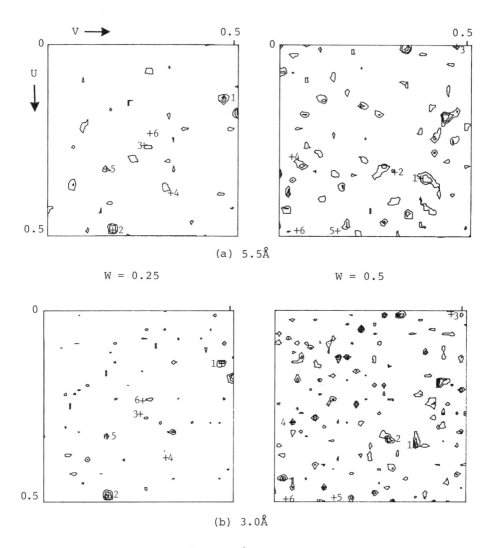

(a) 5.5Å

W = 0.25   W = 0.5

(b) 3.0Å

Fig. 1. Harker sections at 3Å and 5.5Å resolution of the difference
Patterson.   Self Harker vectors calculated from the refined atomic positions
are indicated by a numbered cross on the Harker sections, W = 1/4 and W = 1/2.

atom solutions of the Patterson were determined by computing a symmetry minimum function yielding all potential x,y mercury atom coordinates consistent with the Harker sections at w = 1/4 and w = 1/2. Cross vectors for all pairs of such potential single atom solutions were then searched for in the three-dimensional Patterson. This search took the form of a symmetry minimum function in the Δz coordinate for an atom pair. From 32 potential single atom solutions, all cross vectors for a constellation of four atoms were found by this search. A fifth atom was found by symmetry minimum function searches in the Δz coordinates of the remaining large w = 0.5 Harker vectors which had no significant corresponding w = 0.25 vectors.

The remaining mercury position, vectors for which were not prominent on Harker sections, was found by considering the 583 largest peaks in the Patterson as potential cross vectors between the five known atoms and an unknown position. Simultaneously, a higher order image seeking function was written based on the double sort algorithm of Bricogne[1] by writing a new version of his routine "Generate". Given a subset of known atomic positions this function searched for cross vectors between a known atom and every position in the asymmetric unit (on a 2Å grid). The function determined that no solutions other than the original six atoms were present. In retrospect the function is capable of readily and unambiguously determining the location of all the heavy atoms from the coordinates of the first two found in the Harker search.

The final solution consists of two triangles of atoms 22.7Å and 57.3Å on an edge, the triangles separated by 13Å along the molecular three-fold axis. The stoichiometry of the phenyl glyoxal reaction is expected to be two phenyl glyoxals per arginine.[16] However, the separation of the two triangles seems to be too far apart for covalent attachment to the same arginine and may reflect two substituted arginines per HA$_1$ and HA$_2$ subunit.

Rotation function and the molecular three-fold symmetry axis. A single (sometimes split) prominent peak in the fast rotation functions[12] of the 3Å native, derivative and difference coefficients indicated a non-crystallographic three-fold symmetry axis nearly along the diagonal of the b,c plane (92° from the a-axis, 35.3° from the b-axis and 54.7° from the c-axis). The heavy-atom coordinates establish that this is a 120° non-crystallographic "packing" rotation axis relating two crystallographically identical molecules (such an axis will exist somewhere for any molecules related by a four-fold axis). The molecular three-fold axis, located from the heavy atom coordinates, is nearly

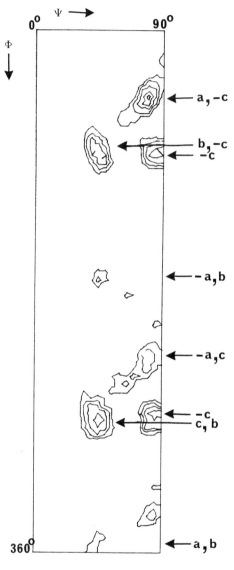

Figure 2. $\kappa = 120°$ Rotation Function
A rotation function using the largest
1000 terms to 10Å resolution[13,14]
shows the non-crystallographic
molecular three-fold symmetry axis
(located near the diagonal of the
$-\hat{a},\hat{b}$ plane) and non-crystallographic
120° "packing symmetry" axes. Polar
angle definitions are given by Rossmann
and Blow (1962).[13] Rotation functions
calculated with radii from 15 to 100Å
(R = 24Å shown) are similar. Planes
(e.g., a, -c) or axes (c) are indicated
on the rotation function.

along the diagonal of the a,b plane (53.4° from the a-axis, 141.6° from the b-axis and 79.9° from the c-axis).

A rotation function[13] based on the 1000 largest 10Å coefficients (Figure 2) shows both the packing and molecular non-crystallographic axes, the molecular axis being much less prominent than the packing axis (further analysis of the rotation function will be presented elsewhere).

Heavy atom parameter refinement and phase calculation. Final heavy atom parameters were determined by alternate cycles of least squares refinement and SIR phasing. All parameters refined well, including occupancy and isotropic temperature factors (Table 2).

The phases of 42,299 reflections used in the refinement (small measurements omitted) were calculated by the SIR method and had an overall figure of merit of 0.34.

Electron density map. An electron density map calculated with the SIR phases clearly indicated one molecule per asymmetric unit. The protein thus occupies only 22% of the total volume of the unit cell giving a small protein/unit-cell volume ratio well outside the normal for protein crystals.[15] The other possibility, that a second set of molecules does not fully occupy another location in the unit cell or is disordered, is not indicated by the Fourier maps.

The electron density map was averaged about the molecular three-fold[1] and the protein (carbohydrate) features were clearly enhanced above background solvent density by the averaging. The SIR map (without anomalous dispersion) is clearly subject to large errors as indicated by the solvent "noise". A comparison of two equivalent regions (4Å thick) of the averaged and unaveraged maps is shown in Figure 3. The connectivity has been increased and the background significantly decreased in the averaged map. On the unaveraged map the close contacts between the molecule and another related molecule can be seen.

DISCUSSION

Molecular shape. The molecule appears to be an elongate trimeric cylinder of approximately 130 Å length with radius varying from 15-38Å. Sections down the molecular three-fold axis often show the subunit boundaries with little density in the centre of the molecule (Figure 3). Other regions have tightly-packed subunits forming a triangular structure with a smaller radius (Figure 4).

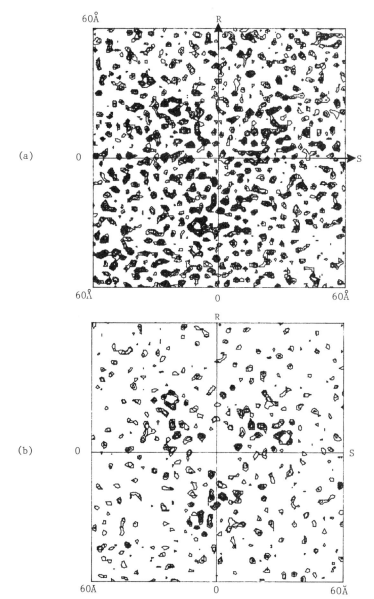

Fig. 3. Electron density maps of the unaveraged (a) and the three-fold averaged (b) SIR map at 3 Å resolution. The maps are viewed down the non-crystallographic molecular three-fold axis as defined in the text. The sections are 4Å thick and 120Å by 120Å centred on the three-fold. The large ring-like features viewed on the outside of each monomer represents artifact density around one triangle of mercury atoms (atoms 3, 4, 6, Table 2). R, S and T are the coordinate axes when viewed down the three-fold axis. The molecule extends from T = -45Å to +85Å. Sections above are T = -14 to -11Å.

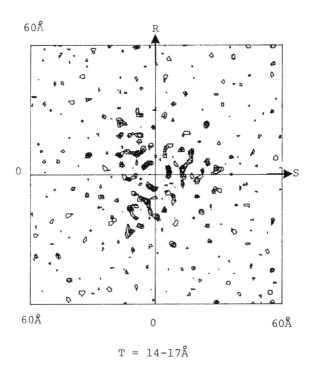

T = 14–17Å

Fig. 4. Electron density of the three-fold averaged map at 3Å resolution in the "thin" end of the molecule where the subunits are more closely packed. The contour level is slightly higher than in Figure 3(b). A slice through the molecule 4Å thick down the non-crystallographic three-fold is shown for T = 14–17Å.

The average azimuthal position of the subunit varies slightly along the length of the three-fold axis. The molecule tends to be thicker at one end (70-80Å diameter), around the heavy atom locations (Figure 3), and thinner (30-50Å) at the other (Figure 4).

Detailed interpretation of the map has not been attempted pending phase refinement by non-crystallographic symmetry averaging.[1]

ACKNOWLEDGMENTS

We are indebted to many members of the Gibbs Structural Group for thoughtful discussions and to Edward Gordon and David Stevens for technical assistance.

REFERENCES

1. Bricogne, G. (1976) Acta Cryst. A32, 832-847.
2. Wiley, D.C. and Skehel, J.J. (1977) J. Mol. Biol. 112, 343-347.
3. Brand, C.M. and Skehel, J.J. (1972) Nature New Biol. 238, 145-147.
4. See this volume.
5. Kilbourne, E. (1969) Bull. Wld. Hlth. Org. 41, 643-645.
6. Monaco, H.L. (1978), Ph.D. thesis, Harvard University.
7. Harrison, S.C. (1968) J. Appl. Crystallogr. 1, 84-89.
8. Crawford, J.L. (1977) Ph.D. thesis, Harvard University.
9. Fox, G.C. and Holmes, K.C. (1966) Acta Cryst. 20, 886-891.
10. Schutt, C.E. (1976) PhD. thesis, Harvard University.
11. Winkler, F.K. et al., (1979) A35, 901-911.
12. Crowther, R.A. (1972) in The Molecular Replacement Method, ed. M.G. Rossmann, pp. 173-178, New York, Gordon and Breach.
13. Rossmann, M.G. and Blow, D.M. (1962) Acta Cryst. 15, 24-31.
14. Tollin, P. and Rossmann M.G. (1966) Acta Cryst. 21, 872-876.
15. Mathews, B.W. (1968) J. Mol. Biol. 33, 491-497.
16. Takahashi, K. (1977) J. Biochem. 81, 395-402.

DISCUSSION

Gething: What effect does the mercury phenyl glyoxyl substitution have on
biological activity?

Wiley: We find no effect on hemagglutinating activity, but so far we have not
done any infectivity assay.

Gibbs: I did not understand how the electron density map had polarity but was
not 3-fold symmetrically superposed.

Wiley: The 3-fold axis of the molecule is not an axis of the crystal, so the
operations of multiple crystals don't average. We can use this redundancy to
get the phases.

Ward: The electron micrographs of Ian Griffith show the same bulging that your
model has.

Wiley: The electron micrographs of Laver and Valatine of HA rosettes show a
bulge at the outer end, which is the only clue at the moment as to which end
is which.

PRELIMINARY STRUCTURAL STUDIES ON TWO INFLUENZA VIRUS NEURAMINIDASES

P.M. COLMAN, P.A. TULLOCH AND W.G. LAVER[+]
CSIRO, Division of Protein Chemistry, 343 Royal Parade, Parkville, 3052,
Melbourne, Australia; [+]Department of Microbiology, John Curtin School of
Medical Research, Australian National University, Canberra, Australia.

INTRODUCTION

Although the phenomena of antigenic drift and shift[1] in influenza virus
present no conceptual difficulties, there is presently no solid basis for
appreciating the extent of structural alteration that is required to enable a
new antigenic variant of the virus to survive where its predecessor could not.
One step towards solving this problem will be the determination of the three-
dimensional structures of hemagglutinin and neuraminidase, the two surface
antigens on the influenza virus particle. In conjunction with the protein and
nucleic acid sequence data which are now becoming extensive (see elsewhere in
this volume), this structural information will point to possible antigenic
determinants on these two molecules. The second and no less important step will
require determining the three-dimensional structures of other hemagglutinins and
neuraminidases of altered antigenicity, in order to study the new conformation
of the antigenic determinants. The necessity for these additional structure
studies arises because there is still no adequate algorithm for translating
amino acid sequence into three-dimensional structure and therefore one cannot
confidently predict the geometrical structure of a chemically altered determinant.

The complementary problem to antigenic changes and their underlying stereo-
chemical aspects, is that of the relationship between the shape and binding
properties of the antibody combining site which is specific for a particular
antigen. There is now a small body of data on the size and shape of antibody
combining sites[2,3] and of the structurally homologous region found in dimers of
immunoglobulin light chains.[4-7] The spatial proximity of the six hypervariable
segments in antibody sequences and the manner in which they delineate a binding
site for hapten, suggest a satisfactory structural basis for the generation of
diverse antibody specificities.[8] The details, however, are less clear. A
study of three closely related light chain dimer fragments[5-7] has shown that an
amino acid substitution at one location in the hypervariable region can alter
the conformation of neighbouring residues and in an immune response such simple
substitutions could lead to greater changes in specificity of the antibody than

would be predicted by a chemical study alone.[7] It is not unlikely that similar effects will cloud attempts to define the structures of altered antigenic determinants in influenza viruses, purely on the basis of sequence changes.

Here we present a preliminary study of two antigenically different but closely related influenza virus N2 neuraminidases.

MATERIALS AND METHODS

Recombinant virus containing NWS (HO) hemagglutinin and either Tokyo/3/67 or Nederlands/84/68 (N2) neuraminidase were incubated with pronase (Calbiochem) at 37°C for 16 hours. Virus cores were removed by centrifugation and neuraminidase heads in the supernatant were crystallised by dialysis against distilled water as previously described.[9,10] Typically, microcrystals appear after this step and they were redissolved in 0.15M NaCl and then centrifuged on sucrose density gradients. Gradual dialysis of this gradient purified material against distilled water yields large crystals (0.5 - 1.0 mm) of Tokyo neuraminidase but only microcrystals of the Nederlands protein. These microcrystals are extremely thin and are therefore ideal objects for study in the electron microscope.

A droplet of crystalline suspension of Nederlands neuraminidase was placed on a carbon coated electron microscope grid and crystallites were allowed to sediment briefly onto the thin carbon substrate. After excess liquid was drawn off, the specimen-support grid was rapidly frozen and then dried under high vacuum. Substrate and adhering crystallites were shadowed with tungsten at an angle of about 60° to the substrate normal and further stabilised with a thin coating of carbon evaporated at normal incidence.

Using standard techniques of optical diffraction and computer image processing[11,12] two-dimensional image averaging was performed on suitable electron micrographs of the shadowed Nederlands neuraminidase crystals.

Three-dimensional X-ray diffraction data for Tokyo neuraminidase have been collected to a resolution of 3.5 Å using rotation cameras and a rotating anode generator. Rotation function analyses[13] of the native data were done on the 5 Å data set. Heavy atom derivatives have been prepared by soaking crystals in ~ 1mM solutions of heavy metal complexes.

RESULTS

1. Nederlands 68 neuraminidase. Wrigley[14] has previously shown that thin crystals of Nederlands neuraminidase show a tetragonal packing of heads when viewed normal to the crystal plate. The reported unit cell dimensions are

$a = b = 98$ Å.[14] There are obvious similarities to the Tokyo neuraminidase crystals (see below) where $a = b = \sqrt{2} \times 98.7$ Å.

It is not possible from a study of either of these crystals normal to the tetragonal plane to determine the full three-dimensional space group. The presence of a body-centred lattice can only be detected by tilting the crystals. Figure 1 shows the relationship between the primitive and body centred lattices that we wish to distinguish. Shadowing the crystals at an oblique angle as described above is an alternative to tilting. Figure 2 is an electron micrograph of part of a shadowed single crystal of Nederlands neuraminidase. White areas indicate where tungsten has coated the surface of the protein in the crystallite and black areas are the shadows cast by the protein to the collimated tungsten beam. Each white structure unit in the micrograph corresponds to a tetrameric neuraminidase head. The direction of shadowing is a few degrees clockwise from the top of the micrograph. The Fourier transform of a selected area of this image is shown in Figure 3 and in Figure 4 is the filtered transform based on unit cell parameters of $a = 145.2$ Å, $b = 145.5$ Å, $\gamma = 91.9°$. There has been some slight distortion of the crystallite in this region. In another area we found $a = b$ with $\gamma = 90°$ as expected for a tetragonal lattice. Clearly the lattice is based upon spacings of $\sim 100 \times \sqrt{2}$ Å and not 100 Å. The reconstructed image (Figure 4) shows that every other row of neuraminidase heads in the crystal is less heavily coated with tungsten, consistent with these rows being deeper in the surface than the others.

Fig. 1. Schematic of body-centred (solid lines) and primitive (dashed lines) unit cells. The motif at the centre of the body-centred cell is out of the plane defined by the motifs at the four corners.

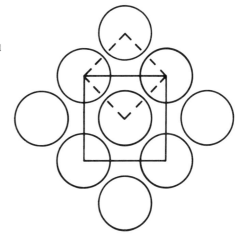

The computer averaged image shows some indication of a cleft dividing the head in a direction parallel to one of the 140 Å lattice spacings. A cleft at 90° to this, if it exists, will have been partly coated with tungsten and will not be prominent. The interpretation of detail of this type in a shadowed object is less straightforward than in the case of a stained object. The feature referred to here could also result from a surface projection at the centre of the head casting its shadow. Insofar as this shadow is not in line with the direction of the tungsten beam, the cleft interpretation is preferable.

2. Tokyo 67 neuraminidase. A characterisation of the Tokyo neuraminidase crystals has already been published.[10] The space group is I422 and the cell dimensions are a = b = 139.6 Å, c = 191 Å, not those given earlier.[10] Assuming a molecular weight of 47,000 for the monomeric subunits of the tetrameric head,[9] the unit cell can accommodate either four or eight heads (i.e. one or two monomers per asymmetric unit) with either 75% or 50% of the cell volume remaining occupied by solvent. These figures vary little if one allows up to 20% carbohydrate content.[15] Crystal density measurements could resolve this question but we have not been prepared to commit sufficient material to this end. Some indication of the packing density can be obtained from a rotation function analysis of the three-dimensional diffraction data. This study shows no evidence of a second monomer in the asymmetric unit and although negative results of this type are equivocal, the implication is that there is only one monomer per asymmetric unit, and four tetrameric heads per unit cell. The tetramers can be accommodated at positions of either circular four fold symmetry or dihedral two fold symmetry and so the point group symmetry of the head remains undetermined at this stage.

Progress towards determining the three-dimensional structure of this protein has been hampered on two fronts. Firstly, the crystals grew from low ionic strength media and dilute solutions of some heavy atom materials dissolve them. Secondly, and more seriously, the crystals can undergo a lattice transition to the space group P422 with little change in cell dimensions. Here the protein formerly located at the body centre of the unit cell is now only approximately so located. This lattice transformation is triggered by some heavy metal compounds, particularly those containing mercury, or by partial dehydration of the crystals.

Sodium tungstate and diamino-dinitro-platinum both bind to Tokyo neuraminidase. The tungstate binding pattern is complex and not yet fully understood but the platinum compound appears to react predominantly at one site. This finding should eventually enable a full three-dimensional structure determination to 3.5 Å resolution.

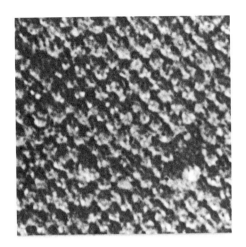

Fig. 2. Electron micrograph of shadowed Nederlands neuraminidase crystal.

Fig. 3. Fourier Transform of a selected area of micrograph in Fig. 2.

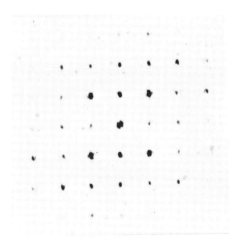

Fig. 4. Filtered Fourier Transform as described in the text.

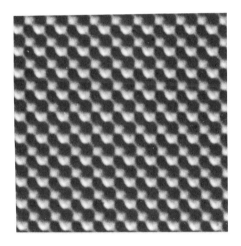

Fig. 5. Image reconstructed from the transform in Fig. 4. Compare with Fig. 1 for interpretation of body-centred lattice.

CONCLUSIONS

Electron microscopy on crystallites of Nederlands neuraminidase has shown
a degree of similarity between these microcrystals and the large crystals of
the Tokyo protein that was not previously apparent. It now seems likely that
the space group of these thin crystals is one of the two space groups
observed for Tokyo neuraminidase. The similar appearance of crystals of Hong
Kong/68 neuraminidase[9] suggests that they too follow this pattern. Isomorphous
crystal forms of these antigenically different neuraminidases would greatly
simplify an eventual comparison of their three-dimensional structures.

ACKNOWLEDGEMENT

We thank Dr. R.D.B. Fraser and Mr. T.P. MacRae for assistance with the image
processing, and Mr. A. Van Donkelaar for technical help.

REFERENCES

1. Webster, R.G. and Laver, W.G. (1975) in The Influenza Viruses and
   Influenza, Kilbourne, E.D. ed., Academic Press, New York, pp.269-314.
2. Poljak, R.J., Amzel, L.M., Avey, H.P., Chen, B.L., Phizackerly, R.P. and
   Saul, F. (1973) Proc. Nat. Acad. Sci. 70, 3305-3310.
3. Segal, D.M., Padlan, E.A., Cohen, G.H., Rudikoff, S., Potter, M., Davies,
   D.R. (1974) Proc. Nat. Acad. Sci. 71, 4298-4305.
4. Schiffer, M., Girling, R.L., Ely, K.R., Edmundson, A.B. (1973) Biochemistry,
   12, 4620-4631.
5. Epp, O., Colman, P.M., Fehlhammer, H., Bode, W., Schiffer, M., Huber, R.
   and Palm, W. (1974) Eur. J. Biochem. 45, 513-524.
6. Fehlhammer, H., Schiffer, M., Epp, O., Colman, P.M., Lattman, E.E.,
   Schwager, P., Steigemann, W., and Schramm, H.J. (1975) Biophys. Struct.
   Mech. 1, 139-146.
7. Colman, P.M., Schramm, H.J. and Guss, J.M. (1977) J. Mol. Biol. 116, 73-79.
8. Kabat, E.A. (1976) in The Immune System, Melchers, F. and Rajewsky, K. eds.,
   Springer Verlag, Berlin, pp.3-18.
9. Laver, W.G. (1978) Virology, 86, 78-87.
10.Wright, C.E. and Laver, W.G. (1978) J. Mol. Biol. 120, 133-136.
11.Klug, A. and DeRosier, D.J. (1966) Nature (London) 212, 29-32.
12.Fraser, R.D.B. and Millward, G.R. (1970) J. Ultrastruct. Res. 31, 203-211.
13.Rossmann, M.G. and Blow, D.M. (1962) Acta. Cryst. 15, 24-31.
14.Wrigley, N. (1979) Brt. Med. Bulletin, 35, 35-38.
15.Laver, W.G. (1973) Adv. Virus Research, 18, 57-103.

GLYCOPROTEINS OF INFLUENZA C VIRUS

HERBERT MEIER-EWERT*, GEORG HERRLER*, ARNO NAGELE*, AND RICHARD
W. COMPANS**

*Virologische Abteilung, Institut für Med. Mikrobiologie, Technische Universität
München, Biedersteiner Str. 29, 8000 München 40/West Germany and **Department of
Microbiology, University of Alabama Medical Center, Birmingham, Alabama, 35294
U.S.A.

INTRODUCTION

Recent studies in several laboratories have shown that influenza C virions share most structural features of other orthomyxoviruses, including a segmented RNA genome and most of the general types of major structural polypeptides.[1-3] The main difference between influenza C viruses and other members of the orthomyxovirus group resides in the glycoproteins of the viral envelope. Hirst's original observation[4] that the red cell receptor for influenza C virions differs from that for type A and B influenza viruses was corroborated by recent studies[1,5] which demonstrated conclusively that the receptor-destroying enzyme activity of influenza C virus is not an α-type neuraminidase. Enveloped viruses that lack neuraminidase generally contain N-acetylneuraminic acid as a component of their membrane glycoproteins and glycolipids.[6,7] The presence of this sugar in the envelope of influenza C virions has been demonstrated by showing that the hemagglutination inhibition activity for type A influenza virus could be abolished by treating influenza C virions with neuraminidase,[8] and also by thin-layer chromatography of ^{3}H-labeled sugars which are released from neuraminidase-treated virions.[9]

Three species of glycoproteins have been detected in influenza C virions by SDS-gel electrophoresis under reducing conditions, and were designated gp88, gp65 and gp30.[1,3,10] The smaller glycoproteins resemble HA_1 and HA_2 of influenza A viruses in that they are linked together by disulfide bonds under reducing conditions to form a glycoprotein with an electrophoretic mobility similar to gp88.[8]

In the present study we have further characterized the viral glycoproteins, and obtained evidence for a large precursor glycoprotein in influenza C virus. The effects of proteases on the biological activities of the viral glycoproteins were studied. We also describe the isolation of biologically active viral glycoproteins.

GLYCOPROTEINS OF INFLUENZA C VIRIONS UNDER REDUCING AND NON-REDUCING CONDITIONS.

Using chick kidney (CK) cells[11] for propagating influenza C virus doubly labeled with ^{3}H-glucosamine and ^{14}C-amino acids, we compared the virion polypeptide patterns under reducing and non-reducing conditions. In the absence of reducing agents two glycoprotein peaks were resolved, as shown in Fig. 1 (upper panel). They are designated gpI and gpII, and exhibit apparent molecular weights of 100,000 and 80,000 when compared with marker proteins of known molecular weights. After reduction with mercaptoethanol, the protein pattern of CK-grown virus corresponded to that previously described for egg-grown virus, with the three size classes of glycoproteins, gp88, gp65 and gp30 (Fig. 1, lower panel). The nonglycosylated viral proteins NP and M have similar electrophoretic mobilities under reducing or non-reducing conditions. When the extent of glycosylation, expressed as the ^{3}H/^{14}C ratio, was calculated for the different species of glycoproteins, it was found that gpI and gp88 are more highly glycosylated than gpII, gp65 or gp30.

To further investigate the relationships between the glycoproteins, gpI and gpII were isolated from an SDS–polyacrylamide gel and reelectrophoresed under reducing conditions. The results (Fig. 2) show that gpI corresponds to gp88, and that under reducing conditions, gpII is cleaved to yield gp65 and gp30. Although treatment of gpI with reducing agents results in an apparent reduction in molecular weight from 100,000 to 82,000, no polypeptide could be discerned in the region of 10,000 to 20,000 daltons (Fig. 3). Thus, the difference in electrophoretic mobility may be due to changes in conformation, produced by the cleavage of intramolecular disulfide bonds.[12]

ANALYSIS OF GLYCOPROTEINS OF INFLUENZA C VIRUS GROWN IN DIFFERENT HOST CELLS.

In order to obtain information about host cell-dependent variation in the patterns of viral glycoproteins, virions grown in embryonated eggs, CK cells and chick fibroblasts (CEF) were analysed by electrophoresis under non-reducing conditions (Fig. 4). Whereas CK-grown virus exhibits similar amounts of gpI and gpII, only traces of gpI can be detected in egg-grown virus, whereas in CEF grown virus gpI was the only detectable glycoprotein. The previous findings that influenza C grown in CEF contains only the gp88 glycoproteins, together with the fact that these virions show only a low level of infectivity, supports the conclusion that gpI corresponds to gp88 and suggests that gpII may be essential for maximal viral infectivity.

EVIDENCE FOR A PRECURSOR GLYCOPROTEIN IN INFLUENZA C VIRUS.

We analysed the peptides of isolated gpI and gpII after extensive trypsin digestion on a cation exchange column. The result in Fig. 5 shows that with few exceptions the profiles obtained from gpI and gpII are identical, which is compatible with the conclusion that the two glycoproteins have a common amino acid sequence.

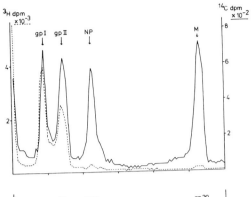

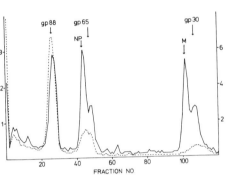

Fig. 1. SDS-polyacrylamide gel electrophoresis of purified influenza C/JHB/1/66 virions grown in CK cells and labeled with (^{3}H)-glucosamine and (^{14}C)-amino acids. The polypeptides and glycoproteins are indicated by arrows and designated as described in the text. Upper panel: electrophoresis under non-reducing conditions; lower panel: electrophoresis under reducing conditions. (From Herrler et al., 1979[10])

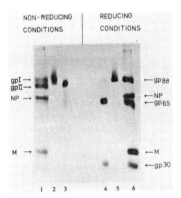

Fig. 2. SDS-polyacrylamide gel electrophoresis of isolated glycoproteins of influenza C/JHB/1/66 grown in CK-cells. (^{3}H)-leucine labeled gpI and gpII bands were isolated and analysed by electrophoresis under reducing and non-reducing conditions. Lane 1 and 6: purified virions; lanes 2 and 5: isolated gpI; lanes 3 and 4: isolated gpII. (From Herrler et al., 1979[10])

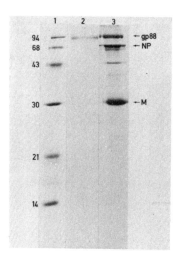

Fig. 3. SDS-polyacrylamide gel electrophoresis under reducing conditions of purified influenza C/JHB/1/66 virions grown in CK cells (lane 3) and of gpI isolated under nonreducing conditions (lane 2). Lane 1: molecular weight markers, from top to bottom: phosphorylase B, bovine serum albumin, ovalbumin, carbonic anhydrase, soybean trypsin inhibitor, lysozyme. Polypeptides were stained with Coomassie brilliant blue.

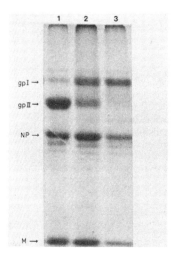

Fig. 4. SDS-polyacrylamide gel electrophoresis under non-reducing conditions of purified C/JHB/1/66 virions grown in different host cells. The proteins were stained with Coomassie brilliant blue. Lane 1: virus grown in embryonated eggs; lane 2: virus grown in CK cells; lane 3: virus grown in CEF. (From Herrler et al., 1979[10])

We also examined the intracellular synthesis of the glycoproteins of influenza C virus in infected CK cells. When CK cells were labeled with ^{3}H-glucosamine for 2 hr at 12 hr p.i., only gpI was detectable (Fig. 6) Even after a chase of 3 hr, most of the virus-specific sugar label was found in the position of gpI. This result indicated that gpI is the primary glycoprotein gene product, which may be cleaved to gpII as a late event in viral assembly. This proteolytic cleavage is apparently host cell dependent, which would account for the host-dependent variation in amounts of gpI and gpII described above.

EFFECT OF TRYPSIN ON INFLUENZA C VIRUS.

The effect of trypsin on the glycoproteins of myxo- and paramyxoviruses and their biological activities is well documented.[14-17] In order to determine whether trypsin also has an effect on the glycoproteins of influenza C virus, we analysed purified CEF-grown virions, which contain almost exclusively gp88, after treatment with various concentrations of trypsin. When ^{3}H-glucosamine labeled CEF-grown virus was treated with trypsin followed by SDS-polyacrylamide gel electrophoresis under reducing conditions, it was found that gp88 is converted to gp65 and gp30 (Fig. 7). Under nonreducing conditions almost complete cleavage of gpI occurs at trypsin concentrations of 0.1 - 10 μg/ml, and gpII is the major cleavage product observed (result not shown). When aliquots of each sample were tested for infectivity titers and protein contents, the results (Table 1) indicated a marked enhancement of specific infectivity at trypsin concentrations of 0.1 to 10 μg/ml, at which gpI had been cleaved into gpII.

TABLE 1   EFFECT OF TRYPSIN ON THE INFECTIVITY OF
INFLUENZA C VIRIONS GROWN IN CEF*

Trypsin concentration (μg/ml)	0	0.01	0.1	1	10	100	1000
PFU/μg protein x 10^{-4}	1.1	1.8	39.7	56	56.6	1.1	1.1

* Purified influenza C/JHB/1/66 virions were treated with various concentrations of trypsin. After pelleting, the virus was assayed for specific infectivity (PFU/μg protein).

From these experiments it can be concluded that the conversion of gpI into gpII is the result of a proteolytic process. The cellular enzyme which catalyzes this cleavage

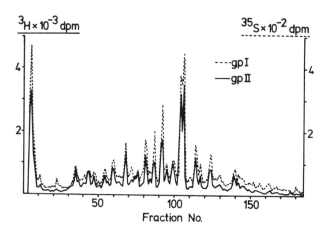

Fig. 5. Tryptic peptide analyses of the gpI and gpII glycoproteins of influenza C/JHB/1/66 virions grown in CK cells, labeled with (^{3}H) methionine and (^{35}S) methionine, respectively. Purified glycoproteins were digested with TPCK-trypsin and neuraminidase. The peptides were eluted from a Durrum DC-1A cation exchange column by a discontinuous gradient of pyridine acetate according to Gentsch and Bishop.[13]

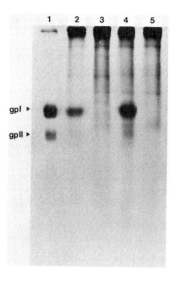

Fig. 6. Analysis of intracellular synthesis of influenza C glycoproteins. CK cells mock-infected or infected with influenza C/JHB/1/66 were labeled with (^{3}H)-glucosamine at 12 hr p.i. After a pulse of 2 hr or after an additional chase of 3 hr, samples were analysed by SDS-polyacrylamide gel electrophoresis under non-reducing conditions. Lane 1: purified (^{3}H)-glucosamine labeled C/JHB/1/66 marker virus; lane 2: infected cells, pulse labeled; lane 3: mock-infected cells, pulse-labeled; lane 4: infected cells, pulse-chase; lane 5: mock-infected cells, pulse-chase. (From Herrler et al., 1979[10])

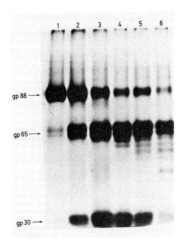

Fig. 7. Effect of trypsin on the glyco-proteins of CEF-grown influenza C/JHB/1/66 virions labeled with (^{3}H)-glucosamine. Purified virions were treated with various concentrations of trypsin. After pelleting, virions were analysed by SDS-polyacrylamide gel electrophoresis under reducing conditions. Trypsin concentrations (μg/ml) were as follows: lane 1: 0; lane 2: 0.1; lane 3: 1; lane 4: 10; lane 5: 100; lane 6: 1000.

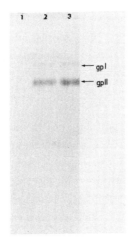

Fig. 8. Glycoproteins of egg-grown influenza C/JHB/1/66 virions isolated by treatment with octylglucoside. The M protein and the RNP-complexes were removed by ultracentrifugation, and the supernatant was analysed by SDS-polyacrylamide gel electrophoresis under non-reducing conditions. Bands were stained with Coomassie brilliant blue. The concentrations of octylglucoside used were: lane 1: 0.2%; lane 2: 1%; lane 3: 5%.

in egg-grown and CK cell-grown influenza C virus may have a similar specificity as that of trypsin.

In Fig. 7 it can be seen that the glycoprotein which migrates in the region of gp65 appears as two bands. The reason for this may be a difference in glycosylation; however, extensive treatment of the glycoproteins with neuraminidase does not abolish the doublet for gp65; thus it is not a result of varying amounts of terminal sialic acid residues.

ISOLATION OF GLYCOPROTEINS FROM INFLUENZA C VIRUS.

Non-ionic detergents have been employed for the isolation of glycoproteins of a number of enveloped RNA-containing viruses.[18-20] Triton X-100 extraction also provides a reliable method to isolate glycoproteins from influenza C virus. However, in contrast to the isolated glycoproteins of other myxoviruses,[13,21] the influenza C glycoproteins did not show hemagglutination activity after the detergent was removed by butanol precipitation. The use of octylglucoside as a detergent offers the advantage that it can be readily separated from the proteins by dialysis. Fig. 8 shows glycoproteins isolated from influenza C virions using octylglucoside. When this preparation of glycoproteins was tested for hemagglutinating (HA) activity after extensive dialysis, an HA titer of 49,000 HAU/ml was found. Electron microscopy of the biologically active glycoproteins revealed heterogeneous lipid vesicles with few glycoprotein spikes adhering to the surface (not shown). The hexagonal arrangement of the surface projections, a characteristic feature of influenza C virion morphology,[3,22] was not observed.

SUMMARY AND CONCLUSIONS

The presence of a precursor glycoprotein which is postranslationally cleaved, to yield two subunits linked together by disulfide bonds, is a characteristic which influenza C virions share with other myxo- and paramyxoviruses. Similarly, the requirement for specific proteolytic cleavage of one or more viral glycoproteins for maximal infectivity is a characteristic shared by these viruses. Influenza C virus, however, seems to be distinct in that only a single glycoprotein gene product has been identified. Further studies of the biological and immunological properties of the isolated viral glycoproteins should demonstrate whether all the known biological functions of influenza C glycoproteins are properties of a single viral glycoprotein.

ACKNOWLEDGMENTS

Research by R. W. C. was support by Grant No. PCM 78-09207 from the National Science Foundation and AI 12680 from the National Institute of Allergy and Infectious Diseases.

REFERENCES

1. Kendal, A. P. (1975) Virology 65, 98-99.
2. Ritchey, M. B., Palese, P., and Kilbourne, E. D. (1976) J. Virol. 18, 738-744.
3. Compans, R. W., Bishop, D. H. L., and Meier-Ewert, H. (1977) J. Virol. 21, 658-665.
4. Hirst, G. K. (1951) J. Exp. Med. 91, 177-185.
5. Nerome, K., Ishida, M., and Nakayama, M. (1976) Arch. Virol. 50, 241-244.
6. Klenk, H. -D., and Choppin, P. W. (1970) Proc. Nat. Acad. Sci. U. S. A. 66, 57-64.
7. Klenk, H. D., Compans, R. W., and Choppin, P. W. (1970) Virology 42,1158-1162.
8. Meier-Ewert, H., Compans, R. W., Bishop, D. H. L., and Herrler, G. (1978) In: Negative Strand Viruses and the Host Cell, (ed. R. D. Barry and B. W. J. Mahy). pp. 127-133.
9. Nakamura, K., Herrler, G., Petri, T., Meier-Ewert, H., and Compans, R. W. (1979) J. Virol. 29, 997-1005.
10. Herrler, G., Compans, R. W., and Meier-Ewert, H. (1979) Virology 99, 49-56.
11. Petri, T., Meier-Ewert, H., and Compans, R. W. (1979) FEMS Microbiol. Lett. 5, 227-230.
12. Dunker, A. K., and Kenyon, A. J. (1976) Biochem. J. 153, 191-197.
13. Gentsch, J. R., and Bishop, D. H. L. (1979) J. Virol. 30, 767-770.
14. Scheid, A., and Choppin, P. W. (1974) Virology 57, 457-490.
15. Klenk, H. -D., Rott, R., Orlich, M., and Blodorn, J. (1975) Virology 68, 426-439.
16. Lazarowitz, S. G., and Choppin, P. W. (1975) Virology 68, 440-454.
17. Nagai, Y. and Klenk, H. -D. (1977) Virology 77, 125-134.
18. Kelley, J. M., Emerson, S. U. and Wagner, R. R. (1972) J. Virol. 10, 1231-1235.
19. Scheid, A., Caliguiri, L. A., Compans, R. W., and Choppin, P. W. (1972) Virology 50, 640-652.
20. Compans, R. W., and Pinter, A. (1975) Virology 66, 151-160.
21. Laver, W. G., and Valentine, R. C. (1969) Virology 38, 105-119.
22. Flewett, T. H., and Apostolov, K. (1967) J. Gen. Virol. 1, 297-304.

(See DISCUSSION on following page)

DISCUSSION

Klenk: What size of peptide is removed during processing?

Meier-Ewart: 10-20,000 MW.

Klenk: Do you know where it is removed from?

Meier-Ewart: No. But a lot of carbohydrate is removed with it.

Palese: We find only 7 RNA segments in flu C.

Meier-Ewart: We have published that there are 7. In some experiments, there are 8 or 9, but these may be due to DI particles.

Scholtissek: Is there polymerase activity in the particles?

Meier-Ewart: So far we have been unable to detect it.

Ertl: Is flu C an orthomyxovirus?

Meier-Ewart: We think so.

SOMATIC CELL HYBRIDS SECRETING HUMAN ANTIBODIES TO INFLUENZA VIRUS

ROBERT L. RAISON, KAREN Z. WALKER, ELIZABETH ADAMS AND ANTONY BASTEN
Immunology Unit, University of Sydney, Sydney, N.S.W., 2006, Australia.

INTRODUCTION

The selection of antigenic variants of influenza virus by growth of the virus in the presence of monospecific antisera has proved to be a powerful tool in the analysis of antigenic variability within a given virus subtype. Recently, three independently mutating antigenic determinants of the A/PR/8/34 haemag-glutinin molecule have been identified using hybridoma derived murine antibodies to select for variants[1,2]. However, the estimated variant frequency of 10^{-24} derived from these studies may be too low to account for the degree of antigenic drift seen in the human population. One reason for this apparent discrepency may be differences in the specificity and repertoire of human and murine antibodies to influenza haemagglutinin. The use of monoclonal human antibodies in such studies may be essential to resolve this problem.

Using the technique pioneered by Kohler and Milstein[3] mouse plasmacytoma lines have been fused with neoplastic human lymphocytes[4] to yield hybrid cell lines secreting human immunoglobulins. We report here the production of anti-body-secreting somatic cell hybrids derived from the fusion of a mouse plasma-cytoma line and human tonsil lymphocytes challenged *in vitro* with influenza virus.

MATERIALS AND METHODS

Virus and haemagglutinin

A/Mem/Bel/72,a recombinant derived from A2/Memphis/102/72 and Ao/Bel/42,was obtained from Dr G. Laver, Dept of Microbiology, Australian National University. Growth of the virus and preparation of purified haemagglutinin was as described by Laver[5].

Preparation of human lymphocytes

Tonsils from children or young adults aged three to 19 years were dissected in RPMI 1640 medium and cell suspensions prepared by forcing the tissue through a sieve. Lymphocytes were prepared by centrifugation through a Ficoll-Hypaque gradient (specific gravity = 1.078 at 20°C). The lymphocyte layer was washed twice and resuspended in RPMI 1640 + 10% FCS (supplemented with penicillin 100 U/ml; streptomycin, 100 μg/ml; gentamycin, 50 μg/ml).

In Vitro stimulation of human lymphocytes

Tonsillar lymphocytes were cultured in flasks at 2×10^6 cells/ml with the addition of 10 µg/ml Mem/Bel virus. The flasks were incubated at 37°C for four to six days on a rocking platform in an atmosphere of 5% CO_2 in air.

Incorporation of ^{3}H thymidine

^{3}H thymidine incorporation of stimulated tonsillar lymphocytes was assessed in 0.2 ml aliquots taken from flask cultures. Labelled thymidine (1 µCi) was added and after 18 hours incubation cells were harvested on a Skatron Cell Harvester and ^{3}H incorporation determined.

Cell fusion and hybrid selection

The murine plasmacytoma line P3/NSI/1-Ag4-1 (NS-1), a non-immunoglobulin secreting line derived from MOPC-21, was obtained from Dr M. Howard, Walter and Eliza Hall Institute, Melbourne. NS-1 (10^7 cells) and human lymphocytes (10^7 to 10^8 cells) were fused in the presence of polyethylene glycol (PEG) M.W. 4000. PEG was added to pelleted cells over a period of one minute, followed by centrifugation for three minutes at 500 xg. Medium (Dubecco's Modified Eagle's, DME) was then added over three minutes, the cells washed and resuspended in DME + 10% FCS and distributed into 48 x 1 ml cultures. Normal mouse peritoneal exudate cells (PEC's) were added at a concentration of 2×10^5 cells/culture as feeder cells. After incubation (37°C, 10% CO_2) 1 ml of double strength HAT medium (2×10^{-4} M hypoxanthine, 8×10^{-7} M aminopterin, 3.2×10^{-5} M thymidine) was added and the cultures fed at two or three day intervals with single strength HAT medium. Hybrid cultures were observed as growth in the culture wells after several days in HAT medium.

Radioimmunoassay

Antibody production in hybrid cultures was determined by solid-phase radioimmunoassay using whole virus or viral haemagglutinin bound to polyvinyl chloride microtitre trays and affinity purified, ^{125}I-labelled goat anti-human immunoglobulins.

Cloning

Hybrid cultures producing specific antibody were cloned by the limit dilution method. Dilutions of 200 cells in 20 ml were distributed in 96 well tissue culture trays. 1×10^5 PEC's were added as feeder cells to each well and the cultures assessed for growth after seven to 10 days.

RESULTS

In Vitro stimulation of human tonsil lymphocytes

Human tonsil lymphocytes were cultured at 2×10^6 cells/ml with the addition of 10 µg/ml whole virus. Culture supernatants were taken at days 0, 4, 5 and 6 and stimulation assessed by incorporation of ^3H thymidine (Fig. 1).

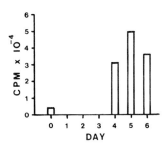

Fig. 1. Incorporation of ^3H thymidine (cpm) by *in vitro* cultured lymphocytes stimulated with influenza virus for 0 to 6 days.

Peak ^3H uptake occurred at day five of *in vitro* stimulation and this correlated with the peak *in vitro* antibody production that was shown, in later experiments, to occur on either day 5 or day 6.

Fusion of human tonsil cells with NS-1

Tonsil lymphocytes from a single patient (S.F.) were stimulated *in vitro* with whole virus. Cells were removed at days 0, 4, 5 and 6 for fusion with NS-1. At each time period, two separate fusions were performed using between 5×10^7 to 10^8 tonsil cells for each fusion. Each fusion yielded hybrid cultures in all 48 tissue culture wells as assessed by growth in HAT medium. Analysis of all primary hybrid cultures revealed a number secreting human antibody to influenza virus. A representative result for a single fusion is shown in figure 2. A varying number of antibody secreting hybrids were obtained at each time period and for the two fusions at that time period (Fig. 3), revealing a correlation between the number of antibody secreting hybrids obtained and the period of *in vitro* stimulation.

Cloning of Hybrid Cultures

A number of the best antibody secreting hybrids were selected for cloning by limit dilution. Several antibody secreting clones were obtained (Table 1).

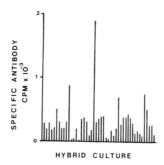

Fig. 2. Specific anti-influenza virus antibody production in supernatants from 48 hybrid cultures derived from a single fusion.

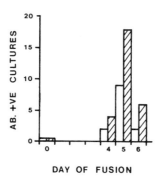

Fig. 3. Specific antibody production by hybrid cultures obtained from
fusions performed at days 0, 4, 5 and 6 of *in vitro* stimulation. The
open and hatched columns refer to two separate fusion experiments performed on each day.

Selected antibody-secreting clones were grown in flask cultures before
storage in liquid nitrogen. Antibody secretion appeared to be lost during this
period of extended culture. However, karyological analysis of some of these
clones revealed mean metaphase chromosome numbers (Table 2) in excess of the
parent mouse tumour line NS-1 (mean = 63) confirming the hybrid nature of these
cloned cell lines.

TABLE 1

YIELD OF ANTIBODY SECRETING CLONES

Fusion	MH4	MH5	MH6	MH9	MH10
No. primary cultures cloned	6	6	5	10	3
No. clones obtained	77	28	35	75	52
No. of antibody-secreting clones frozen	4	4	2	10	5

TABLE 2

KARYOLOGICAL ANALYSES ON SELECTED HYBRID CLONES

Clone	Chromosome Count	
	Mean	Range
A44-1g	83	81-86
B16-6d	73	68-78
B15-8c	74	67-78
B31-3e	76	74-79
A44-1e	84	79-87

Stability of antibody-secreting clones

As shown by the data in Table 1, loss of antibody-secreting capacity of the hybrid clones occurred at two stages. Losses were evident during the cloning procedure and also during the period of growth of clones prior to storage by freezing. Furthermore, upon thawing a number of stored clones, antibody secretion could no longer be detected. Despite the loss of the ability to secrete antibody, human immunoglobulin could be detected on the cell surface of a number of these clones by immunofluorescence.

CONCLUSION

In vitro stimulation of human tonsil lymphocytes with a type A influenza virus facilitated the production of mouse/human hybrid cells secreting human antibodies specific for the challenging virus. Peak hybridoma yield correlated with peak in vitro activity of the stimulated lymphocytes as assessed by uptake of ^{3}H-thymidine and in vitro antibody production. It would therefore appear that the target cell for fusion with the murine tumour line NS-1 is a blast cell actively producing antibody, i.e. a plasma cell. The very low yield of anti-

body secreting cultures obtained from unstimulated lymphocytes (day 0 fusion)
emphasises the importance of *in vitro* priming in obtaining useful mouse/human
hybridomas.

Instability of antibody secreting clones led to the final loss of antibody
production in the clones described here. These losses are probably due to
chromosome instability or overgrowth of the cultures by non-secreting variants.
The latter problems might be overcome by cloning hybrid cultures as early as
possible after fusion and by recloning any antibody-secreting clones several
times to select a more stable antibody-secreting line. It would appear that
the loss of ability to secrete human immunoglobulin does not necessarily involve
loss of the chromosomes carrying structural genes for human immunoglobulin
since human immunoglobulin could still be detected on the cell surface after
antibody secretion had ceased.

In related studies to be reported elsewhere we have obtained apparently
stable mouse/human hybrid clones secreting human immunoglobulin of unknown antibody specificity. Also, clones of mouse/human hybrids which had lost their
ability to secrete specific antibody have been grown *in vivo* as subcutaneous
or ascitic tumours in athymic 'nude' mice of Balb/c origin. These results
indicate the potential for obtaining antibody-secreting hybrids that will
remain stable and can be grown *in vivo* yielding large quantities of antibody.

ACKNOWLEDGEMENT

We are indebted to Ms D. Bartimote for her excellent preparation of this
manuscript.

REFERENCES

1. Gerhard, W., Croce, C.M., Lopes, D. and Koprowski, H. (1978) Proc. Natl.
   Acad. Sci. U.S. 75:1510.
2. Yewdell, J.W., Webster, R.G. and Gerhard, W.U. (1979) Nature 279:246.
3. Kohler, G. and Milstein, C. (1976) Eur. J. Immunol. 6:511.
4. Schwaber, J.F. and Rosen, F. (1978) J. Exp. Med. 148:974.
5. Laver, W.G. (1969) in Fundamental Techniques in Virology, Haber, K. and
   Salzmann, N.P. eds. Academic Press, New York.

DISCUSSION

Gibbs: Have you tried other cell lines, and what happens to the chromosomes
   after fusion?

Raison: We have shown that there are 20 more chromosomes, but have not
   identified which have been lost. Unfortunately, there are not yet available
   any human myeloma cell lines, which would be the best.

ANTIGENIC ANALYSIS OF THE HAEMAGGLUTININ, NEURAMINIDASE AND NUCLEOPROTEIN
ANTIGENS OF INFLUENZA A VIRUSES

G C SCHILD[+], R W NEWMAN[+], R G WEBSTER[++], DIANE MAJOR[+] AND VIRGINIA S HINSHAW[++]
[+]National Institute for Biological Standards and Control, Holly Hill
London NW3 England; [++]Laboratories of Virology, St Jude Children's Research
Hospital, P O Box 318, Memphis, Tennessee 38101, USA

SUMMARY

A comprehensive collection of prototype and other strains of influenza A
virus of human, swine, equine and avian origin were studies in immuno-
double-diffusion tests with antisera to purified haemagglutinin and neuraminidase antigens. These tests were selected because of their ability to reveal
antigenic relationships which may not be apparent by conventional haemagglutination and neuraminidase-inhibition techniques. The antigenic analyses
of strains, based on immuno-double-diffusion tests, permitted the classification of influenza A viruses into twelve groups of H antigens and nine
groups of N antigens.

It was notable that amongst the influenza A viruses of avian origin
there exist H and N antigens representative of each of the five H antigen
groups (H1, H2, H3, Heq1 and Heq2) and four N antigen groups (N1, N2,
Neq1 and Neq2) found amongst human, swine and equine influenza viruses.
Seven H antigenic subtypes (Hav2-Hav6, Hav8 and Hav9) and five N antigen
subtypes (Hav1, Hav2, Hav4, Hav5 and Hav6) have been isolated so far only
from avian species.

Studies of the nucleoprotein (NP) antigens of influenza A virus indicated antigenic differences between strains which appeared to correlate with
host of origin of the viruses.

INTRODUCTION

The present system for the nomenclature of influenza viruses is based
on recommendations of an expert group of the World Health Organization in
1971[1]. The elements of the nomenclature included the host from which the
strain was isolated, the geographical location, strain number and year of
isolation. Influenza A viruses were divided into subtypes based on the
antigenic character of their haemagglutinin (H) and neuraminidase (N)
antigens. The H antigen subtypes of human influenza A viruses were
designated HO, H1, H2 and H3. These subtypes are represented by the human

influenza A viruses prevalent from 1932-1946 (HON1), 1947-1957 (H1N1),
1957-1968 (H2N2, 'Asian') and 1968 to the present (H3N2, 'Hong Kong').
There was one H antigen subtype of swine influenza virus (Hsw1), two H
antigen subtypes of equine virus (Heq1 and Heq2) and eight H antigen subtypes
of avian influenza viruses (Hav1 to Hav8). Since 1971, it has become
apparent that antigenic relationships exist between certain viruses which
were classified into different H antigen subtypes[2,3,4]. These have been
demonstrated by a variety of methods but particularly by immuno-double-
diffusion (IDD) tests in gels with potent, specific antisera to isolated
H antigens[2,3]. IDD tests have been found to be more broadly reactive
than conventional haemagglutination-inhibition (HI) tests[5]. Evidence is
now available to support the designation of two additional H antigen subtypes
amongst recently characterized avian influenza A viruses[6,7].

In the WHO system of nomenclature the N antigens of influenza A viruses
were likewise divided into antigenic subtypes[1]. Among human influenza A
viruses there were two NO antigen subtypes, N1 and N2, represented by the
viruses prevalent from 1932-1956 (HON1 and H1N1) and from 1957 to the present
(H2N2 and H3N2). Among swine influenza viruses there was one subtype (N1),
closely related to the human N1 subtype. Amongst equine influenza viruses
two distinct N antigen subtypes, designated Neq1 and Neq2 were described.
For avian influenza A strains there were eight subtypes of N antigen; two of
these (N1 and N2) were shared with human influenza A viruses, two (Neq1, Neq2)
were shared with equine viruses and four subtypes (Nav1 to Nav4) were
unique to viruses of avian origin. Since that time, evidence for two
additional neuraminidase subtypes among avian subtypes has become available[8,9]

The present paper describes a comprehensive antigenic analysis of prototype strains of influenza A virus of human, swine, equine and avian origin
employing IDD tests with H or N antigen specific antisera. The information
obtained permitted a re-evaluation of the nomenclature of influenza A viruses.
The influenza A viruses so far studied could be grouped into twelve H
antigen subtypes and nine N antigen subtypes.

MATERIALS AND METHODS

Viruses

The influenza A virus strains previously designated[1] as prototype strains
were used in the studies. For some of the studies antigenic 'hybrid'
recombinant influenza viruses were prepared as previously described[10].
The viruses were grown in eggs and purified by sedimentation through sucrose

gradients (10-40% sucrose in 0.15 M NaCl and 0.01 M sodium phosphate, pH 7.4)[11].

Preparation of purified haemagglutinin and neuraminidase antigens

A variety of methods were attempted and the ones most suitable for each particular virus strain were employed. From some reference strains of influenza viruses both the H and N antigens were antigenically stable on treatment of the virus particles with detergents or enzymes to release the surface antigens. To permit separation of H and N antigens from these viruses antigenic hybrid viruses were prepared that possessed either H antigen from A/Bel/42 (HO) virus or N antigen from A/NSW/33 (N1) virus[10]. The following general methods of isolating H and N antigens were used.

(i) Disruption of the virus with suitable detergents and separation of the proteins by electrophoresis on cellulose acetate[12]. A variety of detergents were used (see table 1).

(ii) Enzymatic release of the surface glycoproteins, with selective digestion of one surface antigen[13,14].

Purified nucleoprotein (NP) antigens of influenza A viruses were prepared as described previously[16].

Antisera

For the preparation of potent immune sera, the isolated H, N or NP antigens (50-300 ug) were emulsified in Freund's complete adjuvant, and injected into goats, sheep or rabbits. The animals received two doses of antigen with an interval of 30-40 days. Blood samples were collected 7-14 days after the second injection and the serum was stored at $-20^{\circ}C$.

Serological tests

Immuno-double-diffusion (IDD) tests were performed as described previously[17,18].

RESULTS
Haemagglutinin Antigens

Table 1 shows the results of IDD tests with antisera to the purified H antigens of prototype strains of influenza A viruses. Each serum was tested against a comprehensive collection of prototype virus strains. The criteria for the selection of antisera for use in the test was the production of a well defined precipitin line with the homologous influenza A virus but no

Table 1

Haemagglutinin antigen relationships demonstrated by IDD tests on prototype strains of influenza A virus of human, swine, avian and equine origin

Antiserum to	ANTIGENS																
	HO[a]	H1[b]	H2[c]	H3[d]	Hsw1[e]	Heq1[f]	Heq2[g]	Hav1[h]	Hav2[i]	Hav3[j]	Hav4[k]	Hav5[l]	Hav6[m]	Hav7[n]	Hav8[o]	Hav9[p]	Hav10[q]
HO	+	+s															
H1	+s	+															
H2			+														
H3				+	+s												
Hsw1	+s	+s		+	+												
Heq1						+	+s										
Heq2						+s	+	+									
Hav1							+s	+									
Hav2									+								
Hav3										+							
Hav4											+						
Hav5												+					
Hav6													+				
Hav7														+s			
Hav8															+		
Hav9																+	
Hav10																	+

a A/PR/8/34 (HON1)
b A/FM/1/47 (H1N1)
c A/Sing/1/57 (H3N2)
d A/HK/8/68 (H3N2)
e A/NJ/8/76 (Hsw1N1)

f A/Eq/Prague/56 (Heq1Neq1)
g A/Eq/Miami/1/63 (Heq2Neq2)
h A/FPV/Dutch/27 (Hav1Neq1)
i A/Chick/Germ/49 (Hav2Neq1)
j A/Duck/Eng/56 (Hav3Nav1)

k A/Duck/Czech/56 (Hav4Nav1)
l A/Tern/SA/61 (Hav5Nav2)
m A/Ty/Mass/3740/65 (Hav6N2)
n A/Duck/Ukr/1/63 (Hav7Neq2)
o A/Ty/Ont/6118/68 (Hav8Nav4)

p A/Ty/Wisc/66 (Hav9N2)
q A/Duck/alb/60/76 (Hav10Nav5)

s = spur formation

reaction against influenza B virus together with evidence (based on HI and NI tests) that the antibody present in the serum was directed against H antigen. The majority of H antigen subtypes proposed in the 1971 nomenclature system[1] remain valid, being composed of antigenically unique H antigens, ie not cross-reacting with viruses of other subtype designations. Thus subtypes H2, Nav2, Hav3 (Fig 1), Hav4, Hav5, Hav6 and Hav8 showed no cross-reaction with viruses of other subtypes. Two H subtypes designated since 1971, Hav9[6] and Hav10[7] represented by the virus strains A/turkey/Wisconsin/66 and A/duck/Alberta/60/76 respectively, were also antigenically unique. In contrast, several discrepancies between the 1971 subtype designation and the serological findings were apparent.

1. In the 1971 nomenclature system, human influenza viruses isolated from 1933 to 1956 were divided into subtypes HON1 and H1N1 on the basis of the differences detected between these viruses in H1 tests and on sero-epidemiological grounds. It was clearly shown in our studies employing IDD tests that the H antigens of the subtypes HO and H1 are related. In addition the H antigen of swine (HswlN1) virus strain was shown to possess antigenic determinants shared with haemagglutinins of human strains, HO and H1.

2. The H antigens of human Hong Kong (H3N2) virus, equine (Heq2Neq2) virus and certain avian influenza viruses, eg A/duck/Ukraine/63, (Hav7Neq2) were shown by IDD to be antigenically related.

3. The H antigen of equine (HeqlNeql) virus was found in IDD tests to be antigenically related to those of avian viruses of subtype Hav1 including FPV/Dutch/27 (HavlNeql) and turkey/England/63 (HavlNav3).

4. A/turkey/Wisconsin/66 virus was listed in the 1971 nomenclature system as Hav6N2, although it was not regarded as a prototype strain. However IDD tests failed to show that the H antigen of this virus was related to that of other Hav6 viruses. In Table 2 this virus has been listed as Hav9[6], in agreement with a previous proposed[6] since its haemagglutinin showed no relationships with those of other H antigen subtypes.

Neuraminidase antigens

Table 2 shows the antigenic relationships demonstrated in IDD tests with specific antisera to the purified N antigens of the prototype human, equine and avian influenza viruses. The designation of N1, N2, Neq1, Neq2, Nav1 and Nav4 as unique N antigen subtypes, as described previously in the 1971 nomenclature system appeared to be valid since these N antigens failed to

Table 2

Neuraminidase antigen relationships demonstrated by IDD tests on prototype strains of influenza A viruses of human, equine and avian origin

Antiserum to	ANTIGENS									
	N1[a]	N2[b]	Neq1[c]	Neq2[d]	Nav1[e]	Nav2[f]	Nav3[g]	Nav4[h]	Nav5[i]	Nav6[j]
a N1	+									
b N2		+								
c Neq1			+							
d Neq2				+						
e Nav1					+					
f Nav2						+	+s			
g Nav3						+s	+			
h Nav4								+		
i Nav5									+	
j Nav6										+

Source of antigen & antiserum

a A/PR/8/34(H1N1)
b A/Sing/1/57(H2N2)
c A/Eq/Prague/56(Heq1Neq1)
d A/Eq/Miami/63(Heq2Neq2)
e A/Duck/Eng/56(Hav3Nav1)
f A/Tern/SA/61(Hav5Nav2)
g A/Turkey/Eng/63(Hav1Nav3)
h A/Turkey/Ont/6118/68(Hav8Nav4)
i A/Shearwater/EA/72(Hav6Nav5)
j A/Duck/Memphis/546/74(Hav3Nav6)

s = spur formation

show inter-subtype reactions. However, one major discrepancy between the
1971 nomenclature system and the present findings in respect of N antigens
was apparent. The N antigens of subtypes Nav2 and Nav3 appeared in IDD tests
to be antigenically related. The results of NI tests with antisera to
purified N antigens of those viruses (Webster and Hinshaw unpublished)
provided support of this relationship.

Another discrepancy concerns A/duck/Eng/62 virus which was described in
the literature as Hav4Nav1[24]. The IDD tests failed to show that the N antigen
of this virus is related to that of prototype Nav1 strains, including
A/duck/Eng/56 (Hav3Nav1) and A/duck/Czech/56 (Hav4Nav1), but it did cross
react with viruses containing Neq2. This virus appeared to belong to
subtype Hav4Neq2.

The N antigen of A/Shearwater/E Australia/72 (Hav6Nav5), a virus strain
isolated since the 1971 nomenclature system was developed[8], has been found
to have an antigenically unique N antigen. An additional subtype of neuraminidase, Nav6, of A/duck/Memphis/546/74 virus has been recently proposed[9].
This neuraminidase also appeared to be antigenically unique[7] and no cross-
reactions were detected when this virus was tested against sera to other
neuraminidase subtypes N1, N2, Neq1, Neq2 and Nav1-Nav5.

Antisera prepared against the NP antigens of representative human
(A/PR8/34 and A/Hong Kong/68), swine, equine and avian influenza A viruses
were used in IDD tests to compare the NP antigens of a variety of strains[16].
Evidence of identity of the NP antigens of test strains was taken as the
complete fusion of their precipitin lines whilst 'spurs' between strains
indicated lack of identity. Human influenza A viruses could be separated
into two groups on the basis of their NP antigens. Strains isolated from
1933 to 1942 formed one group whilst strains (H1N1, H2N2 and H3N2) isolated
from 1946 to 1979 formed a second group. Avian influenza A viruses (30
strains of a wide range of subtypes) isolated from 1902 to 1978 were
found to form a homogeneous group in respect of their NP antigens which
were distinguishable from those of viruses of human origin (both NP groups).
The NP of Heq2Neq2 viruses was found to resemble that of avian viruses whilst
that of Heq1Neq1 strains was distinguishable from the NP of both avian and
human viruses. Studies on the NP characteristics of swine influenza A viruses
are incomplete, however, these antigens appear to be clearly distinguishable
from the NP antigens of early and late human influenza A viruses.

DISCUSSION

The results of serological studies on influenza A viruses of human, swine, equine and avian influenza viruses which formed the basis for the 1971 nomenclature system have been extensively reviewed elsewhere[24, 25, 26, 27, 28, 29]. These investigations were mainly based on HI and NI tests with antisera which contained antibodies to both surface antigens H and N. It has since become clear that because of 'steric' inhibition effects with sera containing both antibodies, serological data for the classification of H and N antigens into subtypes should be obtained by the use of specific sera prepared against isolated and purified H and N antigens[5]. HI and NI tests are effective in demonstrating antigenic differences between strains but they do not reveal all antigenic relationships which are detectable by IDD techniques[5]. In contrast, IDD tests are broadly reactive[2, 3, 5, 30] indicating shared antigenic determinants which may not be revealed as cross-reactions in inhibition tests. IDD methods were therefore recommended by WHO[1,31] for the characterization of H and N antigen subtypes.

The results of the haemagglutinin-specific IDD tests described in this paper support the merging of the HO, Hl and Hswl viruses in a single H antigen subtype. Likewise there was clear evidence of the antigenic relatedness of H3, Heq2 and Hav7 and of Heq1 and Hav1.

The merging of groups of H antigens showing relationships in IDD tests would result in their being ten H antigen subtypes amongst human, swine, equine and avian influenza A viruses corresponding to the fourteen subtypes proposed in the 1971 nomenclature system (Table 3). In addition, two avian H antigen subtypes, Hav9 and Hav10, have been characterized since 1971 providing a total of twelve H antigen subtypes.

The data presented supports the designation of nine subtypes of N antigen (table 3) amongst human, swine, equine and avian viruses which react uniquely in neuraminidase-specific IDD tests with the exception of a possible minor cross-reaction between Navl and Nav6. Evidence was obtained to support the merging of two subtypes described in 1971, Nav2 and Nav3, whilst two new subtypes Nav5 and Nav6 have been described since the 1971 nomenclature system was proposed.

The H and N antigen subtypes among the large collections of avian influenza A viruses now available for examination and their ecological distribution has been reviewed[32]. A notable feature of the findings to date is that amongst avian influenza A viruses there exist H and N antigen subtypes antigenically related to each of the antigenic subtypes of influenza virus

Table 3

Proposed grouping of haemagglutinin and neuraminidase antigens based on immuno-double-diffusion tests with specific anti-haemagglutinin and anti-neuraminidase sera

Proposed new designation	Previous subtype designation	Proposed prototype strains
H1	HO H1 Hsw1	A/PR/8/34 A/FM/1/47 A/swine/Wisconsin/15/30
H2	H2	A/Singapore/1/57
H3	H3 Heq2 Hav7	A/Hong Kong/1/68 A/Eq/Miami/1/63 A/duck/Ukraine/1/63
H4	Hav4	A/duck/Czech/56
H5	Hav5	A/tern/South Africa/61
H6	Hav6	A/turkey/Mass/3740/65
H7	Heq1 Hav1	A/equine/Prague/1/56 A/FPV/Dutch/27
H8	Hav8	A/turkey/Ontario/6118/68
H9	Hav9	A/turkey/Wisconsin/66
H10	Hav2	A/chick/Germ/N/49
H11	Hav3	A/duck/England/56
H12	Hav10	A/duck/Alberta/60/76
N1	N1	A/PR/8/34 A/FM/1/47 A/swine/Wisconsin/15/30
N2	N2	A/Singapore/1/57 A/Hong Kong/1/68
N3	Nav2 Nav3	A/tern/South Africa/61 A/turkey/England/63
N4	Nav4	A/turkey/Ontario/6118/68
N5	Nav5	A/shearwater/E.Aust/72
N6	Nav1	A/duck/England/56
N7	Neq1	A/equine/Prague/1/56
N8	Neq2	A/equine/Miami/1/63
N9	Nav6	A/duck/Memphis/546/74

of human, swine and equine origin. The proposed designation of subtypes indicated in table 3 clearly reflect these antigenic relationships which are not apparent in the 1971 nomenclature system.

Minor antigenic differences between the NP antigens of different influenza A virus strains have been reported by Schild et al[16] indicating that this antigen is to some extent capable of variation. The present studies indicated that the NP antigens of avian influenza A viruses form an antigenically homologous group readily distinguished from those of previous and current subtypes of human influenza A virus. This finding is of interest in relation to ecological studies of influenza A viruses and is the first indication of an antigenic 'marker' for host of origin of influenza viruses.

REFERENCES

1. A WHO Expert Committee: A revised system of nomenclature for influenza A viruses (1971) Bull.Wld.Hlth.Org. 45, 119-123
2. Schild, G.C. (1970) Studies with antibody prepared against the purified haemagglutinin of influenza Ao virus. J.gen.Virol. 9, 197-201
3. Baker, N., Stone, H.O. and Webster, R.C. (1973) Serological cross-reactions between the haemagglutinin subunits of HON1 and H1N1 influenza viruses detected with monospecific antisera J.Virol. 11, 137-142
4. Laver, W.G. and Webster, R.G. (1973) Studies on the origin of pandemic influenza III Evidence implicating duck and equine influenza viruses as possible progenitors of the Hong Kong strain. Virology 51, 383-391
5. Schild, G.C. and Dowdle, W.R. (1975) Influenza virus characterization and diagnostic serology. In "Influenza Viruses and Influenza' ed E.D. Kilbourne. Academic Press, NY 316-368
6. Webster,R.G., Tumova, B., Hinshaw, V.S., Lang, G. (1976) Characterization of avian influenza viruses. Designation of a newly recognised haemagglutinin. Bull.Wld.Hlth.Org. 555-560
7. Hinshaw, V.S. and Webster, R.G. (1979) Characterization of anew avian influenza virus subtype and proposed designation of its haemagglutinin as Hav10. J.gen.Virol. In press
8. Downie, J.C. and Laver, W.G. (1973) Isolation of a type A influenza virus from an Australian pelagic bird. Virology 51, 259-269
9. Webster, R.G., Maurita, M. Pridgen, C. and Tumova, B. (1976) Ortho- and paramyxoviruses from migrating feral ducks: Characterization of a new group of influenza A viruses. J.Gen-Virol. 32, 217-225
10. Webster,R.G. (1970) Antigenic hybrids of influenza A viruses with surface antigens to order. Virology 42, 633-642
11. Skehel, J.J. and Schild, G.C. (1971) The polypeptide composition of influenza A viruses. Virology 44, 396-402
12. Laver, W.G. (1964) Structural studies on the protein subunits from three strains of influenza virus. J.molec.Biol. 9, 109-119
13. Brand, C.M. and Skehel, J.J. (1972) Crystalline antigen from the influenza virus envelope. Nature, New Biol. 238, 145-148
14. Wrigley, N.G., Skehel, J.J., Chalwood, P.A. and Brand, C.M. (1973) The size and shape of influenza virus neuraminidase. Virology 51,525-529
15. Haukenes, G., Harboe, A. and Mortensen-Egnund, K. (1965) A uronic and sialic acid free chick allantoic mucopolysaccharide sulphate which combines with influenza HI antibodies to host material I Purification of the substance. Acta path microbiol.Scand. 64, 534-540

16. Schild, C.C., Oxford, J.S. and Newman, R.W. (1979) Evidence for antigenic variation in influenza A nucleoprotein Virology, 93, 569-573
17. Schild, G.C., Winter, W.D. and Brand, C.M. (1971) Serological diagnosis of human influenza infections by immuno-precipitin techniques. Bull.Wld. Hlth.Org. 45, 465
18. Schild, C.C. (1972) Evidence for a new type-specific structural antigen of the influenza virus particle. J.gen.Virol, 15, 99-103
19. Wood, J.M., Schild, C.C., Newman, R.W. and Seagroatt, V. (1977) An improved single-radial-immunodiffusion technique for the assay of influenza haemagglutinin antigen. Application for potency determinations of inactivated whole virus and subunit vaccines. J.Biol.Stand. 5,237-247
20. Laver, W.G. and Webster, R.C. (1972) Studies on the origin of pandemic influenza. II Peptide maps on the light and heavy polypeptide chains from the haemagglutinin subunits of A2 influenza viruses isolated before and after the appearance of Hong Kong influenza. Virology, 48, 444-452
21. Schulman, J.L. and Kilbourne, E.D. (1969) The antigenic relationships of the neuraminidase of Hong Kong virus to that of other human strains of influenza A virus. Bull.Wld.Hlth.Org. 41, 425-428
22. WHO Expert Committee on Respiratory Virus Diseases. Wld.Hlth.Org. Tech.Rep.Ser. No 170 (1953)
23. Aymard, M., Coleman, M,T., Dowdle, W.R., Laver, W.C., Schild, C.C. and Webster, R.G. (1973) Influenza virus neuraminidase-inhibition test procedures. Bull.Wld.Hlth.Org. 48, 199-205
24. Tumova, B. and Schild, C.C. (1972) Antigenic relationships between influenza A viruses of human, porcine, equine and avian origin. Bull.Wld.Hlth.Org. 47, 453-457
25. Pereira, H.C., (1969) Influenza: antigenic spectrum. Progr.Med.Virol. 11, 46-59
26. Easterday, B.C. and Tumova, B. (1972) Avian influenza. In 'Disease of Poultry' (6th Ed) Ed.Hofstrad, M.S. Iowa State University Press, 670-690
27. Webster, R.G., (1972) On the origin of pandemic influenza viruses Curr.Top.Microbiol. Immunol 59 75-81
28. Schild, C.C. and Stuart Harris, C.H. (1976) Influenza viruses of lower animals and birds In 'Influenza , the viruses and the Disease', 78-95
29. Webster, R.G. and Laver, W.C. (1979) Ecology of influenza viruses in lower mammals and birds. Brit.Med.Bull. 35, No.1 29-33
30. Schild, G.C. and Newman, R.W. (1969) Immunological relationships between the neuraminidases of human and animal influenza viruses. Bull.Wld. Hlth.Org. 41, 437-445
31. WHO Expert Group. Reconsideration of influenza A virus nomenclature (1979) Bull.Wld.Hlth.Org. 57, 227-233
32. Hinshaw, V.S., Webster, R.G. and Rodriguez, R.J. (1979) Influenza A viruses: Combinations of haemagglutinin and neuraminidase subtypes isolated from animals and other sources. Arch.Virol. In press.

(See DISCUSSION on following page)

DISCUSSION

Scholtissek: Our hybridisation data agrees with your conclusions.

Gibbs: What is the relationship between 1918 flu and the 1933 strains with regard to NP?

Schild: They are different, but we do not know if this is drift or a new gene.

Rott: Using complement fixation tests, we found minor but significant differences between H0 and H1.

Schild: Did you exclude other antigens - M, P, etc?

Rott: Yes.

COMPARISON OF THE HAEMAGGLUTININ GENES OF HUMAN H2 AND H3 AND AN AVIAN Hav₁
INFLUENZA A SUBTYPE

GEORGE G. BROWNLEE
Medical Research Council Laboratory of Molecular Biology, Hills Road,
Cambridge CB2 2QH, England.

INTRODUCTION

The haemagglutinin of influenza is the major surface protein of the virus.
Changes in its antigenic properties are well known to be associated with the
emergence of new infective strains because they escape the immunity acquired to
earlier strains. Major changes in antigenicity (shift) occur infrequently in
Man at intervals of about 10-15 years. These can now be correlated with the
primary structure of the haemagglutinin as the complete amino acid sequence of
both an H2 and several H3 subtypes is now available[1-4]. Here I will represent
this data of others in an easily accessible if very preliminary form, as well
as comparing it with an avian fowl plague haemagglutinin[5]. I will not present
or discuss a correlation of minor changes in antigenicity with changes in amino
acid sequence (genetic drift) as these are adequately described elsewhere in
this volume[6-8].

RESULTS

Figure 1 shows a computer print-out of the plus (+) strand RNA of the subtypes H2, H3 and fowl plague. Sequences were aligned at the codon (residues
117-119) for the cysteine residue corresponding to amino acid 4 of the mature
HA1 of the H2 and Hav₁ subtypes. Shaded areas correspond to the 5' non-coding
region (or leader) which is followed by the A-U-G specifying the initiator
methionine of the signal peptide. The 3' non-coding region following the
terminator U-G-A or U-A-A is also marked. The gene codes for a single polypeptide chain.

Figure 2 shows another print-out comparing the amino acid sequences numbering
from the first methionine of the signal peptide of the H3 subtype. Occasional
additions (indicated by dashes) were inserted to align the sequences to give
maximal amino acid homology. Although alignment of the three subtypes was made
using the cysteine residues these are, mostly, well conserved and are shown by
dark shading. Light shading is used to indicate the signal peptide and the
peptide region between HA1 and HA2 subunits of the haemagglutinin. The signal
peptides are out of alignment with respect to the initiator methionine residue

```
          10         20         30         40         50         60
                      A  GCAAAAGCAG  GGGUUAUACC  AUAGACAACC  AAAAGCAAAA
AGCAAAAGCA  GGGGAUAAUU  CUAUUAAUCA  UGAAGACCAU  CAUUGCUUUG  AGCUACAUUU
                      AGCAAAAG  CAGGGGUUAC  AAAAUGAACA

          130        140        150        160        170        180
UUGGAUACCA  UGCCAAUAAU  UCCACAGAGA  AGGUCGACAC  AAAUCUAGAG  CGGAACGUCA
UGGGACAUCA  UGCGGUGCCA  AACGGAACAC  UAGUGAAAAC  AAUCACAAAU  GAUCAGAUUG
UUGGACAUCA  UGCUGUAUCA  AAAUGGCACCA  AAGUAAACAC  ACUCACUGAG  AGAGGAGUAG

          250        260        270        280        290        300
ACGGAAUCCC  UCCACAGUGAA  CUAGGGGACU  GUAGCAUUGG  CGGAUGGCUC  CUUGGAAAUC
CUCAUCGAAU  C---CUUGAU  GGAAUAGACU  GCACACUGAU  AGAUGCUCUA  UUGGGGGACC
GGAAAAGAAC  C---ACGUAU  CUUGGCCAAU  GCGGACUGUU  AGGGACCAUU  ACCGGACCAC

          370        380        390        400        410        420
CGAGAGACGG  UUUGUGUUAU  CCAGGCAGCU  UCAAUGAUUA  UGAAGAAUUG  AAACAUCUCC
CU---UUCAG  CAACUGUUAC  CCUUAUGAUG  UGCCAGAUUA  UGCCUCCCUU  AGGUUACUAG
GA---AAUGA  UGUUUGUUAC  CCGGGGAAGU  UUGUUAAUGA  AGAGGCAUUG  CGACAAAUCC

          490        500        510        520        530        540
AUACAACAAC  UGGAGGUUCA  CGGGCCUGCG  CGGUGUCUGG  UAAUCCAUCA  UUUUUCAGGA
UCACUCAGAA  UGGGGGAAGC  AAUGCUUGCA  AAAGGGGACC  UGAUAGCGGU  UUUUUCAGUA
UAAGGACCAA  CGGAACAACU  AGUGCAUGUA  GAAGAUCAGG  GUCUUCA---  UUCUAUGCAG

          610        620        630        640        650        660
ACAACAAUAC  AAGCGGAGAA  CAAAUGCUAA  UAAUUUGGGG  GGUGCACCAU  CCCAUUGAUG
UGCCAAACAA  UGACAAUUUU  GACAAACUAU  ACAUUUGGGG  GGUUCACCAC  CCGAGCACGG
ACAAAAACAC  AAGGAGAAA  UCAGCUCUGA  UAGUCUUGGGG  AAUCCACCAU  UCAGGAUCAA

          730        740        750        760        770        780
CAUUGAACAA  AAGGUCAACC  CCAGGAAUAG  CAACAAGGCC  UAAAGUGAAU  GGACAAGGAG
GAAGCCAGCA  AACUAUAAUC  CCGAAUAUCG  GGUCUAGACC  CUGGGUAAGG  GGUCAGUCUA
AAUAUCAUCA  AUCUUUUGUG  CCGAGUCCAU  GAACACGACC  GCAGAUAAAU  GGCCAGUCCG

          850        860        870        880        890        900
CUGGUAAUCU  AAUUGCACCA  GAGUAUGGAU  UCAAAAUAUC  GAAAAGAGGG  AGUUCAGGGA
AUGGGAACCU  AAUUGCUCCU  CGGGGUUAUU  UCAAAAUGCG  CACUGGGAAA  AGCUCA---A
AUGGGCUUU  CAUAGCUCCA  AAUCGUGCCA  GCUUCUUGAG  G---GGAAAG  UCCAUGGGGA

          970        980        990        1000       1010       1020
CAAUAAAUAC  AACAUUGCCU  UUUCACAAUG  UCCACCCACU  GACAAUAGGU  GAGUGCCCCA
GCAUUCCCAA  UGACAAGCCC  UUUCAAAACG  UAAACAAGAU  CACAUAUGGG  GCAUGUCCCA
CUAUAACAAG  CAGAUUGCCU  UUUCAAAACA  UAAAUAGCAG  AGCAGUUGGC  AAAUGCCCAA

          1090       1100       1110       1120       1130       1140
AAUCAAGA--  ----------  GGAUUGUUUG  GGGCAAUAGC  UGGUUUUAUA  GAAGGAGGAU
GAACUAGA--  ----------  GGCCUAUUCG  GCGCAAUAGC  AGGUUUUCAUA  GAAAAUGGUU
CCAAAAAAG  GGAAAAAGA  GGCCUGUUUG  GCGCUAUAGC  AGGGUUUAUU  GAAAAUGGUU

          1210       1220       1230       1240       1250       1260
AUGCAGCAGA  CAAAGAAUCC  ACUCAAAAGG  CAUUUGAAGG  AAUCACCAAC  AAGGUAAAUU
AAGCAGCAGA  UCUUAAAAGC  ACUCAAGCAG  CCAUCGACCA  AAUCAAUGGG  AAACUGAAUA
CUGCAGCAGA  CUACAAAAGC  ACCCAAUCGG  CAAUUGAUCA  GAUAACCGGA  AAGUUAAAUA

          1330       1340       1350       1360       1370       1380
AGAGAAGACU  GGAGAACUUG  AACAAAAGGA  UGGAAGACGG  GUUUCUAGAU  GUGUGGACAU
AAGGGAGAAU  UCAGGACCUC  GAGAAAUACG  UUGAAGACAC  UAAAAUAGAU  CUCUGGUCAU
AAAAGCAGAU  UGGCAAUUUA  AUUAACUGGA  CCAAAGACUU  CAUCACAGAA  GUAUGGUCUU

          1450       1460       1470       1480       1490       1500
AUGUCAAGAA  UCUGUAUGAU  AAAGUCAGAA  UGCAGCUGAG  AGACAACGUC  AAAGAACUAG
AAAUGAACAA  ACUGUUUGAA  AAAACAGAGG  CGCAACUGAG  GGAAAAUGCU  GAGGACAUGG
AGAUGAACAA  GCUGUAUGAG  CGAGUGAGGA  AACAAUUAAG  GGAAAAUGCU  GAAGAGGAUG

          1570       1580       1590       1600       1610       1620
ACGGGACGUA  UGAUUAUCCC  AAGUAUGAAG  AAGAGUCUAA  ACUAAAUAGA  AAUGAAAUCA
AUGGGACUUA  UGACCAUGAU  GUAUACAGAU  ACGAAGCAUU  AAACAACCGG  UUUCAGAUCA
ACAAUACUUA  UGAUCACAGC  AAAUACAGAU  AAGAAGCGAU  GCAAAAUAGA  AUACAAAUUG

          1690       1700       1710       1720       1730       1740
CAGGUUCUCU  GUCACUGGCA  AUCAUGAUGG  CUGGGAUCUC  UUUCUGGAUG  UGCUCC---A
CAUGCUUUUU  GCUUUGU---  GUAGUUUUGC  UGGGGUUCAU  CAUGUGGGGCC  UGCCAGAAA-
CAUGCUUUUU  GCUUCUU---  GCCAUUGCAG  UGGGCCUUGU  UUUC---AUA  UGUGUGAAGA
```

.... H2
UUCUACU H3
U .... FP

```
          70         80         90        100        110        120
CAAUGGCCAU CAUUUAUCUC AUUCUCCUGU UCACAGCAGU GAGAGGGGAC CAGAUAUGCA
UCUGUCUGGU UCUCGGCCAA GACUUUCCAG GAAAUGACAA CAGCACAGCA ACGCUGUGCC
CUCAAAUCCU GGUUUUCGCC CUUGUGGCAG UCAUCCCCAC AAAUGCAGAC AAAAUUUGUC

         190        200        210        220        230        240
CUGUGACUCA UGCCAAGGAC AUUCUUGAGA AGACCCAUAA CGGAAAGUUA UGCAAACUAA
AAGUGACUAA UGCUACUGAG CUGGUACACA GUUCCUCAAC GGGGAAAAUA UGCAACAAUC
AAGUUGUCAA UGCAACGGAA ACAGUGGAGC GGACAAACAU CCCCAAAAUU UGCUCAAAAG

         310        320        330        340        350        360
CAGAAUGUGA UACGCUUCUA AGUGUGCCAG AAUGGUCCUA UAUAAUGGAG AAAGAAACCU
CUCAUUGUGA UGGCUUUCAA AAUGAGACAU GGGACCUUUU CGUU----GAA CGCAGCAAAG
CUCAAUGCGA CCAAUUUCUA GAAUUUUCAG CUGAUCUAAU AAUC----GAG AGACGAGAAG

         430        440        450        460        470        480
UCAGCAGCGU GAAACAUUUG GAGAAAGUAA AGAUUCUGCC CAAAGAUAGA UGGACACAGC
UUGCCUCGUC AGGCACUUUG GAGUUUAUCA AU--------GA AGGCUUCACU UUGACUGGGG
UCAGAGGAUC AGGUGGGGAUU GACAAAGAAA CA--------AU GGGAUUCACA UAUAGUGGAA

         550        560        570        580        590        600
ACAUGGUCUG GCUG------ ACAAAGGAAG GAUCAGAUUA UCCGGUUGCC AAAGGAUCGU
GACUGAACUG GUUG------ UACAAAUCGA GAAGCACAUA UCCAGUGCUG AAUGUGACUA
AAAUGGAGUG GCUCCAGUCA AAUACAGACA AUGCUUCUUU CCCACAAAUG ACAAAAUCAU

         670        680        690        700        710        720
AGACAGAACA AAGAACAUUG UACCAGAAUG UGGGAACCUA UGUUUCCGUA GGCACAUCAA
ACCAAGAACA AACCAGCCUA UAUGUUCAAG CAUCAGGGAG AGUCACAGUC UCUACCAAGA
CCACCGAACA GACCAAACUA UAUGGGAGUG GAAAUAAACU GAUAACAGUC GGGAGUUCCA

         790        800        810        820        830        840
GUAGAAUGGA AUUCUCUUGG ACCCUCUUGG AUAUGUGGGA CACCAUAAAU UUUGAGAGUA
GUAGAAUAAG CAUCUAUUGG ACAAUAGUUA AACCGGGAGA CAUACUGGUA AUUAAUAGUA
GACGGAUUGA UUUUCAUUGG UUGAUCUUGG AUCCCAAUGA UACAGUUACU UUUAGUUUCA

         910        920        930        940        950        960
UCAUGAAAAC AGAAGGAACA CUUGAGAACU GUGAGACCAA AUGCCAAACU CCUUUGGGAG
UAAUGAGGUC AGAUGCACCU AUUGGCACCU GCAUUUCUGA AUGCAUCACU CCAAAUGGAA
UCCAGAGCGA UGUGCAGGUU GAUGCUAAUU GCGAAGGGGA AUGCUACCAC AGUGGAGGGA

        1030       1040       1050       1060       1070       1080
AAUAUGUAAA AUCGGAGAAG UUGGUCUUAG CAACAGGACU AAGGAAUGUU CCCCAGAUUG
AGUAUGUUAA GCAAAACACC CUGAAGUUGG CAACAGGGAU GCGGAAUGUA CCAGAGAAAC
GAUAUGUAAA ACAGGAAAGU UUAUUAUUGG CAACUGGGAU GAAGAACGUU CCCGAACCUU

        1150       1160       1170       1180       1190       1200
GGCAAGGAAU GGUUGAUGGU UGGUAUGGAA ACCAUCACAG CAAUGACCAA GGAUCAGGGU
GGGAGGGAAU GAUAGACGGU UGGUACGGUU UCAGGCAUCA AAAUUCUGAG GGCACAGGAC
GGGAAGGUCU GGUCGACGGG UGGUACGGUU UCAGGCAUCA GAAUGCACAA GGAGAAGGAA

        1270       1280       1290       1300       1310       1320
CUGUGAUUGA AAAGAUGAAC ACCCAAUUUG AAGCUGUUGG GAAGGAAUUC GGUAACUUAG
GGGUAAUCGA GAAGACGAAC GAGAAAUUCC AUCAAAUCGA AAAGGAAUUC UCAGAAGUAG
GACUCAUUGA GAAAACCAAC CAGCAAUUUG AGCUAAUAGA UAAUGAAUUC ACUGAAGUGG

        1390       1400       1410       1420       1430       1440
ACAAUGCUGA GCUUCUAGUU CUGAUGGAAA AUGAGAGGAC ACUUGACUUU CAUGAUUUCUA
ACAAUGCGGA GCUUCUUGUC GCUCUGGGGA ACCAACAUAC AAUUGAUCUG ACUGACUCGG
ACAAUGCUGA ACUUCUUGUG GCAAUGGAAA ACCAGCACAC UAUUGAUUUG GCUGAUUCAG

        1510       1520       1530       1540       1550       1560
GAAAAUGGAUG UUUUUGAAUU UAUCACAAAU GUGAUAGAUGA AUGCAUGAAU AGUGUAAAA
GCAAUGGUUG CUUCAAAAUA UACCACAAAU GUGACAAUGC UUGCAUAGGG UCAAUCAGAA
GCACUGGUUG CUUUGAAAUU UUUUCAUAAAU GUGACGAUGA UUGUAUGGCU AGUAUAAGGA

        1630       1640       1650       1660       1670       1680
AAGGGGUAAA AUUGAGCAGC AUGGGGGUUU AUCAAAUCCU UGCCAUUUAU UGCUACAGUAG
AAGGUGUUGA ACUGAAGUCA GGAUACAAAG ACUGGAUCCU GUGGAUUUCC UUUGCCAUAU
ACCCAGUCAA AUUGAGUAGU GGCUACAAAG AUGUGAUACU UUUGGUUUAGC UUCGGGGCAU

        1750       1760       1770       1780       1790       1800
ACGGGUCUCU GCAGUGCAGG AUCUGCAUAU GAUUAAUAAG UCAUUUUUAU AAUUAAAA
--GGCAACAU UAGCUGCAAC AUUUUGCAUU GAGUGUAUUA GUAAUUAAAA ACACCCUUGU
ACGGAAACAU GCGGUGCACU AUUUUGUAUAU AAGUUUGGAA AAAAACACCC UUGUUUCUAC
```

Fig. 1. Sequence of the "+" strand of gene 4 of: top line, H2 subtype (A/Jap/307/57); middle line, H3 subtype (A/Mem/107/72); bottom line, Hav$_1$ subtype (fowl plague, Rostock). Dashes are inserted occasionally for improved alignment (see Fig. 2). The 3' terminus of the H2 subtype is incomplete.

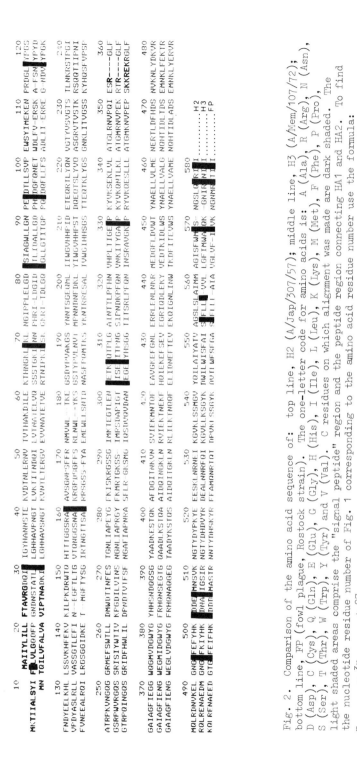

Fig. 2. Comparison of the amino acid sequence of: top line, H2 (A/Jap/307/57); middle line, H3 (A/Mem/107/72); bottom line, FP (fowl plague, Rostock strain). The one-letter code for amino acids is: A (Ala), R (Arg), N (Asn), D (Asp), C (Cys), Q (Gln), E (Glu), G (Gly), H (His), I (Ile), L (Leu), K (Lys), M (Met), F (Phe), P (Pro), S (Ser), T (Thr), W (Trp), Y (Tyr) and V (Val). C residues on which alignment was made are dark shaded. The light shaded areas comprise the "signal peptide" region and the peptide region connecting HA1 and HA2. To find the nucleotide residue number of Fig. 1 corresponding to the amino acid residue number use the formula:

$$n_{Fig. 1} = 3n_{Fig. 2} + 27.$$

because the N-terminal region of H3 is 10 residues longer than that of H2 or Hav$_1$. The HA1-HA2 interpeptide region also differs in one of the three subtypes, it being five amino acids long in Hav$_1$ and only one residue in H2 and H3. But all three cases have either an arginine or lysine residue which would be susceptible to a trypsin-like enzyme, which breaks the peptide bond, thus generating the HA1 and HA2 subunits.

Table 1 shows the extent of overall amino acid sequence conservation expressed as % similarity between the three subtypes. Results are presented for the HA1 and HA2 subunits separately and for the whole haemagglutinin.

TABLE 1

AMINO ACID CONSERVATION OF HAEMAGGLUTININS OF DIFFERENT SUBTYPES

	H2 (A/Jap/57)	H3 (A/Mem/72)	Fowl plague (Rostock)
H3 (A/Mem/72)	36, 49, 42[a]	-	-
Fowl plague (Rostock)	35, 52, 42	39, 66, 49	-

[a] Values are as per cent (100 = identical). The first figure is for HA1 (residues 27-352 of Figure 2), the second figure is for HA2 (residues 358-580) and the third overall (residues 27-580). Computations using unpublished programs of R. Staden counting deleted or inserted positions as mismatches.

The similarity between the HA2 subunit of fowl plague and H3 subtypes (66%) is remarkable and significantly greater than in the other two comparisons. Within HA2 it is well known that the N-terminal region is absolutely conserved (residues 358-368, Figure 2). Another region of absolute identity is between residues 451 and 456. HA1 is less well conserved (between 35% and 39%) but considering that a fair proportion of the changes are to related amino acids, e.g. V $\rightarrow$ I or R $\rightarrow$ K (results not shown) a realistic assessment of sequence similarity would be higher than the figures indicated.

Other regions of similarity have been noted in which "hydrophobicity" rather than any particular amino acid is conserved. Thus the signal peptide is very poorly conserved between the H3 and Hav$_1$ subtypes, even if re-aligned with respect to the initiator methionine. But both these, as well as the H2 subtype, are hydrophobic. Similarly the C-terminal region of the HA2 subunit (residues 548-580) is generally hydrophobic in all three subtypes, consistent with its attachment to the cell membrane in this region.

DISCUSSION

The extent of variation between the haemagglutinins of different subtypes is far too great to correlate any particular region with changes in antigenicity, yet the conservation is extensive enough to indicate that much of the sequence has a "structural" role not readily susceptible to variation in the evolution of influenza. For example, the invariant cysteine residues (excepting those at residues 568, 576 and 579, which have not been studied) are known to be present as disulphide bonds either connecting the HA1 and HA2 subunits or interconnecting separate regions of the HA1 subunit. The function of other conserved regions may only become clear when the three-dimensional structure is known.

ACKNOWLEDGEMENTS

I am very grateful to authors presenting their sequence data at Thredbo for supplying me with unpublished data for correlation and presentation here. It is inevitable in doing this that I will have repeated points made by them, but I hope this brief summary will be valuable to the general reader.

REFERENCES

1. Gething, M.-J., Bye, J., Skehel, J. and Waterfield, M. (1980), this volume.
2. Sleigh, M.J., Both, G.W., Brownlee, G.G., Bender, V.J. and Moss, B.A. (1980), this volume.
3. Min Jou, W., Verhoeyen, M., Devos, R., Saman, E., Huylebroeck, D., van Rompuy, L., Fang, R.X. and Fiers, W. (1980), this volume.
4. Ward, C.W. and Dopheide, T.A. (1980), this volume.
5. Porter, A.G., Barber, C., Carey, N.H., Hallewell, R.A., Threlfall, G. and Emtage, J.S. (1979) Nature 282, 471-477.
6. Moss, B.A., Underwood, P.A., Bender, V.J. and Whittaker, R.G. (1980), this volume.
7. Laver, W.G., Air, G.M., Webster, R.G., Gerhard, W., Ward, C.W. and Dopheide, T.A. (1980), this volume.
8. Both, G.W., Sleigh, M.J., Bender, V.J. and Moss, B.A. (1980), this volume.

Index

N-Acetylneuraminic acid, 357
Aggregation, influenza hemagglu-
    tinin, 21-24
Albumin, antigenic structure of,
    250-53, 257
Antibodies
  binding with hemagglutinin
    fragments, 309-19
  thymus-dependent formation of,
    321
  monoclonal. see Monoclonal
    antibodies
Antigenic drift, 39, 51, 63, 69,
    115, 296
  of Hong Kong strains, 33, 35
    59, 329-37
  monoclonal antibodies in study
    of, 283-91
  in neuraminidases, 125-32
  nucleotide sequences and, 81-88
Antigenicity
  in autoimmune response, 255-57
  lysozyme, 246-50
  myoglobin, 243-46
  see also Antigenic sites
Antigenic shift, 39, 115, 125
Antigenic sites, hemagglutinin,
    21, 47, 51, 206-207, 275
  amino acid sequence changes in,
    257-59, 295, 298-305, 307,
    336-37, 375-81
  carbohydrate component of, 311,
    314-16
  chemical modification of, 299-
    301
  conformational changes, 245-
    46, 252-55, 258, 295, 313,
    321, 351-52
  continuous, 253
  determination of, 242, 246-48,
    268-69
  discontinuous, 253
  formation of, 158-65
  fragments, 309-19, 326-27
  genetic control of, 259-61
  for helper T cells, 321, 322-27

Antigenic sites, hemagglutinin
    (continued)
  monoclonal antibodies for, 273,
    274-80, 282, 284-91, 330-33
  sulphated oligosaccharide, 239
  variation in, 81-88, 285-90,
    389-90
Antisera, adsorption of, 311
Autoimmune reaction, 255-57

Brazil/11/78 strain, 108, 109,
    111, 113

Carbohydrate side chains, hemag-
    glutinin, 12, 17, 33-35, 47,
    213-18
  attachment sites of, 214, 215,
    236
  sulphated, 233-40
  types of, 214, 215, 216, 223,
    224, 233, 235
  variations in, 216-18, 221, 224-
    28
California/10/78 strain, 109, 111,
    114
Cleavage, hemagglutinin, 13-16,
    22, 26, 46, 201-207, 213, 218-
    20, 309, 310, 326-27
Cloned DNA copies, viral, 1-9, 52,
    115-19, 122, 152-54, 369-71
  direct analysis of population
    genes compared with, 81
  nucleotide sequence analysis of,
    5-7, 69-77
  orientation of, 120-22
  primer for, 116, 139, 147, 170
  see also Hemagglutinin
Cloning artifacts, 49, 61
Codon usage, 4, 45
Competitive RNA hybridization,
    106-13
Conformation, antigenicity role
  of, 245-46, 252-55, 258,
    295, 313, 321, 351-52
Conservation of amino acid
  sequence, 59, 191-99, 389-90

Continuous antigenic sites, 252-53
Cyanogen bromide cleavage, 309, 310, 314, 326-27

Diamino-dinitro-platinum, neuraminidase binding with, 354
Diazotized sulphanilic acid, hemagglutinin reaction with, 300-301
Dideoxy sequencing procedure, 126, 135
Dimorphism, influenza, 337
Direct binding assay, 314
Discontinuous antigenic sites, 253
Disulfide bonds
  antigenic activity and, 252, 313
  of influenza A hemagglutinin, 11, 13-16, 24-25, 313
  of influenza C glycoproteins, 357, 358
DNA, viral
  cloning, 1-9, 52, 115-19, 152-54, 369-71
  restriction endonuclease mapping of, 5-7, 69-77
Dodecamer primer, 116, 139, 170

Electron density map, hemagglutinin, 345, 346, 347
Endo-H sensitivity, hemagglutinin, 225
Escherichia coli X1776, 147

1-Flouro-2, 4-dinitrobenzene, hemagglutinin interaction with, 299-300
Fowl plague virus hemaggultinin
  amino acid sequence of, 5-8, 9, 46, 67-68, 385-89
  carbohydrate side chain s of, 17
  cleavage sites of, 218
  cloning of, 160-62
  codon usage in, 45
  genetic expression of, 162-65, 167, 168
  nucleotide sequences of, 40-45
  structure of, 32

FW/50 strain, competitive hybridization with, 107, 108

Glycopeptides,
  hemagglutinin, 214, 215, 223-28, 233
  influenza C vivions, 357-64, 366
Glycosylation
  hemagglutinin, 33, 210, 213
  viral mutation and, 228-31

Heavy chain, 310
  see also Hemagglutinin, HA_1 chain
Helper T cells, 321, 322-27
Hemagglutinin, 21, 39, 48, 51
  amino acid homologies in subtypes, 145
  amino acid sequencing of, 1-8, 12, 17, 22-23, 46, 103, 257-59, 295-305, 336-37
  antigenic sites of. see Antigenic sites, hemaglutinin
  biosynthesis of, 8-9, 11, 33, 97-102, 203
  carbohydrate side chains of, 12, 17, 33-35, 311, 314
    attachment sites of, 214, 215, 236
    types of, 214, 215, 216, 223, 224, 233
    variations in, 216-18, 221, 224-28
  chemical modification of, 299-301
  cleavage of, 13-16, 21, 22, 26, 46, 59, 120, 201-207, 213, 218-20, 309, 310, 314, 326-27
  disulphide bonds of, 11, 13-16, 24-25, 313
  fowl plague viral gene for, 40-45
  fragments of, 309-19, 326-27
  glycosylation of, 213-18, 228-31
  HA_1 chain of, 25, 26, 336
    glycopeptides of, 214, 216, 223-28, 233
    molecular weight of, 28-29, 101-102

Hemagglutinin (continued)
  HA$_1$ chain (continued)
    structure of, 25, 26, 29-33,
      35-36
  HA$_2$ chain of,
    amino acid dequence of, 57, 58-
      59
    glycopeptides of, 216, 226
    nucleotide sequence of, 40-45,
      56-59
    structure of, 21-25, 26, 35-36
  hydrophobic regions of, 9, 46, 58-
    59, 68, 207, 389
  infectivity of, 201-203
  membrane insertion, 101-102,
    201, 213, 228
  micropeptide mapping of, 333-35
  migration, 229
  molecular weight of, 28-29, 97
  monoclonal antibody study of,
    274-80, 282, 284-91, 295-305
  nucleotide sequence of, 103, 139-
    45, 172-74, 175-76
  pathogenicity of, 204-208
  receptor for, 211
  secondary structure of, 35-36
  seqences from 3' ends, 139-45
  strain differences in, 77-78, 79
  x-ray crystallographic study of,
    339-48
Hemoglobin, antigenic sites of, 254
H1N1 strains, 105, 107-13, 147,
  149-56
H2N1 strains, 12, 17
H2N2 strains, 1-9, 17, 23, 42-44
H3N2 strains
  antigenic variants of, 81-88, 105,
    107-13, 283-305
  HA$_1$ chain of, 25-33
  structure of, 21-25, 35-36
Hong Kong/1/68 strain, 81-88, 283-
  305
Hybridization, molecular, 191-98

Infectivity, 201-203

Influenza A virus
  antigenic variation in. see
    Antigenic sites
  cloning nucleotide sequences of,
    1-5
  naturally occurring recombinants
    of, 105-13
  nomenclature for, 373-74
  restriction mapping of, 5-7, 8
  see also Hemagglutinin
Influenza C virus, glycoproteins
    of, 357-64, 366
Immune response
  auto-, 255-57
  genetic control of, 259-61
  hereogeneity of, 261-62
  see also Antigenicity and
    Antigenic sites
Immuno-double-diffusion tests,
    373-74
Immunoglobulin--G-antigen
    complexes, 314-15, 317, 318
Interchain bonds, hemagglutinin,
    13-16, 24-25, 252, 313

Japan/305/57 strain, 1-9, 23

Lectin affinity, hemagglutinin,
    225-26
Light chain(HA$_2$), 310
  see also Hemagglutinin, HA$_2$
    chain
Lysozyme
  antigenic structure of, 241, 243,
    246-53
  immune response to, 260-62
  surface-simulation synthesis
    of antigenic sites of, 265-68

Matrix gene, influenza, 137-38
Membrane insertion, hemagglutinin,
    101-102, 201
Memphis/1/71 strain, 283, 285-
    305
Memphis/1/79 strain, 109, 111
Memphis/10/78 strain, 129

Memphis/102/72 strain
  antigenic properties of, 309-19
  cloning of, 69-72
  comparison with NT/60, 83-85, 87
  comparison with fowl plague
    virus, 42-44
  nucleotide sequence of, 71, 73-77,
    129, 130
  sulphated oligosaccharide of,
    233-40
  variants of, 81-88, 331
Memphis/110/76 strain, RNA
  hybridization with, 108
Methyl mercury hydroxide
  treatment, 150-51, 156
Micropeptide mapping, hemagglutinin,
  330, 333-35
Mismatching of base pairs, 191,
  192, 194, 195-97
Molecular hybridization, 191-98
Monoclonal antibodies
  in antigenic drift study, 283-91,
    295, 298-99, 301-305, 330-33
  in antigenic structure study, 273,
    274-80, 282
  for hemagglutinin carbohydrate
    component, 311
  hyridoma-derived murine, 367-72
Mouse-human hybrid cells, antibodies
  from, 367-72
Mutations, influenza, 51, 63, 329-37
  in amino acid sequence of hemag-
    glutinin, 295-305
  of binding strains, 33
  in conserved and variable gene
    parts, 87-88, 197-99
  of lab strains, 77-78, 79
  point, 283-84
  rate of, 146
Myeloma protein M-603, 264-65
Myoglobin
  antigenic structure of, 241, 243-46,
    251-53, 254, 255-56
  immune response to, 259-62

Neuraminidases
  amino acid sequence of, 125-32,
    377-81
  cloned DNA copies from, 117-18
  homologies in subtypes of, 128-
    32
  nucleotide sequences from 138-
    39, 177-78
  N-termini of, 132, 134
  RNA coding for, 91-95
  variants of, 354-56
Nomenclature, influenza virus,
  373-74
NT/60/68 strain
  dimorphism in, 337
  hemagglutinin of, 83-88
  variants of, 329-37
Nucleotide homology, 191-99,
  389-90
Nucleotide sequencing, 39, 40-45,
  71, 73-77
NWS/33 strain, 127-28, 129

Pathogenicity, hemagglutinin,
  204-206
pBR322 DNA, 149, 152, 158-59
Penetration, viral, 202-203, 207,
  210-11
PR/8/34
  antigenicity of, 274-80, 282
  hemagglutinin of, 171-74, 175, 176
  neuraminidase gene of, 174, 177-
    78
Proteases, action on hemagglutinin
  chains, 218-20, 222
Protein A, Staphylococcus aureus,
  314

Qld/70 strain, 331, 336
Qu/7/70 strain, 85-86, 87

Receptor, hemagglutinin attachment
  to, 211
Reconbinants, nautrally occurring,
  105-13

Restriction enzyme mapping, 82,
   118, 120
   of fowl plague virus, 4, 41
   of Memphis virus, 71, 72
   of Victoria virus, 53, 55-56, 65
Reverse phase high pressure
   liquid chromatography, 226-28
Rio de Janeiro/7/78 strain, 108,
   111, 112-13
RNA, influenza virus
   3/ end sequence of, 135, 137-38,
      169-78
   5' termini of, 121-23, 181-87
   -RNA hybridization, 105, 106-13
   overlapping genes in, 91-95
RNA polymerase II, host, 181-87

Secondary anti-hemagglutinin
   antibody, 322-24
Self-priming, 77, 79
Shanghai/9/79, 109, 111
Signal sequences, 174, 179, 385
Singapore/333/79 strain, 109, 111
Sodium tungstate, neuraminidase
   binding to, 354
Sulfation, hemagglutinin glyco-
   peptide, 225
Surface-simulation synthesis, 242,
   262-68
Synthetic DNA primer, 147, 148

Tetranitromethane, 300
Texas/1/77, 108, 109, 110
30D strain, 87, 88
34C strain, 87, 88
T lymphocytes, 321
Tryptic peptide analysis, 333-35,
   358, 362, 363
Tryptophan operon, plasmid
   construction based on, 157, 158
29C strain, 86-88

Udorn/72 strain, 115-16, 117
USSR/90/77 strain, 108, 109, 110
   cDNA from, 147, 149-51, 156
   cloning of, 152-54

Vaccine production, 157
Victoria/3/75 strain hemagglutinin
   amino acid sequence of, 57, 58-59,
      65-68
   cloning of gene, 52, 54-55, 64-65
   hydrophobic regions of, 58-59
   nucleotide sequencing of, 53-54,
      56-59
Virus penetration, 202-203, 207,
   210-11
Vitamin K_1 OH, surface-simulation
   synthesis of combining site
   residues, 263-64

World Health Organization
   nomenclature system, 373-74,
      380-81
WSN/33 strain
   henagglutinin gene sequence of,
      174, 175, 176, 223-28
   neuraminidase gene sequence of,
      174, 177-78

X-ray crystallography
   for hemagglutinin structure,
      339-48
   for neuraminidase structure,
      352-56
X-31 strain, 331, 336
   hemagglutinin gene sequence of,
      1-9, 69-71, 174, 175, 176
   neuraminidase gene sequence of,
      174, 177-78

r